ADVANCES IN

Family Practice Nursing

Editor-in-Chief
Linda J. Keilman, DNP, MSN,
GNP-BC, FNAP, FAANP

Associate Editors
Melodee Harris, PhD, APRN,
GNP-BC, AGPCNP-BC

Sharon L. Holley, DNP, CNM,
FACNM, FAAN

Ann Sheehan, DNP, CPNP, FAANP

ELSEVIER

PHILADELPHIA   LONDON   TORONTO   MONTREAL   SYDNEY   TOKYO

Editor: Kerry Holland
Developmental Editor: Akshay Samson

Editorial Office:
Elsevier
1600 John F. Kennedy Blvd,
Suite 1800
Philadelphia, PA 19103-2899

International Standard Serial Number: 2589-4722
International Standard Book Number: 978-0-443-34379-7

ADVANCES IN
Family Practice Nursing

CONTRIBUTORS

KHALED ALOMARI, PhD, NP, RN, Assistant Dean, DNP and PLN Programs, West Coast University, Irvine, California

MEI BAI, PhD, RN, Registered Nurse, University of Arkansas for Medical Sciences, Little Rock, Arkansas

SARAH E. BARTON, DNP, CNM, C-EFM, Certified Nurse-Midwife (Private Practice), Rutland Women's Health, Rutland, Vermont

MARY CATHERINE CARPENTER, MSN, CNM, Certified Nurse-Midwife (Private Practice), MaineHealth, Thomaston, Maine

SHANNON COLE, DNP, APRN-BC, Assistant Professor, Vanderbilt University School of Nursing, Nashville, Tennessee

STEPHANIE DEVANE-JOHNSON, PhD, CNM, FACNM, Associate Professor, School of Nursing, Vanderbilt University, Nashville, Tennessee

JULIA DUNHAM-THORNTON, MSN, RN, ANP-BC, AGPCNP-BC, Immersive Simulation Facilitator, Grand Canyon University, College of Nursing Healthcare Professions, Albuquerque, New Mexico

MARY E. FLYNN, DNP, PPCNP-BC, CPNP-AC, Pediatric Nurse Practitioner Program Director, Assistant Clinical Professor, Conway School of Nursing, The Catholic University of America, PNP Pediatric Hospitalist Children's National Hospital, Washington, DC

MELODEE HARRIS, PhD, APRN, GNP-BC, AGPCNP-BC, Associate Professor, University of Arkansas for Medical Sciences, College of Nursing, Little Rock, Arkansas

QUEEN HENRY-OKAFOR, PhD, FNP-BC, PMHNP-BC, Associate Professor, Vanderbilt University School of Nursing, Nashville, Tennessee

SHARON L. HOLLEY, DNP, CNM, FACNM, FAAN, Associate Professor of Nursing, Director of Didactic Education, Nurse-Midwifery Pathway, University of Alabama at Birmingham School of Nursing, Birmingham, Alabama

LINDA J. KEILMAN, DNP, MSN, GNP-BC, FNAP, FAANP, Associate Professor, Michigan State University, College of Nursing, East Lansing, Michigan

CHRISTIE KELLER, DNP, APRN, PMHNP-BC, Clinical Instructor, University of Arkansas for Medical Sciences, College of Nursing, Little Rock/Fayetteville, Fayetteville, Arkansas

PAM LaBORDE, DNP, APRN, TTS, Assistant Professor, University of Arkansas for Medical Sciences, College of Nursing, Little Rock, Arkansas

MARY LAUREN PFIEFFER, DNP, FNP-BC, Associate Professor, Vanderbilt University School of Nursing, Nashville, Tennessee

MARGARET LOVE, DNP, APRN, FNP-BC, ACHPN, Clinical Instructor, University of Arkansas for Medical Sciences, College of Nursing, Little Rock, Arkansas

ANN MATTISON, MSN, CPNP- PC, CPNP-AC, APRN, Advanced Practice Registered Nurse, Well Baby Nursery, Children's Mercy Kansas City, Children's Mercy Hospital, Kansas City, Missouri

STEPHANIE MITCHELL, DNP, CNM, CPM, Certified Nurse Midwife, Certified Professional Midwife, Birth Sanctuary, Gainesville, Alabama

ELIZABETH G. MUÑOZ, DNP, CNM, FACNM, Assistant Professor of Nursing, Nurse-Midwifery Pathway, School of Nursing, University of Alabama at Birmingham, Birmingham, Alabama; Carle Foundation Hospital, Urbana, Illinois

LAUREN NICHOLS, DNP, CPNP-AC, Pediatric Nurse Practitioner, Pediatric Home Ventilator Program C.S. Mott Children's Hospital, University of Michigan Health, Ann Arbor, Michigan

CATHERINE O'BRIEN, DNP, CNM, Certified Nurse-Midwife, Tri-Cities Community Health, Pasco, Washington

GEORGE BYRON PERAZA-SMITH, DNP, GNP-BC, AGPCNP-C, CNE, FAANP, Dean, West Coast University, Irvine, California

ANN MARIE RAMSEY, MSN, CPNP-PC, Pediatric Nurse Practitioner, Pediatric Home Ventilator Program C.S. Mott Children's Hospital, University of Michigan Health, Ann Arbor, Michigan

SARA RAY, MSN, FNP-C, Advanced Practice Registered Nurse, Department of Otolaryngology, Children's Mercy Kansas City, Children's Mercy Hospital, Kansas City, Missouri

CHARLOTTE C. RENSBERGER, MSN, APRN, PNP-PC, Pediatric Nurse Practitioner, Bronson Children's Hospital, Kalamazoo, Michigan

LAILA SHAD, DNP, CNM, Part-Time Lecturer, California State University, Fullerton, School of Nursing, Fullerton, California

TAYLOR STEELE, DNP, RN, CPN, Assistant Professor, University of Arkansas for Medical Sciences, College of Nursing, Little Rock, Arkansas

JANNYSE TAPP, DNP, FNP-BC, Assistant Professor, Vanderbilt University School of Nursing, Nashville, Tennessee

JANICE TAYLOR, DNP, APRN, AGPC-BC, GNP-BC Assistant Professor, University of Arkansas for Medical Sciences, College of Nursing, Little Rock, Arkansas

CRISTY TOBUREN, MSN, CPNP- PC, APRN, Pediatric Nurse Practitioner, Well Baby Nursery, Children's Mercy Kansas City, Children's Mercy Hospital, Kansas City, Missouri

TERESA WHITED, DNP, APRN, CPNP-PC, Associate Dean of Academic Programs and Accreditation, Associate Professor, University of Arkansas for Medical Sciences, College of Nursing, Little Rock, Arkansas

TRISHA WILLIAMS, MSN, CPNP- PC, Advanced Practice Registered Nurse, Department of Otolaryngology, Children's Mercy Kansas City, Children's Mercy Hospital, Kansas City, Missouri

ALEXIS L. WOODS BARR, MS, PhD, Postdoctoral Research Associate, Department of Health and Human Behavior, Gillings School of Public Health, University of North Carolina at Chapel Hill, Chapel Hill, North Carolina

ADVANCES IN
Family Practice Nursing

CONTENTS   VOLUME 7 • 2025

Adult/Gerontology

Neuropsychiatric Symptoms and Mental Health Disparities in Older Adults
Linda J. Keilman, Melodee Harris, George Byron Peraza-Smith, and Khaled Alomari

Neuropsychiatric symptoms (NPS) are common in older adults living with dementia. Early recognition of NPS contributes to timely diagnosis of neurocognitive disorders and improved access to effective treatments. However, dementia is not recognized, not diagnosed, and under-treated or not treated in 75% of dementia cases in the world's population. Socioeconomic constraints, cultural stigmas, limited access to quality care, and language barriers pose significant challenges for marginalized populations including racial-ethnic minorities living with dementia. Nurse practitioners play a vital role in the recognition of NPS, diagnosis, and treatment of neurocognitive disorders in older adults with mental health disparities and inequities.

Musical Interventions and Older Adults Experiencing Sleep Disturbances in Long-Term Care

Julia Dunham-Thornton and Melodee Harris

Approximately 50% of the older adult (OA) population experience poor sleep quality due to various sleep disorders. The percentage increases within OAs who are residing in long-term care facilities. Poor sleep quality is associated with an increased risk for multiple health complications including falls, which is the leading cause of morbidity and mortality in the elderly. This article will explore the nonpharmacologic therapy for listening to personalized music and/or binaural auditory beat music and the potential effect of reducing insomnia experienced by OAs.

Psychological Adaptation to Newly Diagnosed Advanced Cancer: Implications for Older Adults

Mei Bai and Melodee Harris

Cancer patients represent a heterogeneous population. Older adults are generally thought to respond to stress in a more adaptive fashion; nonetheless, adaptation varies across individuals and contexts. We explain that assessing one's strength and overall well-being as well as other determining factors may be equally important as assessing distress. Instead of attempting to diagnose and treat maladaptation or mental disease/disorder, we ask what constitutes adaptation, how to assess psychological adjustment in the context of cancer, and how to optimize older adults' efforts toward that end.

Depression and Older Adults: A Guide for Assessment, Diagnosis, and Management

Christie Keller

Depression often remains undetected and untreated among older adults. Variations in symptom manifestation and subsyndromal symptoms are common among older adults and may be overlooked, complicating diagnosis and leading to inadequate treatment. Untreated depression can increase morbidity and mortality and result in prolonged recovery times, functional disabilities, medical complications, and cognitive decline. Primary care providers play an essential role in the identification, treatment, and management of depression in this population through the incorporation of pharmacologic and nonpharmacological interventions.

Understanding End-of-Life Care for the Older Adults: Assessment, Management, and Ethical Considerations

Margaret Love

End-of-life (EOL) care differs significantly in older adults due to prevalence of chronic conditions, impaired reserve or less functional, cognitive, and limited social support at baseline. A holistic, family-centered approach addresses physical, cognitive, and emotional challenges through comprehensive assessment. Effective communication facilitates determination of services that meet the needs of older adults while aligning care with preferences to enhance comfort and reassurance for caregivers. Awareness of advanced care planning, latest resources such as telemedicine, and guidelines aid robust caregiver support, reduce burdens, and foster ethical, compassionate care that balances patient goals with holistic care at EOL for the older adult.

Resilience in Older Adults: Evaluation and Implications for Poststroke Recovery 87
Janice Taylor

This article explores the resilience and poststroke recovery journey of Mrs B, a 77-year-old female with left-sided hemiplegia and mild cognitive impairment following an ischemic stroke. It highlights the multifaceted challenges of physical, cognitive, emotional, and social recovery while emphasizing the critical role of resilience. Interventions included optimizing medical management, rehabilitation, caregiver support, and reintegration into her church and music teaching activities. Collaborative care and resilience-building strategies resulted in improved functionality, mood, and independence. This study underscores the importance of assessing resilience in stroke recovery and tailoring interventions to promote adaptation and quality of life.

Battling Frailty in Older Adults: The Critical Role of Advanced Practice Registered Nurses in Assessment, Management, and Prevention 95
Pam LaBorde and Melodee Harris

Frailty is a geriatric syndrome and a global health concern for older adults. Although aging is a risk factor, frailty can occur in younger adults. There is no global definition of frailty. Although there are many validated screening tools, there is no gold standard for the assessment of frailty. The 5 criteria for frailty include weight loss, exhaustion, slowness, low activity level, and weakness. Frailty is complex and often overlaps with comorbidities. Frailty can be prevented. Nurses are leaders on the interdisciplinary team to assess, diagnose, manage, and prevent frailty in older adults.

Women's Health

Fragmented Care: Midwifery in a Landscape of Variable Accessibility to Pregnancy Care   109

Stephanie Mitchell, Laila Shad, Catherine O'Brien, and
Elizabeth G. Muñoz

Certified nurse-midwives, in the United States, practice in
different communities and health systems. The way
patients interface with midwives and their health systems
is determined by the accessibility of healthcare resources.
The disparities in the American healthcare system mean
that patients experience systemic fragmentation of
resources. While prenatal care can be inconsistent across
different levels of healthcare access, the culture of
midwifery remains consistent. This article explores cases
representing how midwives impact care in pregnancies
with complications in both high-resource and low-
resource settings.

Interpreting Bone Density Screenings and Treatment for Osteopenia and Osteoporosis

Mary Lauren Pfieffer, Queen Henry-Okafor, Shannon Cole, and Jannyse Tapp

Osteopenia and osteoporosis are progressive skeletal disorders characterized by decreased bone mineral density and compromised bone strength, predisposing individuals to an increased risk of fracture. The prevalence is increasing as our aging population is increasing in the United States. Regular bone density tests are recommended for postmenopausal women, men over 70, and individuals with risk factors. Bone mineral density measurement via dual-energy X-ray absorptiometry (DXA) remains the gold standard for diagnosing osteoporosis and osteopenia. DXA helps classify bone health status and guide clinical decision-making regarding prevention and treatment strategies. Treatment includes a mixture of lifestyle modifications and pharmacologic treatment.

Episiotomy: Indications, Techniques, and Postpartum Care Considerations 139

Sharon L. Holley, Sarah E. Barton, and
Mary Catherine Carpenter

Episiotomy—a surgical incision in the perineum during the second stage of labor—is used to reduce severe perineal trauma and expedite delivery. Routine use is discouraged by World Health Organization, American College of Obstetrics and Gynecology, and International Federation of Gynecology and Obstetrics due to increased risks of severe perineal injury. Indications for performing include prolonged second stage, rigid perineum, and certain fetal conditions. Complications include additional perineal trauma, dyspareunia, and infection. Informed consent is essential. Further research is needed on long-term effects. This article reviews evidence, techniques, and recommendations for episiotomy, emphasizing restrictive use and individualized care.

Understanding Intersectionality in African American Breastfeeding: Insights for Health Care Professionals

Alexis L. Woods Barr and Stephanie Devane-Johnson

The article presents a comprehensive analysis of the historic context, including the legacy of slavery and forced wet-nursing, and its ongoing impact on perceptions of breastfeeding in African American communities. It also addresses the persistence of health care disparities across socioeconomic strata, emphasizing the need for an intersectional approach in health care delivery. Key implications for health care professionals are discussed, including strategies for providing culturally congruent care, engaging family members in breastfeeding education, and addressing systemic barriers. It emphasizes the importance of recognizing and challenging personal biases, using inclusive language, and connecting patients with culturally-relevant resources and support networks.

Pediatrics

Managing the Pressure: Pediatric Blood Pressure Screening and Management in Primary Care

Teresa Whited and Taylor Steele

Blood pressure evaluation is a key part of every well-child visit beginning at age 3 or sooner if the child has risk factors. Evaluation for hypertension (HTN) is based on age/gender percentiles until 13 years of age. Ambulatory blood pressure monitoring and evaluation for secondary causes of HTN is a key part of the diagnostic process. Management of HTN includes lifestyle modification, medication management, and sports participation considerations.

Updated (New) Hyperbilirubinemia Guidelines for the Primary Care Provider

Mary E. Flynn

Many newborns will develop some degree of jaundice in the first week of life. Most bilirubin levels are consistent with physiologic jaundice of the newborn and are expected to resolve without treatment. Bilirubin levels that exceed the level of physiologic jaundice in the first few weeks of life warrant close follow-up and/or treatment. The American Academy of Pediatrics published new guidelines that include the prevention, risk assessment, monitoring, and treatment of infants with hyperbilirubinemia. These guidelines replace the 2004 guidelines with updated hospital management of hyperbilirubinemia and include guidance for follow-up and management in outpatient settings.

Caring for Children with Trisomy 18 in the Primary Care Setting

Ann Marie Ramsey and Lauren Nichols

Trisomy 18 is a rare chromosomal abnormality associated with multiple congenital anomalies. Previously, trisomy 18 was fatal; however, developing medical treatment and technologies have inspired parents to choose life-prolonging care. This has resulted in a significant increase in this population requiring comprehensive care across acute, subspeciality, and primary care domains. Although respiratory and cardiac conditions represent the most acute early life problems, these children are also at risk for multisystem problems. This article provides a comprehensive review of pathophysiology of trisomy 18, care guidelines, and emerging evidence to guide clinical care and direct ongoing surveillance.

Diagnosing and Treating Disorders of the Gut–Brain Interaction in Pediatric Patients

Charlotte C. Rensberger

Disorders of gut–brain interaction, formerly known as functional gastrointestinal disorders, are a group of chronic disorders frequently diagnosed in children around the world with no organic cause for their symptoms. While these conditions are usually considered to be benign, patients and their families are often worried about the longevity of symptoms and possible underlying organic diseases that could be causing them. In pursuit of a diagnosis, many patients undergo unnecessary procedures and testing looking for a cause. This article intends to help pediatric primary care providers recognize, diagnose, treat these disorders, and determine when to refer to a specialist.

A Dose of Prevention is Worth a Pound of Cure: Respiratory Syncytial Virus Immunity for a Safer Community

Ann Mattison and Cristy Toburen

Respiratory syncytial virus (RSV) is the leading cause of lower viral respiratory tract infection in infants and young children worldwide. It can cause mild-to-severe illness in children. Treatment of the disease is supportive. In 2023, the US Food and Drug Administration approved 2 immunization products to decrease the disease burden. Beyfortus (Nirsevimab) is used in infants and young children to prevent RSV-associated lower respiratory tract infections. Abrysvo (RSVpreF) is given to pregnant women to protect infants after delivery.

Common Pediatric Ears, Nose, and Throat Referrals 239
Trisha Williams and Sara Ray

It is pivotal for patient care that primary care providers (PCPs) are up to date on the current practice guidelines for referral to surgical specialty and other specialty clinics. Having patients participate in medical management of a given disease process prior to referrals and understanding indications for surgical intervention as well as risks and benefits of surgical procedures are vital in directing patient care prior to a specialty clinic. Pediatric ears, nose, and throat are one of the most common surgical specialties that PCPs refer to. Often for diagnoses such as acute suppurative otitis media, tonsillitis, tonsil hypertrophy with/without snoring, and epistaxis.

Advances in Family Practice Nursing 7 (2025) xxiii–xxv

ADVANCES IN FAMILY PRACTICE NURSING

PREFACE

Sharing the Knowledge and Expertise of Advanced Practice Nurses in Providing Care Across the Lifespan

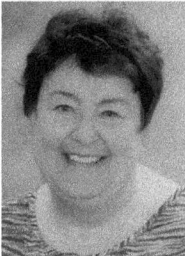

Linda J. Keilman, DNP, MSN, GNP-BC, FNAP, FAANP
Editor

O n January 22 of this year, the cofounder of the nurse practitioner (NP) profession, Dr Loretta C. Ford, left this earth after being present for 104 years. Due to her futuristic vision and advocacy, there are currently more than 385,000 NPs in the United States, providing care for all human beings in a multitude of settings. Dr Ford developed the Unification Model of Nursing that emphasizes the intersectionality between nursing education, research, scholarship, and advanced clinical practice. The authors presenting their work in this seventh issue are advanced practice nurses (APNs), who provide quality care to specific populations from conception through the end of life. Each author has the lived experience of Dr Ford's vision in that they have advanced education as a nurse and have or currently provide holistic, comprehensive care to all age groups. This issue is dedicated in appreciation to

https://doi.org/10.1016/j.yfpn.2025.02.002
2589-420X/25/© 2025 Published by Elsevier Inc.

Dr Ford as a visionary and mentor for all APNs, everywhere. I like to think she would be proud of each author who has shared their passion and dedication with us through their professional work.

In the Pediatrics section, there is information about common ear-nose-throat conditions that may need to be referred to, how to manage blood pressure screening and appropriately treating if there are abnormalities, as well as who to best care for children born with trisomy 18. The reader will also learn about preventing respiratory syncytial virus through vaccination and immunity, discover the new hyperbilirubinemia guidelines, and understand the importance of diagnosing and treating disorders of the gut-brain interaction.

Continuing to Women's Health, you will learn about some of the access issues leading to inequities and disparities of receiving quality pregnancy care in the United States. Would you be surprised to know that, in 2022, for every 100,000 live births in the United States, 22 women died? What do you know about the indications, techniques, and postpartum care considerations for episiotomies? Tear, incision, or forego? Some insights into understanding the intersectionality of African American breastfeeding are proposed as well as considerations for interpreting bone density screenings and treatment for osteopenia and osteoporosis.

Do you listen to music when trying to fall asleep at night? You might be interested in the interventions provided to older adults related to sleep disturbances. Depression is a condition that is underdiagnosed, underreported, and undertreated in older adults, often chalked up to normal aging, which is inaccurate; learn how to ethically assess, diagnose, and manage the condition. Research demonstrates that older adults who exhibit more resilience characteristics do better in poststroke recovery. What about those newly diagnosed with cancer, what is their psychological adaptation to the disease? Once you read the articles, you might see benefits for many conditions based on resiliency factors. Mental health disparities are common in the United States but perhaps are harder felt by older adults experiencing neuropsychiatric symptoms—read the article and see what you think. APNs have a significant role in preventing frailty in older adults—what can you do proactively? And finally, when we have done the best we can for older adults, they are moving toward the end of their life journey. How can you assist in providing a peaceful, comfortable death for the individual and their loved ones? You might find some helpful information you can apply to your clinical practice.

I leave you by sharing a wonderful quote from Dr Ford at the age of 103 that I hope will have meaning for you and give you renewed purpose as well! Thank you for reading our issue!

> It fills my heart with immense pride to see how far the nurse practitioners have come . . . remember that each of you has the power to make a profound impact on the lives of your patients. Embrace the opportunity to learn, to grow, and to inspire one another. Never forget that the essence of our work is rooted in compassion, knowledge, and unwavering

dedication to providing the highest quality of care. Together, we are the heartbeat of healthcare.

—Dr Loretta C. Ford (2024 at the American Association of Nurse Practitioners Annual Conference)

Linda J. Keilman, DNP, MSN, GNP-BC, FNAP, FAANP
Michigan State University
College of Nursing
East Lansing, MI 48824, USA

E-mail address: keilman@msu.edu

Adult/Gerontology

Advances in Family Practice Nursing 7 (2025) 1–21

ADVANCES IN FAMILY PRACTICE NURSING

Neuropsychiatric Symptoms and Mental Health Disparities in Older Adults

Linda J. Keilman, DNP, MSN, GNP-BC, FNAP, FAANP[a],*,
Melodee Harris, PhD, APRN, GNP-BC, AGPCNP-BC[b],
George Byron Peraza-Smith, DNP, GNP-BC, AGPCNP-C,
CNE[c], Khaled Alomari, PhD, NP, RN[c]

[a]Michigan State University, College of Nursing, 1355 Bogue Street, A126 Life Sciences, East Lansing, MI 48824, USA; [b]University of Arkansas for Medical Sciences, College of Nursing, 4301 West Markham Street, Little Rock, AR 72205, USA; [c]West Coast University, 151 Innovation Drive, Irvine, CA 92617, USA

Keywords
- Neuropsychiatric • Dementia • Mental health • Health disparities
- Health inequities • Marginalized • Older adult

Key points
- Neuropsychiatric symptoms are common in older adults living with dementia.
- Stigma surrounding neurocognitive disorders prevents older adults for accessing health care.
- Neuropsychiatric symptoms are often overlooked and untreated in older adults living with dementia.
- Marginalized older adults are more vulnerable to poor mental health outcomes.
- There is limited research about neuropsychiatric symptoms and mental health disparities.

INTRODUCTION

Did you know that worldwide, someone–somewhere, develops dementia every 3 seconds? [1] And, based on this number, that equates to approximately 10 million individuals diagnosed with dementia yearly? Perhaps more importantly is understanding that dementia is not diagnosed in 75% of dementia

*Corresponding author. E-mail address: keilman@msu.edu

https://doi.org/10.1016/j.yfpn.2025.02.001

Abbreviations

AD	Alzheimer's disease
AD/ADRD	Alzheimer's disease and other related dementias
FTD	frontotemporal dementia
GDS	Geriatric Depression Scale
HTN	hypertension
MCI	mild cognitive impairment
MMSE	Mini Mental Status Examination
MoCA	Montreal Cognitive Assessment
NACC	National Alzheimer's Coordinating Center
NP	nurse practitioners
NPI	Neuropsychiatric Inventory
NPS	neuropsychiatric symptoms
NTG-EDSD	National Task Group-Early Detection Screen for Dementia
PCP	primary care provider
QoL	quality of life
SLUMS	St. Louis University Mental Status Examination
T2DM	Type 2 diabetes

cases in the world's population [1]. Imagine the tremendous global impact nurse practitioners (NP) could make if cognitive screening of older adults were an integral component of every assessment during every appointment when caring for this population! This paper aims to address how to mitigate mental health disparities, stigma, and cultural differences that play a role in the early recognition of neuropsychiatric symptoms and diagnosis of neurocognitive disorders.

Neuropsychiatric symptoms (NPS) are common with Alzheimer's disease and other related dementias (AD/ADRD) [2,3]. Up to 97% of individuals diagnosed with AD are affected by NPS [2]. Common NPS related to dementia are apathy, depression, sleep disorders, hallucinations, delusions, psychosis, agitation, and aggression [2,3].

Mental health disparities impact the physical and mental well-being of older adults. Memory loss is a more obvious symptom in the initial stages of a dementia. Depression, anxiety, agitation, and other NPS are often unrecognized as warning signs associated with dementia in older adults [2]. Socioeconomic constraints, cultural stigmas, limited access to quality care, and language barriers pose significant challenges for marginalized populations including racial-ethnic minorities, lower incomes, and lesbian, gay, bisexual, transgender, questioning plus older adults [2,4]. The stigma around older adults with a mental or behavioral health condition adds to these barriers, promoting discrimination that discourages health-seeking behaviors and worsens health care inequities [4–6].

The following case illustrates the intersection of NPS and mental health disparities of an older adult with mental illness, cultural differences, and limited finances and social support.

Case report

Mala is a 61-year-old Cambodian-American female who functioned fairly well when she first moved into a small apartment within a senior housing complex. Mala moved into the apartment 5 years ago after quitting her job in a cafeteria due to back pain. Mala experiences life-long bipolar disorder, mild intellectual disability, and undiagnosed early-stage frontotemporal dementia (FTD). Mala immigrated to the United States from Vietnam when she was a teenager. Before her bipolar disorder was adequately treated, Mala's symptoms resulted in alienation from her siblings who did not understand her mental illness or that she needed professional help at an early age. Overall, Mala could safely live independently and worked hard all her life in food services.

At age 54 years old, Mala married for the first time to Ray (a white American) who also had intellectual disabilities. Ray was 23 years younger than Mala. She and Ray met at a church fellowship, and they were a perfect match. Ray had the habit of not taking care of his bills, and he would wear the same clothes day after day. Although resources were limited, Mala took over their simple finances and helped Ray with his activities of daily living. Ray accepted Mala's mental illness, and they overcame their cultural differences. Mala spoke in her native Khmer or Vietnamese language when she did not know how to express herself in English. Ray could communicate with Mala despite language barriers. They helped each other live independently until Ray passed away 3 years ago. Mala insisted on living alone as she did not want to leave the home she had created with Ray. Mala began hoarding mail, clothing, empty potato chip bags, napkins, plastic forks, and anything that remotely reminded her of Ray.

In addition to her mental health diagnoses and undiagnosed FTD, Mala has a history of several chronic medical conditions, including Type 2 diabetes (T2DM), hypertension (HTN), hypercholesterolemia, and glaucoma. She had not yet applied for Medicare disability benefits, which limited her access to health care. She did not understand how to access additional enabling resources such as food banks, or assistance for utilities. Mala's age, symptoms of grief, depression, and bipolar disorder overlapped with NPS and further delayed a referral and diagnosis of FTD by her primary care provider (PCP). Her own self-neglect, after Ray's passing, resulted in worsening T2DM, glaucoma, HTN, and increased NPS. Over time, Mala's church friends noticed personality changes. She was apathetic and more irritable. Often, she would not answer the phone, missed church services, and self-isolated in a dark room. She lived on chips and snack cakes which she ate continuously while watching the Price is Right on television. She gained weight. Every Wednesday, Mala's church friends stopped by to clean her apartment and bring groceries. Mala became terribly angry if her friends attempted to bring healthier food choices. As time went on, Mala began frequently calling the police because she thought people were trying to break into her apartment. One night, Mala was so anxious and paranoid that she thought someone had entered her home and poisoned her food. She called the ambulance and was transferred to the hospital for observation. Subsequently, Mala's NPS progressed. After consultation with a gerontological nurse practitioner, Mala was diagnosed with FTD.

Mental health disparities

Mental health disparities refer to gaps in mental health status, mental health outcomes, treatment access, and quality among minority or marginalized groups [4,7,8]. As in Mala's case, mental health disparities result from multifaceted factors including compromised physical health, limited access to care, inadequate chronic condition treatment, socioeconomic barriers, cultural stigmas, communication barriers, inadequately trained staff, insufficient supportive services, limited public awareness, and paucity of research. Older adults living with dementia and other related cognitive impairments exhibiting NPS often encounter additional health disparities in their physical health, especially if they have difficulty adequately communicating their needs. Like Mala, there are often comorbid chronic conditions with co-existing mental health disorders. In the case for many older adults, chronic conditions are inappropriately prioritized by health care professionals (HCPs). Symptoms such as depression or anxiety remain inadequately addressed for prolonged periods of time. In fact, this juncture of chronic physical disorders and mental health disorders potentiate NPS leading to poor health outcomes.

Neuropsychiatric symptoms

Addressing mental health disparities in older adults with dementia or NPS requires a multifaceted approach. NPS must be distinguished from similar characteristics associated with mental illnesses [9]. NPS herald neurocognitive disorders [9]. Decreased stigma and early recognition of NPS contributes to timely diagnosis of neurocognitive disorders, improved access to effective treatments and NPS management, cultural sensitivity training for HCP, community education initiatives, and the development of accessible, equitable, and diverse support resources [6,9]. Mala's friends were bewildered by her personality changes and the NPS of FTD; even her PCP missed these early NPS.

Mental illness in older adults

Mental health conditions, including depression, anxiety, dementia, and NPS, are common among older adults. The prevalence of any mental illness is 13.9% for adults 50 years and 3% of older adults report a serious mental illness [10]. Contrary to stereotypical beliefs, developing a mental health disorder is not a part of the expected or normal (usual) age-related changes.

Mental illness in older adults is intricately linked with their physical health and functionality, often exacerbating existing health conditions leading to overall poorer outcomes and diminished quality of life (QoL). Despite the significant burden of mental health issues on older adults, they are often hesitant to seek mental health services [11,12]. The reluctance of older adults to seek mental health services is intensified among racial-ethnic, gender, and sexual minority groups. As with ageist negative effects, these diverse minority groups often face adverse mental health outcomes due to factors such as limited access to quality care, cultural prejudices against mental health treatment, discrimination, and an overarching lack of awareness about mental health. In Mala's case, her family did not recognize her early symptoms of mental illness. Mala's earliest symptoms were deemed irrelevant which led to isolation from those who might help her the most including family, friends, and even HCP.

Stigma and mental illness
Mental illness or psychiatric disorders continue to carry a heavy burden of stigma. The destructive and discriminatory attitudes, beliefs, and stigmas toward those with psychiatric or mental health disorders negatively impact the individual's overall health and well-being [6]. Individuals seeking help with mental health issues are often considered weak or even dangerous [5,6]. Stigma compounds health disparities in already marginalized groups, such as those living with dementia or older adults with limited income. According to the US Centers for Disease Control and Prevention, health disparities occur when preventable differences in the burden of disease, injury, or violence are borne by socially marginalized populations, preventing them from achieving optimal health [13].

Cultural stigma
Mala encountered cultural stigmas and communication barriers. Cultural stigma surrounding NPS and mental health issues may often hinder carers from accessing the assistance and support services they critically need. Globally, there are cultures that have deep-rooted stigmas, misperceptions, and misconceptions associated with mental health and psychiatric care-related issues. Negatively held societal beliefs may lead to feelings of shame or fear of judgment, discouraging older adults and carers from speaking openly about their struggles or challenges, furthering isolation, and decline. Negative cultural stigmas related to dementia or mental health conditions contribute to delays in care and impede older adults and carers from seeking treatment. As language and comprehension can be impacted by dementia or NPS, older adults often receive inadequate information in an accessible manner or may face challenges in expressing their needs. Furthermore, communication barriers, whether they stem from language differences, low health literacy, or the complexities of navigating the health care system, can further complicate the process. Carers often feel overwhelmed or under-informed, uncertain about where to turn, or how to effectively advocate for mental health treatment and services. Cultural differences must be considered. In Mala's case, mental illness may be interpreted and explained according to her religion, Buddhism, prevalent in Vietnam and Cambodia.

Cognition, communication, and neuropsychiatric symptoms
Older adults with mental health disparities, like Mala, have unique needs [9]. Older adults with cognitive impairment often have multiple chronic conditions leading to complex health needs [14]. For HCP, mental status assessments are essential for identifying and tracking NPS and helping to distinguish between

mental and cognitive health issues. When combined with the older adult's health history and mental status assessments, it enables the creation of individualized treatment/management plans and allows providers to monitor changes over time.

Mental status and neuropsychiatric symptoms. A comprehensive approach to care is crucial for addressing mental health disparities among older adults experiencing NPS. Mental status is the mental state or snapshot of an individual's psychological functioning and includes the person's overall emotional and cognitive well-being, encompassing elements such as mood, awareness, orientation, and alertness. A mental status examination is a structured assessment used to evaluate the behavioral and cognitive functioning of an older adult.

Assessment of mental and cognitive status is crucial for HCP assessing older adults presenting with NPS. This examination aids in differentiating between various diagnoses, such as medical conditions, dementia, delirium, depression, parkinsonian disorders, and anxiety, among others. Mental and cognitive assessment results are useful when determining treatment and disposition. A well-documented mental status examination serves as a valuable reference for comparing future assessments with past ones. This practice assists HCP in gauging the progression of an older adult's symptomatology and in determining whether they are ameliorating or deteriorating.

A mental status examination is conducted in conjunction with a thorough medical and mental health history. Table 1 provides information on 4 commonly used screening tests for mental status. The structured mental status examination includes evaluating an individual's appearance and general behavior, level of consciousness, mental alertness, motor activity, speech, mood and affect, thoughts and perceptions, attitude and insight, and cognitive function including language, memory, constructional ability, and abstract thinking.

Mental status and mental health services among diverse populations. As in Mala's case, a mental/cognitive assessment must be culturally appropriate. The Montreal Cognitive Assessment (MoCA) is widely used and available in many languages [17,18]. While there is no MoCA version for Khmer, there is a Vietnamese version. Mala may benefit from an interpreter. The MoCA is similar to the Mini Mental Status Examination (MMSE) and St. Louis University Mental Status Examination (SLUMS) [19,20]. The MoCA has a broader range than the MMSE with an advantage for distinguishing mild cognitive impairment (MCI) [22]. One systematic review showed that the MoCA has a better capacity to detect neurocognitive disorders than the MMSE [23].

Mala's symptoms consistent with FTD were not only confounded by the co-existing bipolar disorder, but also by her intellectual disability. The National Task Group-Early Detection Screen for Dementia (NTG-EDSD) is a 30-item screening to detect dementia in persons with intellectual disabilities [24]. Mala could benefit by the NTG-EDSD screening to distinguish between intellectual disabilities and dementia. A mental status examination is conducted in conjunction with a thorough health/medical and mental health history. Table 1

Table 1
Cognitive screening tests for mental status [15]

Screening test for cognition	Description

Mini-Mental State Examination (MMSE) [15,16]	• Assesses mental status
	• 11-questions that assess 5 areas of cognitive functioning: orientation, registration, attention & calculation, recall, & language
	• Screening tool for cognitive decline
	• Is *not diagnostic* of dementia!
	• Since 1975, commonly used in clinical & research settings to screen for cognitive changes & impairment, especially in older adults.
	• Tracks cognitive changes or progress over time with repeated use; marker for when to refer for comprehensive neuropsychological testing.
	• Useful in determining overall functional independence.
	• Test-retest reliability; 0.80–0.95.
	• Limitations:
	  ◦ Low education levels = poor specificity
	  ◦ Individuals with vision or hearing issues, low English language literacy, those with communication disorders may score low even though cognitively intact.
	• Copyrighted; forms must be purchased; there is restriction from freely reproducing the full content.

Montreal Cognitive Assessment [15,17,18] Certification information available at: https://mocacognition.com	• Published 2005 • Screening tool for mild cognitive impairment • Assesses 6 cognitive domains including memory, executive functions, attention, language, visuospatial skills, & orientation • Available in over 100 languages & dialects • Cross-cultural consideration: research conducted with English-speaking populations; may consider if you feel appropriate for use in non-English speaking populations • More sensitive in identifying subtle cognitive decline vs MMSE • Free 1-h training is suggested prior to administration & scoring
Saint Louis Mental State Examination (SLUMS) [19,20] Available at: https://www.slu.edu/medicine/internal-medicine/geriatric-medicine/aging-successfully/assessment-tools/mental-status-exam.php	• 11 questions • Screens for cognitive deficits over time • Attention, recall, orientation, calculation, registration, language, working memory, visual spatial, executive function • Video available for instruction • Not a final diagnostic tool for dementia • Similar to the MoCA & MMSE • Can be administered by many health care professionals • Available in many languages

(continued on next page)

Table 1
(continued)

Screening test for cognition	Description
MiniCog [21] Available at: https://mini-cog.com/ download-the-mini-cog-instrument/	• Three steps • Recall, registration, clock drawing • Complete in 3 min • Minimal training • Not a final diagnostic tool for dementia

provides information on 4 commonly used screening tests for mental status. The structured MMSE includes evaluating an individual's appearance and general behavior, level of consciousness, mental alertness, motor activity, speech, mood and affect, thoughts and perceptions, attitude and insight, and cognitive function including language, memory, constructional ability, and abstract thinking. At this time, the MMSE is copyrighted and is no longer as widely used [15,16]. The SLUMS is similar to the MMSE [19,20]. The SLUMS is also available in many languages. Finally, the MiniCog is a short screening for cognition that can be completed in about 3 minutes [21]. The MiniCog tests for recall, registration, clock drawing, and executive function [21]. None of the cognitive screening tools are diagnostic for dementia (see Table 1).

Assessment of mental and cognitive status is crucial for HCP assessing older adults presenting with NPS [24] (Table 2). The Neuropsychiatric Inventory (NPI) Questionnaire addresses delusions, hallucinations, agitation/aggression, depression, dysphoria, anxiety, elation/euphasia, apathy/indifference, disinhibition, irritability/lability, aberrant motor behavior, sleep, and appetite/eating [25]. The scoring for NPI includes symptoms, frequency, and severity of NPS.

Overall, mental and cognitive assessment aids in differentiating between various diagnoses, such as medical conditions, dementia, delirium, depression, parkinsonian disorders, and anxiety, among others. Results are useful when determining treatment and disposition. A well-documented mental status examination serves as a valuable reference for comparing future assessments with past ones. This practice assists HCP in gauging the progression of an older

Table 2
Cognitive screening for intellectual disability [24]

National task group early detection screen for dementia	
• Activities of Daily Living (ADL)	• Adult's self-reported problems
• Language & Communication	• Changes observed by others
• Sleep & Wakefulness	• Chronic conditions
• Ambulation	• Medications
• Memory	• Demographics
• Behavior & Affect	• Can be completed by anyone
	• Complete between 15 and 60 min

NTG-EDSG: https://www.dhs.wisconsin.gov/publications/p01622m.pdf.

adult's symptomatology and in determining whether they are ameliorating or deteriorating. Table 3 describes the general mental status areas of consideration as well as the specific cognitive domains that should be assessed.

Mental health services are tailored to address the psychological and emotional well-being of aging individuals across varied racial, ethnic, socioeconomic, and cultural backgrounds. Ensuring mental health equity, irrespective of background, is a pressing concern for adults as they age. Addressing the mental health needs of diverse older adult populations requires a multifaceted, multidisciplinary approach. HCPs play a crucial role in recognizing, diagnosing, and referring older patients to appropriate care. Addressing these mental health and other disparities is essential to ensure that older adults with dementia-related disorders and NPS receive comprehensive, compassionate, and appropriate care throughout the trajectory of their illness. Assessment tools such as the Geriatric Depression Scale (GDS) need to be culturally appropriate [26]. For Mala, there is a Vietnamese version of the GDS [27].

Psychosoical factors
The interinfluence of determinants of health, experiences of discrimination and oppression, and the paucity of access to care combine to delay diagnosis and prompt treatment for those with dementia-related conditions [28]. This is especially evident in undertreated and underserved communities [4]. Older adults with NPS who are confronted with health disparities and finite resources usually have limited treatment options available or lack access to affordable options for long-term care, which is crucial for those with advanced dementia or those experiencing NPS. Of the 40 million individuals worldwide requiring palliative and hospice services, only 14% can access them, highlighting the significant challenges to access [29]. Access for older adults exhibiting NPS compounds timely and effective access.

According to the National Council on Aging and reports by the US Census Bureau, over 17 million older adults over 65 years of age are economically insecure with incomes below 200% of the federal poverty level [30]. Poverty indicators are significant risk factors for declines in mental health and lead to poor outcomes for older adults with NPS. Socioeconomic inequalities also have detrimental effects on older adults with NPS [2]. Socioeconomic disparities limit access to quality health care, necessary medications and treatments, and supportive services which may exacerbate or worsen mental health disparities [4].

INTERSECTION OF NEUROPSYCHIATRIC SYMPTOMS AND DISPARITIES
Research outcomes using the National Alzheimer's Coordinating Center (NACC) data and other data bases can help to provide the foundation for what is known about NPS symptoms and mental health disparities [31–34]. Data using the NACC repository data on MCI and AD/ADRD can offer insight into NPS and mental health disparities. It is important to take racial-ethnic

Table 3
Mental status assessment/examination of the older adult [15]

Mental status domain	Assessment/examination
General Areas of Consideration *Appearance:* Provides insight into the individual including values, social status, personality, functioning, level of independence, etc.	• What is the overall appearance or presentation? • Includes age, race, hair, facial features, make-up, grooming, expression, posture, eye contact, piercings, tattoos, clothing (appropriate for season), shoes, jewelry, assistive devices (glasses, hearing aid, braces, cane, crutches, wheelchair, etc.), body build, distinguishing characteristics, deformities, odor of breath/body, gender.
Level of Consciousness OR *Arousal/Awareness:* Measure of responsiveness to you & environmental stimuli	• Are they alert, attentive, able to follow instructions; cooperative, sleepy, lethargic, unresponsive? • Able to understand what you are saying? • Able to hear you? • Able to see you?
Attention & Concentration *Attention:* ability to stay focused on the situation & filter out distractions *Concentration:* maintaining focus over time; staying on task	• Is the individual able to the following: ○ Focus & resist distraction? ○ Sustain attention over time? ○ Complete a thought? ○ Think clearly & problem-solve? ○ Count backward by 7's? ○ Spell a word forward & backward?
Attitude & Insight *Attitude:* emotional demeanor & ability to engage in conversation; cooperate; includes facial expression, body language, & vocalizations *Insight:* understanding purpose of current situation & self-awareness	• What are the verbal & nonverbal cues you are observing (eye contact, tone of voice, body language, fasciculations, body movements?) • Is the individual friendly, cooperative, helpful, apathetic, indifferent, and guarded hostile? • What is the older adult's level of cooperation or ability to follow directions? • Is there ambivalence or uncertainty? • How willing is the individual to engage in telling their story or engaging in meaningful conversation? • Does the individual demonstrate understanding of their symptom(s) & impact on health & quality of life? ADLs?

Orientation:
Awareness of own identity & current surroundings

Affect & Mood
Affect: observation of an individual's ability to present themselves in a specific time & place; expression of emotion
Mood: individuals self-description of how they are currently feeling; underlying atmosphere or tone

- Aware of the following:
  - o Self (own person) & others
  - o Place (current location)
  - o Time (current)
- For affect, YOU observe the following:
  - o Facial expression
  - o Eye contact; presence of tears
  - o Tone of voice
  - o Body posture & movements (wringing of hands, tapping feet, crossing/un-crossing legs, etc.)
  - o YOU might document as follows: appropriate to the situation; exaggerated; flat; blunted; labile, euthymic (normal); dysphoric (depression, guilt, anxiety); euphoric (pathologic elevated sense of well-being) with descriptive terms [15]
- For mood, YOU might ask:
  - o How are you feeling today?
  - o On a scale of 1–10 with 10 the best mood ever, how are you feeling right now? How about most of the time?
- You are looking for pattern & congruency about what YOU observe & what they tell you they are feeling.
- Do verbal & nonverbal findings correlate to one another?

Cognitive Areas of Consideration
Language:
The goal is to use lay language that ensures clear communication & respects the individual's comfort in discussing personal health issues; how do they best learn?; how can you convey to them what YOU want them to understand regarding their health care?

- What is the individual's primary language (speaking, reading, writing)?
- Ask, "what language do you prefer to use in discussing your health care?"
- Does the individual formulate & communicate clear ideals or thoughts?
- Are they having challenges with expressing or understanding?
- How many words can the individual list that start with a certain letter within 1 min?

(continued on next page)

Table 3
(continued)

Mental status domain	Assessment/examination
Judgment: The ability to make sound decisions based on values & what matters most to the individual.	• Generally, YOU need to ask simple questions of what the individual would do in a specific situation. • Are they able to effectively solve a problem (eg, "If you found a driver's license on the ground, what would you do?") • How does the individual handle a minor household emergency, such as the air conditioner breaking down?

Memory:
Short-term: temporarily store & recall information from a few seconds to a few minutes; working memory
Long-term: the brains way of storing information over long periods of time; recall of past events; capacity, retrieval; *types* = explicit or declarative; implicit or nondeclarative; *subtypes* = episodic (personal experiences), semantic (general knowledge), procedural (skills & habits) [17]
	• Ask the older adult to do the following:
	  ○ Recent recall: name 3 items & then after 3 min ask the person to repeat (eg, car, nickel, pony)
	  ○ Remote recall: identify a memory from childhood or an event that occurred earlier in life
	  ○ Repeat a name, address, or short sentence after engaging in another task
	  ○ Personal past events that occurred in childhood or in the far past
	• Utilization of screening tools: described in Table 1.

Visuospatial Perception: Ability to understand & interpret visual information related to spatial relationships.
Issues with this domain can indicate parietal lobe brain dysfunction.
Proficiency is the ability to perceive & manipulate objects & shapes in space.
	• Use of tasks such as the following:
	  ○ Ability to copy or draw an object, such as a diamond, an overlapping pentagon, or a 3-dimensional cube
	  ○ Correctly draw a clock indicating a specific time; look for correct numbers in symmetric spacing with 2 hands—1 shorter than the other pointing to the hour; generally, use 2:50 [19]
	  ○ Reproduce a block design
	  ○ Write a short sentence
	  ○ Mark on a map the most direct route to go from one place to another

Praxis:
The ability to perform complex motor movements
Ideomotor: perform intentional, learned motor movements or simple gestures [5]
Ideational: ability to plan, design, and execute sequence of motor actions to interact with objects [5]

Executive Function (EF)
OR
Abstract Reasoning (AR)
EF: the skills used to manage daily tasks of life & living (planning, problem-solving, adapting to new situations; high level skills)
AR: involves higher order reasoning; allows individuals to think about the big picture or situation as a whole & envisioning the future

- How well can the older adult do the following:
  o Perform increasingly complex motor tasks (eg, demonstrate using an object [hairbrush, fork, hammer, etc]) = ideomotor praxis
  o Follow a sequenced set of actions (eg, "Take this paper, fold it in half & place it in the envelope") = ideational praxis
  o Follow actions such as "touch your nose, then your shoulder, then your knee" [5]
- Does the older adult do the following:
  o Accurately balance a checkbook
  o Recall a sequence of mixed numbers or letters of the alphabet in ascending order
  o Interpret similarities & differences (eg, watch-ruler; pen-pencil)
  o Understand idioms (eg, warm-hearted)
  o Logically interpret proverbs (eg, "a rolling stone gathers no moss")
  o Recognize numerical patterns (eg, 3-9-15-21)
- Screening tools such as the following:
  o Trail Making Test; Clock Drawing Test

minorities into consideration because early diagnosis is essential to treatment and planning, especially in this older adult population.

Prevalence of neuropsychiatric symptoms

Little is known about the prevalence of NPS, cognition, and race [32,34]. NPS are common with the diagnosis of dementia. One retrospective study using NACC data compared characteristics of 1528 Black persons living with dementia (27%) and 11,267 White persons living with dementia (36%) [33]. Compared with community samples, the data showed that although there is a decrease in the prevalence for Black persons living with dementia, there are comparable or worse risk factors, cognitive impairment, functional limitations, and NPS than their White counterparts [33]. The increase in NPS is in spite of a decreased prevalence of dementia in Black persons [33].

Diagnosis of dementia in marginalized populations

The diagnosis of dementia for Black and Hispanic/Latino/a older adults is often missed or delayed; early diagnosis of dementia in Black persons is delayed [35]. Dementia is twice as high for Black persons and there is a one and one-half times the risk for dementia in the Hispanic/Latino/a population [35]. Delays in diagnosis are also a delay in treatment and health care inequalities [33].

Neuropsychiatric symptoms characteristics and risks

NPS associated with agitation, irritability, lability, motor disturbances, abnormal nighttime behaviors, and changes in appetite occur more frequently in Black persons than White persons living with dementia [33]. Black persons present with more hallucinations and delusions than White persons [33]. One study comparing Hispanic/Latino/a and non-Hispanic White older adults showed that hallucinations were disproportionally higher in Hispanic/Latino/a older adults [32].

An exploratory cross-sectional retrospective using NACC data compared Asian, Black, and White populations living with FTD [36]. The study showed that Black persons with a diagnosis of FTD had more agitation, delusions, and depression [36]. Compared with White populations, Black persons living with a diagnosis of FTD experienced less apathy. Asian populations experience a greater frequency of apathy, nighttime behaviors, and changes in appetite and eating when compared with White populations with FTD [36]. A cross-sectional study showed that Black persons living with Huntington's disease experienced more psychiatric symptoms as an initial presentation; motor and psychiatrics symptoms are most common [37].

There are scarce data to document gender differences and NPS in very old Hispanic/Latino/a adults [38]. Data from the Hispanic Established Epidemiologic Study of the Elderly revealed gender differences in NPS for Mexican-American community dwelling adults 80 years and older [38]. Compared with women, men experienced greater odds of agitation and aggression, while women demonstrated higher odds of depression and anxiety [38].

Severity of neuropsychiatric symptoms

Across all racial-ethnic groups with NPS, there is a higher risk of disease progression toward cognitive impairment [34]. However, Black/African Americans experience a greater risk of cognitive impairment than Hispanic/Latino/a or Asian groups [34]. There are higher levels of NPS severity for Black persons [33]. A cross-sectional study of persons living with Huntington's disease showed that social structural determinants of health contributed to disability in minority populations [37]. Higher education was associated with less advanced disease and less disability [37]. Black persons living with Huntington's disease experienced more disability ($P= <0.001$) than White non-Hispanic populations [37]. In Mexican-American adults 80 years and older, severity of NPS did not show any statistical differences by gender, except for anxiety in women [38]. Data from the Texas Alzheimer's Research and Care Consortium showed difference in severity due to ethnicity in AD, but not in those with a diagnosis of MCI [32].

Inequalities and neuropsychiatric symptoms

One observational study in Spain found that inequalities in NPS were gender related with more women receiving antidepressants [39]. Another study showed that social determinants of health led to more disability for persons living with Huntington's disease [37]. NPS are under-reported in data bases, even though NPS are especially burdensome to persons living with a diagnosis of dementia and their loved ones and contribute to stress and institutionalization [38]. Out of 30,544 participants with a diagnosis of dementia, 12% of cases reported a diagnosis of dementia and related NPS [39]. While the aim of the study was to specifically identify inequalities by gender and socioeconomic status and dementia related NPS, poor record keeping was a significant barrier [39].

Racial bias and neuropsychiatric symptoms

The extent of racial bias on the severity and course of disease on racial-ethnic minority populations is unknown [33]. Decreased enrollment of racial-ethnic minorities is common across all clinical trials [39]. From a research perspective, enrollment of racial-ethnic minority populations into research trials is critical to learning more about health disparities for diagnosis and treatment [33]. Persons living with dementia and NPS have lower socioeconomic status and depend on the system, resulting in higher allocation of health care costs [39]. Reliable tools such as the NPI to document NPS are needed to help monitor the symptoms and progression [25]. Culturally appropriate screening and treatment is needed [40]. More qualitative studies may be helpful in determining perspectives of marginalized older adults such as persons living with Huntington disease [37].

Impacts of disparities on neuropsychiatric outcomes

HCP working on the front lines of primary care play a pivotal role in recognizing and addressing mental health issues in older adults. A critical challenge to be cognizant of is the existence and persistence of mental health disparities and their impact on treatment and outcomes. Mental health disparities, rooted in socio-economic, racial, ethnic, and geographic differences, have profound effects on NPS outcomes, including both QoL and the severity of symptoms. Understanding these impacts will enable HCP to provide comprehensive care that considers the broader disparities, including mental conditions influencing older adult overall health.

Mental health disparities often result in the emergence or complication of comorbid conditions. The lack of timely care and the stresses stemming from disparities can lead to physical health issues like HTN, T2DM, or substance use disorder. HCP must be particularly vigilant about these potential comorbidities, as they add layers of complexity to the older adults' care and treatment. Mental health disparities not only increase the severity of NPS but also substantially impact the older adult's QoL. Older adults from marginalized communities, who already encounter multiple socio-economic challenges, might find their conditions exacerbated by the stresses of poverty, food insecurity, discrimination, functional decline, or outright limited access to quality care. This unremitting cycle of stress means that the mental health condition amplifies these stresses derived from disparities, and these stresses, in turn, aggravate the NPS. For example, an older adult with significant anxiety who struggles with housing instability and food insecurity due to socio-economic disparities may find their anxiety and NPS worsen in the face of these external pressures. The combined effect of the mental condition and external stresses reduces the individual's ability to function, cope with NPS, or engage in meaningful relationships, further diminishing the older adult's QoL.

Disparities in mental health care, such as limited access to timely and quality services, result in significant delays in diagnosis and treatment. These mental health disparities also exacerbate mental health conditions and NPS due to inadequate and delayed interventions and treatment. In older adults confronting such barriers, NPS and other conditions often escalate unchecked. For instance, depression, when untreated or inadequately treated due to mental health disparities, can progress to more severe forms, including major depressive disorder or even suicidal ideation. Similarly, older adults with dementia from underserved communities might experience more severe NPS, and psychosis, exacerbated by a failure of early intervention and treatment. When older adults present with significant NPS due to delayed or inadequate care, it places an added burden on HCP and the health care system. Older adults experience a downward spiral of requiring more intensive interventions, longer treatment durations, and significant transitional care, which can strain their already limited resources. Table 4 outlines some of the challenges and solutions regarding the impact of mental health disparities on managing NPS.

Research

There are considerable research gaps on culturally responsive approaches to mental health interventions specifically designed for older adults from diverse backgrounds. Older adult racial-ethnic minority populations are frequently underrepresented in clinical studies on NPS which can lead to limited applicability

Table 4
Challenges and solutions of mental health disparities in managing neuropsychiatric symptoms [4,8,10,12]

Challenges	Solutions
Delayed diagnosis due to lack of access to mental health care.	• Implement community outreach programs to raise awareness & provide early screening services.
Increased severity of conditions like dementia, depression, and anxiety due to delayed treatment.	• Establish telehealth services to reach older adult patients in remote or underserved areas, ensuring timely intervention.
Older adult patients' reluctance due to cultural stigma associated with mental health, ageism, & biases.	• Develop culturally tailored psychoeducation campaigns to normalize discussions around mental health & aging.
Inadequate resources for comprehensive care in marginalized communities.	• Allocate funds & resources to community mental health clinics & support centers.
Lack of culturally aware care leading to mistrust & reduced adherence to treatment.	• Train health care providers in cultural sensitivity & hire diverse health care team members.
Comorbidities due to untreated neuropsychiatric conditions.	• Adopt an integrated care approach, combining mental health & primary care services.
Strain on existing mental health services due to high demand from untreated cases.	• Collaborate with community organizations & health care settings to expand mental health services & support structures for older adults.

of evidence and leads to ineffective strategies to address mental health disparities in these communities [2,33,36,37]. Including a more diverse range of participants in research studies will improve understanding of the unique challenges faced by marginalized groups and lead to more effective interventions that address disparities in mental health care. Research that does not represent all populations leads to HCP lack of a thorough understanding of mental health disparities, continuing inequities, and widening health outcome gaps among aging individuals [33,36].

Further research is needed to examine the mental health disparities and conditions with NPS. However, older adults from racial-ethnic minority and marginalized groups who have AD/ADRD and NPS are often underrepresented in clinical trials, which affects the generalizability of research findings [33,36]. One of the National Institutes on Aging strategic research directives through 2025 is to better understand health disparities related to aging and develop strategies to improve the health status of older adults in diverse and marginalized groups [8].

IMPLICATIONS FOR NURSE PRACTITIONERS PRACTICE

The world is experiencing a major demographic shift where people are living longer [1]. There are many reasons for this increased life expectancy. Longer life means an increased risk for developing health conditions and diseases that are common in older adults. The loss of biodiversity, depleted water supplies, food systems that are diminishing, and environmental toxins are changing the face of global health [41]. A total of 25% of individuals aged 65 and older report anxiety or depression [42].

NPs working with older adults can recognize warning signs of cognitive decline, perform simple cognitive testing over time, and recognize changes that impact ALD and instrumental activities of daily living, well-being, and QoL. Knowing the person and what matters most to them is also extremely important. The earlier a diagnosis of cognitive changes is made, the earlier the best interdisciplinary team can be on board, managing symptoms using nonpharmacologic interventions and appropriate medications. Know yourself! What are your strengths and level of competence in caring for older adults? Where do you need to gain knowledge and expertise? Experience and education related to concepts of aging, normal aging, and deviations from normal are important aspect of treating the whole person based on their values, needs, and wants. If you don't know, be knowledgeable about the resources and supports that are available in your community. There are over 6 hundred Area Agencies on Aging in every state in the United States, and some of the territories. This is a great organization for you to familiarize yourself with in your community. They have a lot to offer and are good partners for those NP caring for older adults. The better you know your older adult patient, and their family of choice, the better you will understand the individual's story and the better you will feel in helping them travel their aging path with quality and care.

CLINICS CARE POINTS

- Older adults are living longer. According to the World Health Organization, by 2030, 1 in 6 people will be 60 years and older.
- The United Nations has reported the global population of those 65 years and older will increase from the current 761 million to 1.6 billion by 2050.
- It is imperative that health care professionals and providers caring for older adults are educated to understand the aging process and the potential mental health issues and conditions that become more prevalent the longer a person lives.
- Neuropsychiatric symptoms can lead to carer burden, nursing home placement, increase in morbidity and mortality, and skyrocketing health care costs—for the individual, their family, and health systems.
- Older adult mental health disparities derive from multifactorial biological, physical, and psychosocial environments accrued over one's entire lived experience.
- Social determinants of health impact the well-being and quality of life of older adults. It is important to understand and document an individual's socioeconomic status, level of education, their neighborhood and built environment, health literacy, and ability to access quality health care.
- Globally, older adults have traditionally been relegated to a powerless position (marginalized) within groups and societies.

- Marginalization of older adults can negatively impact mental and physical health, sense of self, well-being, social engagement, and quality of life.
- The role of the NP working with older adults should be to perform cognitive assessment screening with every visit and document changes over time. This will lead to earlier diagnosis of dementia and NPS while also providing peace of mind and improving quality of life.

Disclosure

The authors have nothing to disclose.

References

[1] Alzheimer's Disease International. Numbers of people with dementia. Date unknown. Available at: https://www.alzint.org/about/dementia-facts-figures/dementia-statistics/. Accessed January 31, 2025.

[2] Pless A, Ware D, Saggu S, et al. Understanding neuropsychiatric symptoms in Alzheimer's disease: challenges and advances in diagnosis and treatment. Front Neurosci 2023;5: 1–13.

[3] Press D. Management of neuropsychiatric symptoms of dementia. 2023. Available at: https://www.uptodate.com/contents/management-of-neuropsychiatric-symptoms-of-dementia. Accessed January 31, 2025.

[4] United Way. Health disparities: creating health care equity for minorities. Available at: https://unitedwaynca.org/blog/healthcare-disparities/. Accessed January 31, 2025.

[5] American Psychiatric Association. Stigma, prejudice, and discrimination against people with mental illness. 2023. Available at: https://www.psychiatry.org/patients-families/stigma-and-discrimination. Accessed January 31, 2025.

[6] Ahad AA, Sanchez-Gonzalez M, Junquera P. Understanding and addressing mental health stigma across cultures for improving psychiatric care: a narrative review. Cureus 2023;15(5):e39549:PMID: 37250612; PMCID: PMC10220277.

[7] Safran MA, Mays RA Jr, Huang LN, et al. Mental health disparities. Am J Public Health 2009;99(11):1962–6, PMID: 19820213; PMCID: PMC2759796.

[8] National Institute of Health. Minority health and health disparities strategic plan 2021-2025. Available at: https://www.nimhd.nih.gov/docs/nimhd-strategic-plan-2021-2025.pdf. Accessed January 31, 2025.

[9] Wolinsky D, Drake K, Jolene B. Diagnosis and management of neuropsychiatric symptoms in Alzheimer's disease. Curr Psychiatry Rep 2018;20(12); https://doi.org/10.1007/s11920-018-0978-8.

[10] National Institute of Health. Mental illness. Available at: https://www.nimh.nih.gov/health/statistics/mental-illness. Accessed January 31, 2025.

[11] Machenzie CS, Scott T, Mather A, et al. Older adults' help-seeking attitudes and treatment beliefs concerning mental health programs. 2008;16(2):1010-1019. Available at: https://www.ncbi.nlm.nih.gov/pmc/articles/PMC2735824. Accessed January 31, 2025.

[12] World Health Organization. Mental health of older adults. 2023. Available at: https://www.who.int/news-room/fact-sheets/detail/mental-health-of-older-adults. Accessed January 31, 2025.

[13] CDC what is health equity?. 2017. Available at: https://www.cdc.gov/health-equity/what-is/index.html. Accessed January 31, 2025.

[14] Wittenberg GF, McKay MA, O'Connor M. Exploring the association between multimorbidity and cognitive impairment in older adults living in the community: a review of the literature. HHCMP 2022;34(1):52–62.

[15] Newman G. How to assess mental status. Merck Manual 2023. Available at: https://www.merckmanuals.com/professional/neurologic-disorders/neurologic-examination/how-to-assess-mental-status. Accessed January 31, 2025.

[16] Rosenzweig A. The mini-mental state exam for Alzheimer's: understanding MMSE scoring. VeryWellHealth 2024. Available at: https://www.verywellhealth.com/mini-mental-state-exam-as-an-alzheimers-screening-test-98623. Accessed January 25, 2025.

[17] Wood J, Weintraub S, Coventry C, et al. Montreal Cognitive Assessment (MoCA) performance and domain-specific index scores in amnestic versus aphasic dementia. J Int Neuropsychol Soc 2020;26:927–31.

[18] MoCA cognition. Available at: https://mocacognition.com. Accessed January 31, 2025.

[19] Tariq SH, Tumosa N, Chibnall JT, et al. The Sait Louis University Mental Status (SLUMS) Examination for detective mild cognitive impairment and dementia is more sensitive than the Mini Mental Status Examination (MMSE)-a pilot study. Am J Geriatr Psych 2006;14: 900–10.

[20] Saint louis university. Available at: https://www.slu.edu/medicine/internal-medicine/geriatric-medicine/aging-successfully/assessment-tools/mental-status-exam.php. Accessed January 31, 2025.

[21] MiniCog. Available at: https://mini-cog.com. Accessed January 31, 2025.

[22] Trzepacz PT, Hochstetler H, Wang S, et al. Relationship between the Montreal cognitive assessment and Mini-mental State Examination for assessment of mild cognitive impairment in older adults. BMC Geriatr 2015;107:1–9.

[23] Siqueira GSA, Hagemann PDMS, Coelho DDS, et al. Bertolucci PHFCan MoCA and MMSE be interchangeable cognitive screening tools? a systematic review. Gerontol 2019;59(6): e743–63.

[24] National Task Group. NTG-EDSD. Available at: https://www.dhs.wisconsin.gov/publications/p01622m.pdf. Accessed February 1, 2025.

[25] Cummings JL, Mega M, Gray K, et al. The Neuropsychiatric Inventory: comprehensive assessment of psychopathology in dementia. Neurology 1994;44:2308–14.

[26] Kim G, DeCoster J, Huang C, et al. A meta-analysis of the factor structure of the Geriatric Depression Scale (GDS): the effects of language. Int Psychogeriatr 2013;25(1):71–81.

[27] Nguyen TV, Nguyen KT, Nguyen PM, et al. Vietnamese version of the geriatric depression Scale (30 items): translation, cross-cultural adaptation, and validation. Geriatrics (Basel) 2021;6(4):116, PMID: 34940341; PMCID: PMC8701202.

[28] Balls-Berry JE, Babulla GM. Health disparities in dementia. Continuum 2022;28(3): 872–84. Available at: https://www.ncbi.nlm.nih.gov/pmc/articles/PMC9924306/. Accessed January 29, 2025.

[29] WHO. Palliative care. Available at: https://www.who.int/news-room/fact-sheets/detail/palliative-care. Accessed January 25, 2025.

[30] National Council on Aging. Get the facts on economic security for seniors. 2023. Available at: https://www.ncoa.org/article/get-the-facts-on-economic-security-for-seniors. Accessed February 1, 2025.

[31] NACC. About NACC. Available at: https://naccdata.org/nacc-collaborations/about-nacc. Accessed October 24, 2023.

[32] Salazar R, Dwivedi AK, Royall DR. Cross-ethnic differences in the severity of neuropsychiatric symptoms in person with mild cognitive impairment and Alzheimer's disease. J Neuropsychiatry Clin Neurosci 2017;29(1):A6–78.

[33] Lennon JC, Aita SL, Del Bene VA, et al. Black and White individuals differ in dementia prevalence, risk factors, and symptomatic presentation. Alzheimer's Dement 2022;18:1461–71.

[34] Babulal GM, Zhu Y, Trani JF. Racial and ethnic differences in neuropsychiatric symptoms and progression to incident cognitive impairment among community-dwelling participants. Alzheimers Dement 2023;(8):3635–43, PMID: 36840665; PMCID: PMC10440214.

[35] Alzheimers Association. Fact sheet. Race, ethnicity, and Alzheimer's. 2020. Available at: https://aaic.alz.org/downloads2020/2020_Race_and_Ethnicity_Fact_Sheet.pdf. Accessed January 29, 2025.

[36] Jin HA, McMillan CT, Yannatos I, et al. Racial differences in clinical presentation in individuals diagnosed with frontotemporal dementia. JAMA Neurol 2023; https://doi.org/10.1001/jamaneurol.2023.3093.

[37] Mendizabal A, Singh AP, Perlman S, et al. Disparities in Huntington disease severity: analysis using the ENROLL-HD dataset. Neurol Clin Pract 2023;13(6):e200200.

[38] Milani SA, Cantu PA, Berenson AB, et al. Gender Differences in neuropsychiatric symptoms among community-dwelling Mexican Americans aged 80 and older. Am J Alzheimers Dis Other Demen 2021;36:15333175211042958.

[39] Mar J, Arrospide A, Soto-Gordoa M, et al. Dementia-related neuropsychiatric symptoms: inequalities in pharmacological treatment and institutionalization. Neuropsychiatr Dis Treat 2019;15:2027–34.

[40] Act on Alzheimer's. Cultural competence and awareness. Available at: https://actonalz.org/cultural-competence. Accessed February 1, 2025.

[41] Cornell University. Our planet, our health: addressing the public health impacts of human-induced environmental change. Cornell K. Lisa Yang Center for Wildlife Health. Date Unknown. Available at: https://wildlife.cornell.edu/our-work/our-planet-our-health#:~:text=Disease%20patterns%20are%20changing%20as,toxins%2C%20and%20collapsing%20food%20systems. Accessed January 26, 2025.

[42] Cameron K. Why we must address the rising mental health needs of our growing older adult population. National Council on Aging, Behavioral Health for Professionals 2023. Available at: https://www.ncoa.org/article/why-we-must-address-the-rising-mental-health-needs-of-our-growing-older-adult-population/. Accessed February 1, 2025.

Advances in Family Practice Nursing 7 (2025) 23–36

ADVANCES IN FAMILY PRACTICE NURSING

ELSEVIER
MOSBY

Musical Interventions and Older Adults Experiencing Sleep Disturbances in Long-Term Care

Check for updates

Julia Dunham-Thornton, MSN, RN, ANP-BC, AGPCNP-BC[a],*,
Melodee Harris, PhD, APRN, GNP-BC, AGPCNP-BC[b]

[a]Grand Canyon University, College of Nursing Healthcare Professions, Albuquerque, NM, USA;
[b]College of Nursing - University of Arkansas for Medical Sciences, Little Rock, AR, USA

Keywords
- Dementia • Insomnia • Long-term care facilities • Older adults
- Musical intervention • Sleep

Key points
- Music has been known to have therapeutic benefits, including the potential to improve sleep quality.
- Musical interventions have gained more attention as a tool for older adults with insomnia, particularly those in long-term care facilities.
- Holistic approaches such as music can be helpful for Older Adults to decrease or eliminate complications related to medications used for sleep.

INTRODUCTION

Sleep is a physiologic process that is essential for maintaining good health [1]. Poor sleep is estimated to effect 72% of older adults (OAs) living in long-term care (LTC) [2]. OAs can experience trouble falling asleep, staying asleep, or early in the morning arousals [3]. Many factors increase the risk for sleep disturbances in the OA such as changes in physical health, medications, cognitive decline, environmental stressors, and a decrease in physical or social activity contribute to sleep disturbances [4]. Poor sleep quality can influence the health

---

*Corresponding author. Grand Canyon University – Albuquerque, 6200 Jefferson Street Northeast, Suite 300, Albuquerque, NM 87109. E-mail address: Julia.DunhamThornton@gcu.edu

https://doi.org/10.1016/j.yfpn.2024.12.001

Abbreviations

CBT-i   cognitive behavioral therapy
LTC   long-term care
OA   older adult
SCN   suprachiasmatic nucleus

of the older adult, leading to an increased risk for depression, cognitive decline, fatigue, and a decreased quality of life [4–7].

LTC environment itself is a big contributor to lack of sleep [8]. OAs can have sleep issues due to excessive time in bed, noise from staff and other residents, light, or incontinence issues that require frequent staff to provide care [9,10]. OAs can have sleep issues due to excessive time I bed, noise from staff and other residents, light, or incontinence issues that require frequent staff assessments to provide care. [11]. Withdrawal from antipsychotic agents can also temporarily interfere with the resident sleep patterns [11].

Music has long been known for its therapeutic benefits for anxiety, depression, including the potential to improve sleep quality [12–17]. Music as an intervention can be effective for those who have difficulty with pharmacologic treatments or those residents who may seek a more holistic treatment approach [12]. Calming music has been found to reduce sleep onset latency, allowing the resident to fall asleep sooner [17]. Subjectively, music can improve sleep quality, reducing the times a resident will awaken during the night and increase the overall sleep duration [15–17].

For those residents who experience anxiety and depression, music has been shown to reduce behaviors such as agitation and somnolence as they are also linked to sleep disturbances [12–14,18]. OAs can be provided with education about the importance of listening to music as part of their sleep hygiene routine, this would include the importance of a regular bedtime, reducing caffeine intake, and creating a sleep friendly environment [12,17]. Education needs to be provided on sleep hygiene practices for the resident, family, and the LTC staff [19–21]. The education should focus on health practices and environmental factors that may restrict the residents' ability to initiate or maintain sleep [19–21]. These measures, although they sound simplistic, are initiated to develop good sleep patterns and decrease environmental factors that may interfere with getting a good night's sleep. Guidelines incorporate sleep hygiene, evidenced-based measures from sleep physiology, sleep and circadian rhythms, and pharmacology [21–24]. This is why it is so important to introduce the intervention, particularly since there are no adverse outcomes in resident care (Box 1) [24].

INSOMNIA
The problem
OAs have reduced circadian rhythm behaviors that include sleep [25]. As a result, OAs have changes in sleep timing, duration, and consolidation, which

Box 1: Sleep hygiene adapted for residents in long-term care

- Get up at the same time each day, including the weekends.
- Get bright light (optimally natural sunlight) first thing in the morning.
- Limit nap times to 15 to 30 minutes. No napping after 3 PM
- Encourage participation in social activities even if tired.
- Have a consistent schedule for meals, medications, and other activities.
- Establish a bedtime routine that will help with relaxation such as a warm bath, small snack, reading, or listening to soft music.
- Avoid screen time, which includes tablets and the TV.
- Avoid stimulants such as caffeine within 6 to 8 hours before bedtime.
- Sit up—do something relaxing until you feel sleepy again.
- Avoid clock watching

Adapted from AASM (2024). Improving your sleep in five simple steps, retrieved from … Sleepeducation.org/improve-your-sleep-in-five-steps/ [24].)

decrease sleep and fragments total sleep time. Because of the changes in sleep such as poor quality and duration, cognitive performance may suffer [26]. The suprachiasmatic nucleus (SCN) is considered to be the internal pacemaker of the circadian system [25]. The SCN signals both directly and indirectly to many brain regions, clock function, and aging may be linked by the various different physiologic functions at the level of the SCN [25]. Clock activity in other areas of the brain and in peripheral tissues may also change with aging [25]. Even in healthy OAs, sleep is compromised [25].

Insomnia as defined by the Diagnostic and Statistical Manual of Mental Health Disorders, Fifth Edition, Text Revision (DSM-5TR) (2022) is a disorder characterized by resident complaints about a dissatisfaction with sleep quality and quantity and it is associated with 1 or more of the following symptoms: (1) difficulty initiating sleep, (2) difficulty maintaining sleep that is accompanied by frequent awakenings or problems with returning to sleep after awakenings, and (3) early morning awakening and inability to return to sleep [26]. Sleep problems also cause clinically significant distress or impairment in social, behavioral, or other important areas identified by the resident [27]. Difficulty sleeping that occurs at least three nights per week for a period of three months even with plenty of opportunities to sleep [27]. An Insomnia disorder also does not occur with other sleep-wake disorders, substance, or co-existing mental health diagnosis that may explain why the patient would have insomnia [27].

DSM_5-TR (2022) criterion for episodic insomnia are symptoms that last at least 1 month, but less than 3 months. Persistent insomnia are when symptoms occur 3 months or greater; and recurrent if there are 2 or greater episodes within a 1 year period [27]. Advanced practice registered nurses in LTC primarily rely on a thorough patient interview, sleep diary analysis, observation of sleep patterns by clinical staff, and assessment of daytime symptoms to assess and diagnose insomnia [28,29]. The advanced practice registered nurse must also take into account the resident's ability to communicate as well as potential cognitive impairments, while ruling out other medical conditions that could contribute to the resident's complaint of sleep difficulties, like pain or side effects from medications. Multiple comorbidities can be linked to the diagnosis of insomnia [28]. Psychiatric disorders are the most common to be associated with insomnia, such as anxiety, depression, and psychosis [28,29]. Sleep disturbance is also associated with hormone level alterations, blood pressure, and numerous comorbid conditions such as hyperthyroidism, cancer, heart failure, gastroesophageal reflux disease, chronic pain due to arthritis, and restless leg syndrome [28,30].

The LTC environment presents many challenges for residents experiencing insomnia as versus their community-dwelling counterparts [8]. Sleep itself can be affected by environmental factors like noise, lighting, room temperatures, room sharing, and nighttime care activities due to frequent incontinence [7,8,10]. Also, residents may seldom leave their rooms, thus having limited exposure to bright light, which can contribute to circadian rhythm dysfunction [9,10]. Environmental noises and incontinence issues result in sleep disruption of residents [7,8,10]. Nursing staff may have limited experience with bundling of care, which can result in loss of sleep [7]. Long-term residents also have issues related to the amount of time they spend in bed, are physically inactive, and have limited social contact with other residents during the daytime [8,9]. This leads to concerns about napping, which can lead to decreased sleep at nighttime and alter the sleep–wake cycle [10]. Emotional distress, isolation, loneliness, and loss of independence lead to significant social changes that impact resident sleep patterns [8,10]. Sleep difficulties are often secondary to other comorbid conditions [10]. Residents in LTC often have multiple medical conditions, which can also affect sleep patterns, such as depression, dementia, chronic pain, incontinence, heart failure, and respiratory diseases [10]. It is estimated that 60% to 90% of residents in LTC have some form of dementia or cognitive impairment, which also contributes to sleep fragmentation and daytime sleepiness [31]. These residents also take medication to manage both medical and psychiatric illness, which interfere with sleep [10].

Sleep assessment/screening

Nurse practitioners need to become familiar with taking a good medical history as well as a sleep history asking pertinent questions about comorbidities that may affect sleep, such as chronic pain [28,29,32]. Medications: are they prescription or over-the-counter or both? Although these are residents in LTC, do they have a history of recent alcohol or substance abuse? Are they still physically active and able to ambulate either independently or do they need assistance? Additional components to the history and physical are observing and asking appropriate questions about mood, concentration, and the residents' ability to function on a daily basis. A sleep assessment including a sleep history should be a priority of the advanced practice nurse. Residents, family, and LTC nursing staff can provide invaluable insights about sleep health. The history will also include observations of both daytime and nighttime sleep and a physical examination [28,29,32]. If indicated, a sleep diary, actigraphy, and questionnaires, such as the Pittsburgh Sleep Quality Index, Epworth Sleepiness Scale, Restless Legs Syndrome Questionnaire, STOP-Bang for Obstructive Sleep Apnea, may be required [21,28,32–37]. Polysomnography is not usually indicated for residents in LTC centers unless obstructive sleep apnea or parasomnias are suspected but is often not well-tolerated due to the nature of chronic illness or cognitive impairment [35,37]. Wrist actigraphy is an effective in monitoring treatment responses and to screen for circadian rhythm disorders [38]. The sleep diary can be collected over 1–2 weeks [8,39]. Important data to capture for the advanced practice provider is (1) time resident went to bed, (2) when the resident fell asleep, (3) total amount of sleep time, and (4) amount of awakenings during the night and what time the resident woke up [21,39]. Symptoms collected will provide valuable information on the severity of insomnia experienced and screen for other sleep disorders. Sleep diaries are also important to determine the effectiveness of prescribed therapies (Box 2) [21,39].

Treatments for insomnia
Current treatments of insomnia include prescribed and over-the-counter medications as well as psychological and behavioral therapies, and holistic or

---

Box 2: Insomnia diagnostic toolbox for the advanced practice registered nurse

Sleep diaries
- This can be completed by either the resident or the caregiver; record sleep times, wake times, naps, and notable sleep disturbances over time
- Helps identify patterns and potential factors that contribute to sleep issues

Observation of sleep patterns
- LTC staff can monitor sleep patterns during the night, including sleep onset, wakefulness, and movements throughout the night
- Note daytime sleepiness and frequent napping

History of present illness
- Differential diagnosis to rule out other medical conditions that can cause sleep disturbances, such as pain, restless leg syndrome, respiratory issues, or urinary problems
- Review current medications that may affect sleep

Neurobehavioral assessment
- Does the resident have dementia? Sleep disturbances may be related to cognitive decline and different management may be needed.
- Use institution specific assessment tool if no formal diagnosis of dementia.

complementary therapies. In the LTC centers, initiation of melatonin or other prescribed therapies are utilized for insomnia. Cognitive behavioral therapy (CBT-i) is usually not initiated due to lack of therapists in the LTC environment. Alternative and complementary therapies are limited within the LTC setting due to availability of nursing staff to implement these strategies.

Pharmacologic management

Pharmacologic therapy may be considered if the resident is not responsive to nonpharmacologic and behavioral interventions. Nonpharmacologic interventions should not be replaced by only medication, but enhanced with medication to promote a healthy night's sleep [20]. Benzodiazepines are prescribed medication for treating sleep concerns for OAs in LTC. The unproven effectiveness of these medications in treating sleep-related complaints and also concerns of adverse events related to these medications such as cognitive impairment and increased risk for falls make this an unattractive choice for those in LTC [40]. Morin and Buysse [21,22] have steadily seen the use of benzodiazepines decrease, but trazodone use has steadily increased, which is an off-label use for the medication. Melatonin agonists have fewer adverse events in OAs but do not have a specific dose for insomnia. Melatonin has been found to have a small effect on sleep onset, with little effect on wakefulness during sleep or total sleep time [22]. Orexin receptor antagonists (suvorexant, lemborexant, and daridorexant) are the newest agents that are clinically indicated for insomnia. Clinical trials have shown that these agents are effective for both sleep onset and sleep-maintenance symptoms [21,22]. Hypnotic agents are still prescribed for women, OAs, and non-Hispanic White patients. The Beers criteria, which provide guidance on medications that may be deemed inappropriate for residents aged greater than 65 years, includes benzodiazepine receptor agonists and heterocyclic drugs, but excludes doxepin, trazodone, or orexin antagonists [40].

Nonpharmacologic management of insomnia: what do the guidelines say?

Nonpharmacologic approaches are considered first-line therapies in the treatment of insomnia. CBT-i is considered the most effective mind body intervention for insomnia. CBT-i consists of several interventions, which include sleep hygiene, relaxation training, stimulus control therapy, sleep restriction therapy, and cognitive therapy [41]. Treatment is continually being evaluated through the use of sleep diaries completed by the patient during treatment [41]. Treatment usually lasts for 4 to 8 sessions [41]. CBT-i can have a significant cost but can also be offered in group sessions as a cost-effective therapy and has been shown to have clinical benefit for OAs with insomnia [41]. Another identified obstacle to CBT-i therapy is there is a lack of well-trained professionals to conduct these interventions that may make it harder to access in LTC centers, where it is commonplace to have one psychiatric professional who is not on site daily [41].

So what are the differences between music therapy and a musical intervention and why is knowing the terminology so important? Music therapy is defined by the American Music Therapy Association as a clinical and evidenced-based modality offered by a licensed musical therapist [42]. Individualized clinical goals are set with the patient and involve actively listening to music [42]. Manzella [43] defined a musical intervention as passive listening offered as a prerecorded selection of music, or active listening of music that is chosen by the resident. Actively listening to music offers a patient-centered approach, allowing the resident to have a voice in their care [42]. If the patient is cognitively impaired family and friends can assist in appropriate music choices [44].

A musical intervention as a nonpharmacologic therapy

A 2015 Cochrane analysis found that listening to music improves sleep quality and is not only safe but also easy to administer [13]. Research involving a music intervention has steadily increased. Music has been found to affect OAs on many levels, just not sleep. It is hypothesized that improvements in sleep quality are seen because music with a slow rhythm relaxes the older adult [12]. What are some of the physiologic benefits that music provides the older adult? Music has been found to reduce anxiety and depression [12–14]. Potential physiologic mechanisms for these changes are thought to occur in the sympathetic nervous system and levels of the stress hormone cortisol [13,45,46]. Also, music has been found to have the power of distraction [47]. One study suggests that music can provide a focus for the person and serve as a point of distraction to minimize stressful thoughts and improve sleep [13,47,48].

What are some beginning steps in providing a musical intervention (Box 3)? [43] A personalized music approach will be important, if the resident is able to do so, they can assist in building a play list. If the resident is cognitively impaired, a family member or friend may be able to give insight into musical

---

Box 3: Initiating a musical intervention for patients in long-term care

Allow resident to pick their own music if no cognitive impairment or allow for family involvement with cognitive impairment

MP3/ Smart Phone/Tablet with headphones—particularly for binaural beats music

Play music at a volume that is comfortable for the resident.

Stop the music if the patient demonstrates a negative reaction (becomes agitated). Try a new music style for next intervention.

Residents with dexterity issues or blindness may need assistance from LTC staff

Adapted from Manzella M. Holistic nursing reflections on music and medicine. American Holistic Nurses Association, 2024;44(3):18–19 [43].

preferences. The intervention can be delivered by an iPad, smart phone, or MP3 player. There are many options if a personalized play list is not chosen, there are many companies who have sleep music via an app store on any cell phone, tablet, or computer (Table 1) [49].

In one study, the music was approximately 60 to 80 bpm, with a slow stable rhythm, low-frequency tones, and absence of strong percussion or lyrics [44,50]. Instrumental music is preferred for its sleep-inducing effect [44,50]. The resident can use headphones for the intervention, note headphones will definitely be needed for binaural beats music [49]. The volume should be adjusted to a comfortable level based on their ability to hear sounds. A music intervention should last anywhere from 30 to 60 minutes at bedtime [44]. Consistent with other studies, testing intervention effectiveness, includes a trial of more than 1 month, should be completed to see if sleep quality improves [17,51,52]. Greater than 4 weeks was determined the minimal time it takes to form a new habit [17,51,52]. In one study, compared with less than 1 month, music interventions with a duration of more than 1 month showed greater improvements in sleep quality [17]. It is also important to ensure that the musical [53] intervention occurs at the same time each evening when nighttime medications are given. Residents should not be put to bed for the convenience of nursing staff in the early evening (6–7 PM) [10]. Also, if the resident should become agitated or stressed, the intervention should stop and a different music style would be chosen [44].

Binaural beats/dynamic binaural beats music

Binaural beats music is a noninvasive nonpharmacologic type of music intervention that offers a newer approach to emotional well-being. The therapy is easy to initiate and does not require an order by the advanced practice nurse [48]. The intervention can be nurse conducted in the LTC center [54,55]. However, dynamic binaural beats music is not advised for persons with seizures

Table 1
Examples of app-driven music [49]

App-driven applications	Type of music	Free version	Subscriptions	Platforms
Calm	Modern music and soothing sounds	Yes	Annual	iOS and Android
BetterSleep	Autonomous sensory meridian response (ASMR) tones	Yes	Monthly/ annual/ lifetime	iOS and Android
Brainwaves	Binaural tones	No	Annual	iOS/Android/PC
Brain.fm	AI-generated music	No	Annual	iOS/Android/PC
Headspace	Sleep music	Yes	Monthly/ annual	iOS/Android/ Web Alexa/ Google Assistant

Adapted from Bhandari M. (2023) [49]. 9 best binaural beats apps for Android, iOS & PC1 free & paid. Retrieved from - https://Earlystagemarketing.com.

[49]. This therapy works by playing 2 slightly different frequency tones, one in each ear [56,57]. The brain recognizes this combined third tone, known as a binaural beats [48]. Binaural beats have been investigated for their potential effects to enhance sleep quality [54]. Dynamic binaural beats incorporate a dynamic changing carrier frequency differences between the left and right ears [56,57]. This effects the reticular activating system, which alters the electrical potentials of the thalamus and cerebral cortex, which changes the brain wave frequency [48]. The concept is termed frequency following response, in which intervals of neural activity will synchronize with the cycle of the stimulus [48,58,59]. The result is the entrainment or synchronization affects the listener's mental, physical, or emotional state [54,56]. Binaural beats music has been found to have a physiologic impact, influencing brain waves and blood pressure [54]. Research has also identified that low-frequency theta binaural beats music can enhance sleep quality [54,57]. This occurs through the entrapment of the theta wave [57]. It is also hypothesized that listening to binaural beats music have reduce the hyperarousal state and contribute to sleep induction [57]. Binaural beats music may provide better sleep quality and decrease depressive symptoms in OAs in LTC [54]. Future studies will have to be completed to understand the exact mechanism of action that binaural beats have on the brain as well as multifrequency interventions and how they would affect OA's sleep quality [54,57].

Challenges and resident considerations

Music as an intervention is both safe and beneficial. However, there are several challenges that the nursing staff may have to take into consideration. Residents who may have a hearing impairment may need simple adjustments such as adjusting the volume to the appropriate level or using headphones. Residents' preferences may also differ culturally as well, so adjustments may need to be made to reflect preferences. Lastly, not all residents may adapt to listening to music at first, so this may require some experimentation with different genres of music.

Music interventions, like most nonpharmacologic interventions, have not been supported by local or national policymakers. Interventions such as these, although lower cost, have no form of reimbursement from Medicare/Medicaid [55]. This strategy is reliant on volunteers and donations for electronic devices if not provided by family members. Future strategies will have to be developed by long-term care administrators and policymakers to get music in the hands of the OA in the LTC center [55].

SUMMARY

Research has demonstrated the potential benefits that a musical intervention can have on the OA with insomnia. Music interventions can be easily implemented without a costly investment of both training and materials for LTC staff. Listening to music can improve sleep quality for those experiencing insomnia. More research still needs to be completed to investigate how listening to music can affect other factors such as effect on specific insomnia types and daytime dysfunction due to lack of sleep. Music interventions for OAs can be easily implemented by either the resident or staff member as a non-pharmacologic intervention to decrease insomnia in the OA.

CASE STUDY

Maria is a 72 year old who has experienced insomnia for the past 6 months. Maria states, "My sleep problems started when I moved to this place." She resides in the LTC center in the Memory care unit due to a recent diagnosis of early onset dementia. Maria's past medical history includes hypertension, diabetes, and osteoarthritis. Current medications include acetaminophen 1000 mg orally once daily, metformin 500 mg, orally twice daily, amlodipine 5 mg orally once daily, clonazepam 0.25 mg orally twice daily for anxiety (my "nerve pill"), and Aricept 10 mg orally at night. Maria has a daughter who frequently visits but is unable to care for her mother in her home.

The nurse practitioner is visiting with Maria as she has been complaining to the nursing staff about problems with falling asleep, staying sleep, and she complains of not feeling rested in the morning. The nurse practitioner would like to work on Maria's sleep hygiene practices and introduce music at bedtime to promote relaxation and cognitive distraction. Maria can pick the music she prefers to listen to for a period of 30 to 60 minutes, 3 to 5 times per week. The music intervention will be delivered from her iPad/headphones and a play list that will be developed by her family. Maria will start her bedtime routine at about 9 PM each evening. Maria will give this a try for 2 months.

Long-term care staff training

Although the benefits of music have been widely published, many LTC centers may not be aware of the potential benefits as related to OAs and insomnia. If the use of music as an individual therapy has not been utilized in the LTC center, staff training may be warranted. Education may need to be provided about insomnia and the OA in regards to sleep hygiene as well as the musical intervention. Staff need to be educated on initiating the musical intervention when the patient receives her Aricept dose at night. It is important to start the routine then and not trying to put the patient to bed at 6 or 7 PM Other important factors are to ensure that the resident has her MP3 and headphones readily available. If the resident is unable to place the headphones on herself, the nursing staff would need to assist her. The music should play for a period of 30 to 60 minutes. It will be important to maintain a sleep diary even for this intervention to determine effectiveness. Charting will include if the patient fell asleep after the intervention and stay asleep with no nighttime awakenings. For staff the next day, it will be important to ask Maria if she feels rested after the night. The intervention will go on for the duration of 2 months, so education by the nurse practitioner about the importance of good documentation will be needed.

Results

After 1 month of listening to her personalized music, Maria reported feeling more relaxed and calm. She reported she fell asleep faster and had less nighttime awakening. Maria began to feel more refreshed in the morning. The LTC staff during nighttime resident checks noted Maria had fewer sleep disturbances and a decrease in nighttime awakenings. When family members visited, Maria was in a much better mood and appeared to be more alert. The family members also verbalized they were thankful for a holistic therapy that did not add any more medications to Maria's current care routine.

Conclusion

This case study demonstrates the potential for a musical intervention to improve a resident's quality of sleep and reduce insomnia in OAs in LTC. Having a nurse practitioner who is willing to try a nonpharmacologic approach that is easily accessible and cost-effective may provide a promising alternative to traditional sleep medications with side effects.

CLINICS CARE POINTS

- OAs with insomnia can benefit from utilizing music for relaxation and inducing sleep. This therapy can be used to complement CBT-i.
- Music interventions can be easily implemented without a costly investment to implement in LTC facilities.
- Geriatric advanced practice nurses can utilize holistic therapies such as a music intervention in their clinical practice. This can potentially have positive effects on the sleep health of residents in LTC facilities.
- Future research needs to be conducted to establish what type of music is most effective for OAs with insomnia.

Disclosure

The authors declare that there are no commercial or financial conflicts of interest associated with the content of this article. They have not received external financial support for the preparation or publication of this article.

References

[1] Crowley K. Sleep and sleep disorders in older adults. Neuropsychol Rev 2011;21(1): 41–53.
[2] Valenza MC, Cabrera-Martos I, Martín-Martín L, et al. Nursing homes: impact of sleep disturbances on functionality. Arch Gerontol Geriatr 2013;56(3):432–6.
[3] Brewster GS, Riegel B, Gehrman PR. Insomnia in the older adult. Sleep Med Clin 2018;13(1): 13–9.
[4] Mukherjee U, Sehar U, Brownell M, et al. Mechanisms, consequences and role of interventions for sleep deprivation: focus on mild cognitive impairment and Alzheimer's disease in elderly. Ageing Res Rev 2024;100:1–15.
[5] National Institute of Health, What do we know about healthy aging? Available at: https://www.nia.nih.gov/health/healthy-aging/what-do-we-know-about-healthy-aging (Accessed 30 November 2024).
[6] Whibley D, Braley TJ, Kratz AL, et al. Transient effects of sleep on next-day pain and fatigue in older adults with symptomatic osteoarthritis. J Pain 2019;20(11):P1373–82.
[7] Frie B, Graham C, Alissa A, et al. Environmental toolkit to promote quality sleep in long-term care: a quality improvement initiative. JLTC 2021;339–47.

[8] Kim DE, Yoon JY. Factors that influence sleep among residents in long-term care facilities. Int J Environ Res Publ Health 2020;17:1889.

[9] Martin JL, Webber AP, Alam T, et al. Daytime sleeping, sleep disturbance, and circadian rhythms in the nursing home. Am J Geriatr Psychiatr 2006;14:121–9.

[10] Ye L, Richards K. Sleep and long-term care. Sleep Med Clin 2018;13(1):117–25.

[11] Ruths S, Straand J, Nygaard HA, et al. Antipsychotic withdrawal on behavior and sleep/wake activity in nursing home residents with dementia: a randomized, placebo-controlled, double-blinded study the Bergen District Nursing Home Study. J Am Geriatr Soc 2004;52: 1737–43.

[12] Trahan T, Durrant SJ, Mullensiefen D, et al. The music that helps people sleep and the reasons they believe it works: a mixed methods analysis of online survey reports. PLoS One 2018;13(11):E026531.

[13] Jespersen KV, Pando-Naude V, Koenig J, et al. Listening to music for insomnia in adults. CDSR 2022;8; https://doi.org/10.1002/14651858.CD010459.pub3:Art No: CD010459.

[14] Yu AL, Lo SF, Chen PY, et al. Effects of group music Intervention on depression for elderly people in nursing homes. Int J Environ Res Publ Health 2022;19(15):9291.

[15] Kligler B, Teets R, Quick M. Complementary/Integrative therapies that work: a review of the evidence. Am Fam Physician 2016;94(5):369–74.

[16] Chang E, Lai H, Chen P, et al. The effects of music on the sleep quality of adults with chronic insomnia using evidence from polysomnographic and self-reported analysis: a randomized control trial. Int J Nurs Stud 2012;49:921–30.

[17] Chen CT, Tung HH, Fang CJ, et al. Effect of music therapy on improving sleep quality in older adults: a systematic review and meta-analysis. J Am Geriatr Soc 2021;69(7):1925–32.

[18] Ridder HMO, Stige B, Qvale LG, et al. Individual music therapy for agitation in dementia: an exploratory randomized controlled trial. Aging Ment Health 2013;17(6):667–78.

[19] Hedges C, Gotelli J. Managing insomnia in older adults. Nurse Pract Am J Prim Health Care 2019;44(9):16–24.

[20] Hensley JG, Beardsley JR. Insomnia treatment in the primary care setting. Adv Fam Pract Nurs 2020;2:125–43.

[21] Morin CM, Buysse DJ. Management of insomnia. NEJM 2024;391:247–58.

[22] Sateia MJ, Buysse DJ, Krystal AD, et al. Clinical practice guideline for the pharmacologic treatment of chronic insomnia in adults: an American Academy of Sleep Medicine clinical practice guideline. J Clin Sleep Med 2017;13(2):307–49.

[23] AASM Sleep Education, 2024, Available at: https://sleepeducation.org/improve-your-sleep-in-five-simple-steps/ (Accessed 23 Novemeber 2024).

[24] Schutte-Rodin S, Broch L, Buysse D, et al. Clinical guideline for the evaluation and management of chronic insomnia in adults. J Clin Sleep Med 2008;4(5):487–504.

[25] Mattis J, Sehgal A. Circadian rhythms, sleep, and disorders of aging. Trends Endocrinol Metabol 2016;27(4):192–203.

[26] Kim JH, Elkhadem AR, Duffy JF. Circadian rhythm sleep-wake disorders in older adults. Sleep Med Clin 2022;17(2):241–52.

[27] American Psychiatric Association. 2022. Diagnostic and statistical manual of mental health disorders (5th edition, text rev). https://doi.org/10.1176/appi.books.9780890425787.

[28] Resnick B. Sleep issues. In: Geriatric nursing review syllabus: a core curriculum in advanced practice geriatric nursing. 7th edition. New York (NY): America Geriatrics Society; 2022.

[29] Resnick B. Assessment. In: Geriatric nursing review syllabus: a core curriculum in advanced practice geriatric nursing. 7th edition. New York (NY): America Geriatrics Society; 2022.

[30] Resnick B. Depression and other mood disorders. In: Geriatric nursing review syllabus: a core curriculum in advanced practice geriatric nursing. 7th edition. New York (NY): America Geriatrics Society; 2022.

[31] Mukamel DB, Saliba D, Ladd H, et al. Dementia care is widespread in us nursing homes; facilities with the most dementia patients may offer better care. Health Aff 2023;42(6): 795–803.

[32] Patel D, Steinberg J, Patel P. Insomnia in the elderly: a review. J Sleep Med 2018;14(6): 1017–24.

[33] AASM. (n.d.). American academy of sleep medicine. Screening questions – sleep history & physical Available at: https://aasm.org/resources/medsleep/(harding)questions.pdf (Accessed 26 November 2024).

[34] Buysse DJ, Reynolds IIICF, Monk TH, et al. Pittsburgh Sleep Quality Index: a new instrument for psychiatric practice and research. Psychiatr Res 1989;28(2):193–213.

[35] Kapur VK, Aukley DH, Chowdhuri S, et al. Clinical practice guidelines for diagnostic testing for obstructive sleep apnea: an American Academy of Sleep Medicine clincal practice guidelines. J Clin Sleep Med 2017;13(3):479–504.

[36] Chung F, Subramanyam R, Liao P, et al. High STOPBang score indicates a high probability of obstructive sleep apnoea. Br J Anaesth 2012;108(5):768–75.

[37] Celikhisar H, DasdIlkhan DG. Comparison of clinical and polysomnographic characteristics in young and old patients with obstructive sleep apnea syndrome. Aging Male 2020;23(5): 1202–9.

[38] Smith MT, McCrae CS, Cheung J, et al. Use of actigraphy for the evaluation of sleep disorders and circadian rhythm sleep-wake disorders: an American Academy of Sleep Medicine clinical practice guideline. J Clin Sleep Med 2018;14(7):1231–7.

[39] Carney CE, Buysse DJ, Ancoli-Israel S, et al. The consensus sleep diary: standardizing prospective sleep self-monitoring. Sleep 2012;35:287–302.

[40] By the 2023 American Geriatrics Society Beers Criteria® Update Expert Panel. American Geriatrics Society 2023 Updated AGS Beers Criteria® for potentially inappropriate medication use in older adults. J Am Geriatr Soc 2023;71(7):2052–81.

[41] Edinger JD, Arndt JT, Bertisch SM, et al. Behavioral and psychological treatments for chronic insomnia disorder in adults: an American Academy of Sleep Medicine clinical practice guideline. J Clin Sleep Med 2021;17(2):255–62.

[42] American Music Therapy Association, What is the difference between music therapy and a music intervention? Available at: 2024. https://musictherapy.org (Accessed 26 October 2024).

[43] Manzella M. Holistic nursing reflections on music in medicine. American Holistic Nurses Association 2024;44(3):18–9.

[44] Petrovsky DV, Bradt J, McPhillips MV, et al. Tailored music listening in persons with dementia. Am J Alzheimer's Dis Other Dementias 2023;38:1–14.

[45] Koelsch S, Fuermetz J, Sack U, et al. Effects of music listening on cortisol levels and propofol consumption during spinal anesthesia. Front Psychol 2011;2:58.

[46] Nilsson U. The effect of music intervention in stress response to cardiac surgery in a randomized clinical trial. Heart Lung: J Crit Care 2009;38(3):201–7.

[47] Hernández-Ruiz E. Effect of music therapy on the anxiety levels and sleep patterns of abused women in shelters. J Music Ther 2005;42(2):140–58.

[48] Gantt MA, Dadds S, Burns DS, et al. The effect of binaural beat technology on the cardiovascular stress response in military seÖrvice members with postdeployment stress. J Nurs Scholarsh 2017;49(4):411–20.

[49] M. Bhandari, 9 best binaural beats apps for Android, iOS & PC I free & paid Available at: 2023. https://earlystagemarketing.com/binaural-beats-apps/ (Accessed 9 November 2024).

[50] Lai HL. Music preference and relaxation in Taiwanese elderly people. Geriatr Nurs 2004;25(5):286–91.

[51] Chan MF. A randomized controlled study of the effects of music on sleep quality in older people. J Clin Nurs 2011;20(7–8):979–87.

[52] Dickson GT, Schubert E. Music on prescription to aid sleep quality: a literature review. Front Psychol 2020;11:1695.

[53] Safi AJ, Hodgson NA. Timing of activities and their effects on circadian rhythm in the elderly with dementia: a literature review. J Sleep Disord Ther 2014;3(5).

[54] Lin PH, Fu SH, Lee YC, et al. Examining the effects of binaural beat music on sleep quality, heart rate variability, and depression in older people with poor sleep quality in a long-term care institution: a randomized controlled trial. Geriatr Gerontol Int 2024;24:297–304.

[55] Amano T, Hooley C, Strong J, et al. Strategies for implementing music-based interventions for people with dementia in long-term care facilities: a systematic review. Int J Geriatr Psychiatr 2021;1–13.

[56] Yang SY, Lin PH, Wang JY, et al. Effectiveness of binaural beat music combined with rhythmical photic stimulation on older people with depressive symptoms in long-term care institution: a quasi-experimental pilot study. Aging Clin Exp Res 2024;36(1):86.

[57] Lee E, Bang E, Yoon IY, et al. Entrapment of binaural auditory beats in subjects with symptoms of insomnia. Btain Sci 2022;12:339.

[58] Smith JC, Marsh JT, Greenberg S, et al. Human auditory frequency-following responses to a missing fundamental. Science 1978;201:639–41.

[59] Garcia-Argibay M, Santed MA, Reales JM. Efficacy of binaural auditory beats in cognition, anxiety, and pain perception: a meta-analysis. Psychol Res 2019;83(2):357–72.

Advances in Family Practice Nursing 7 (2025) 37–48

ADVANCES IN FAMILY PRACTICE NURSING

ELSEVIER
MOSBY

Psychological Adaptation to Newly Diagnosed Advanced Cancer: Implications for Older Adults

Mei Bai, PhD, RN[a],*,
Melodee Harris, PhD, APRN, GNP-BC, AGPCNP-BC[b]

[a]University of Arkansas for Medical Sciences, 4301 West Markham Street, Mail Slot 547-17, Little Rock, AR 72205, USA; [b]College of Nursing, University of Arkansas for Medical Sciences, 4301 West Markham Street, Slot #529, Little Rock, AR 72205, USA

Keywords

• Adaptation • Cancer • Older adults • Mental health • Quality of life

Key points

• Cancer diagnosis regardless of stage has been seen as a crisis in life.
• Older adults are not immune to the threat of cancer.
• Not every cancer patient is prone to the psychological impact of cancer diagnosis and the majority of cancer patients can successfully handle its impact without becoming mentally disordered.
• Assessment of adaptation and adjustment (as opposed to maladaptation and mental disorders) may facilitate efforts toward maximizing quality of life outcomes for older adults diagnosed with cancer.
• Future innovative research is needed to develop and test measures of psychological adjustment/adaptation in the context of cancer targeting at older adults.

INTRODUCTION

Although age remains to be the strongest determinant of cancer risk [1], cancer diagnosis introduces immediate threat to life regardless of age. From initial diagnosis, treatment, recurrence to progression (or decline), each phase in the cancer trajectory has distinct stressors [2,3]. The process of coping to address different threats produced by cancer at different phases varies with the adaptation requirements of these threats [4]. The time at the initial diagnosis has been

*Corresponding author. E-mail addresses: mei.bai@aya.yale.edu; mbai@uams.edu

https://doi.org/10.1016/j.yfpn.2024.12.002
2589-420X/25/

Abbreviations

PROMIS   Patient-Reported Outcomes Measurement
                                                Information System
QoL   quality of life

viewed as a crisis when feelings, thoughts, and concerns are exacerbated [3,5–8]. The stress associated with cancer diagnosis [9] especially advanced stage [10,11] imposes a significant negative impact on individuals' quality of life (QoL). Paradoxically, however, only a very small portion of cancer patients are found to be mentally disordered due to cancer and the majority are able to maintain or achieve an even higher level of mental functioning. The purpose of this article is to promote an approach of assessment focusing on psychological adaptation potential as opposed to mental disorder for patients newly diagnosed with advanced cancer with implications for older adults.

CASE EXAMPLES

The Case Examples are a summary of responses that may be typical of encounters with older adults who are adapting to a new diagnosed of late stage (or advanced) cancer [12].

Cancer is my reality now.

I am not going to let cancer get me down.

I am a Christian. I find purpose in my faith in God.

I treasure every moment, even taking out the trash.

My family is my highest priority. This is not about me.

Cancer makes me a better human being.

I know I am 75 years old with cancer, but I feel like I am still 45 years old!

Cancer? I think about it when I have to…I have a lot going on in my life besides cancer.

I will be honest. Sometimes it's really hard.

I found peace.

THE CONCEPT OF PSYCHOLOGICAL ADAPTATION

Human beings have the will and capacity to change inner balance *as well as* the external environment (Hartmann, 1939) [13]. This idea is conveyed by the term adaptation, often interchangeably used with adjustment and coping. Adaptation is based on evolutionary concepts, primarily on the notion that living organisms will do what is necessary to struggle to survive; it is a process in which a person continually attempts to maximize the fit between his or her needs and the environment [14]. Inherent in the concept of adaptation is the belief that an individual strives to maintain for oneself a state of equilibrium [14–16] through a constant series of adaptive maneuvers and characteristic problem-solving activities.

In response to many situations throughout a life span, the individual may possess adequate adaptive or reequilibrating mechanisms. However, in a state of crisis, the habitual problem-solving activities are not adequate and do not lead rapidly to the previously achieved balanced state; tension rises and stimulates the mobilization of previously hidden strengths and capacities [17,18]. They actively struggle to surmount difficulties, and they strive to survive physically and psychologically, attempting to adapt to their environment or to change it [19].

This universal adaptation potential may be able to explain the low rates of depression consistently reported in patients living with cancer [20,21]. A recent meta-analysis on interview-defined mood disorders (including depression, anxiety, and adjustment disorder) in patients with cancer yielded the pooled prevalence of 29.0% in palliative care settings and 38.2% in nonpalliative care hospital settings with no association observed between mean age or gender and prevalence of depression or anxiety [22]. Of note, longitudinal studies that offered both prevalence and remission information of depression or other mood disorders suggested distress among patients with a cancer diagnosis as transient [23,24]. Rayner and colleagues [25], for example, found that 69% (27/39) of patients (predominantly older adults) receiving palliative care who were diagnosed with major depressive disorder at baseline had remitted 4 weeks later. Depression remission was also observed in a sample of people with advanced cancer despite deteriorating functions or assignment conditions [26]. Of note, levels of anxiety and depression varied widely by age as well as cancer type and gender [20].

Pitfall of distress screening
Measurement instruments frequently used to screen distress such as the Distress Thermometer [27] or the Hospital Anxiety and Depression Scale [28,29] use thresholds or cutoff scores for screening the intensity of the distress. The cutoff values, however, are not a reliable approach to distinguish adaptive and maladaptive responses because of the considerable overlap between manifestations of patient's response [30]. In a state of crisis, people may suffer from chronic or temporary symptomatology or pathologic patterns of behavior. These 2 conditions have to be conceived of and evaluated separately by primary care providers. That is, whether it is a normal process of adaption/response or represents a mental illness [18], which has been a challenge, especially confronted by repeated threats to life [31].

A mental disorder, such as anxiety disorder or major depressive disorder, is defined as a syndrome characterized by clinically significant disturbance in an individual's cognition, emotion regulation, or behavior that reflects a dysfunction in the psychological, biological, or developmental processes underlying mental functioning [32]. A mental disorder interferes with adaptation, leading to significant distress and disability [30]. Although no screening tools exist allowing us to reliably diagnose mental disorders, certain warning signs or risk factors have been identified that should alert health professionals of the possibility of mental disorder [33].

As Spitzer and Endicott [34] noted, one cannot simply define disorder in terms of dysfunction because dysfunction itself is a concept that requires analysis. And it has been the argument of that symptom or dysfunction alone is neither necessary nor sufficient for diagnosing mental disorder [35,36]. Instead, overall well-being seems to be more determining. According to Wakefield [35], a disorder is justified "only if enduring changes occur inside the person that generalize to other environments" (p.240) and "if there is no harm to the person's overall well-being, there is no disorder." [36].

Intensity and length of the distress symptoms may help differentiate normal reactions from potential disorders, however, raising threshold or adding clinical significance criteria (as used in psychiatric interviews by a trained researcher or health professional) may not solve false positive (that is, incorrectly indicates the presence of a disorder condition) problem, if context (or other contextual factors) remains more of an idea [36]. Baumeister and colleagues [37], for instance, has cautioned against pathologizing normal human adaptive process (such as fight-or-flight response) with special note to the response to a diagnosis of serious illness, as being diagnosed with a life-threatening illness may manifest excessive symptoms and require an extended period of time for recovery that mimic depressive illness.

Alternative approach for assessment focusing on psychological adaptation

While effort was largely directed to assessing, screening, and diagnosing mental disorders among cancer patients, professionals are cautioned not to rely too much on distress screening tools because, although often useful, they are never a substitute for clinical judgment [38]. Also, the frequently used coping and adjustment instruments may not focus on assessment of key aspects of positive functioning. For instance, the mental adjustment to cancer scale [39,40] is dominated by items representing negative functioning and may not be able to validly assess positive functioning.

It must be pointed out that although adaptation is an appealing orientation for mental health in ordinary daily living, under some circumstances (for example, psychological defense mechanisms or Hawthorne effect), it could operate to prevent reporting (see Ryff & Keyes, 1995) [41] or becoming aware of this underlying distress and disturbance. Therefore, it is possible to find individuals who are mentally ill by some other criterion (such as observations or formal interviews), yet who nevertheless report themselves as nondepressed [42].

Adaptation at any given point in time is determined by an interplay of the biological, social, and psychological factors that are impinging at that moment and in the recent and distant past. What really matters is not so much the presence or absence of symptoms or dysfunction, but more importantly the subjective sense of strength, confidence, and well-being [35]. Outcome variance determined by individual-level factors, however, is context-dependent. Contextual factors here referred to temporal and social context.

Table 1 summarizes the outcome and contextual variables for assessment of psychological adaptation that is informed by prior theoretic and psychometric work. It was our hope to aid health professionals to evaluate the coping resources for adaptation and risks for developing mental disorders.

Outcome variables
- Self-esteem
  It has been emphasized that the adequacy of adaptation is a function of the relationship between external demands and a person's resources for dealing with them; satisfactory self-picture or self-esteem must be maintained [43].
- Overall functioning or global QoL
  Clinicians are encouraged to make contact and get information relevant to overall functioning [19].
- Psychological well-being
  Important to one's psychological well-being are a sense of purpose, realizing their given potential, what is the quality of their ties to others, and whether they feel in charge of their own lives [17,41].
- Psychosocial impact of illness: positive aspect (Patient-Reported Outcomes Measurement Information System [PROMIS], 2020) [44].

Individual-level factors
- Personality
  Certain features of personality may be more important than others. It has been noted that we react to dying or life-threatening events in ways consistent with previous manner of living and especially previous pattern of handling life's demands [45].
- Beliefs
  Our response to the world will depend on our conception of it, our beliefs, and attitudes (Adler, 1964) [46].
- Life goals
  As in Gestalt psychology the organization of the whole figure will determine how the parts will be perceived, the organization of the whole person will influence all his partial functions taking to attain one's goal [46].
- Early life experiences
  According to Adler [46], the inner psychological world of the individual, which had such far-reaching consequences, was not objectively caused, but was ultimately the individual's own creation, and that the individual's course of life received its direction not from relatively objective drives, but from his highly subjective goals and values. Moreover, the history of adaptation in younger years has been found to be best predictors of adaptation in old age including a trusting relationship with others, a sense of autonomy, a clearly defined, positively valued identity, and previously confronted adversity without succumbing to it [47].

Contextual factors
- Temporal factors
  The time dimension in the adaptation entails assessment and evaluation of patient's response over a reasonably long period of time as strategy in response to crisis is not created instantly but develops over time [43].
- Support from others (NIH TOOLBOX, 2023) [48].
- Good marital relationship was found to be positively associated with easier adjustment to dying [45].

Risk factors for mental disorders
- Preexisting psychiatric history such as major depression, anxiety, or other [33].
- Prolonged symptoms including feelings of sadness, anxiety, and insomnia [33].

Table 1
Assessment of psychological adaptation in the context of cancer

Variable	Content description	Method
Outcome variables		
Self-esteem	• Trust in self-handling upsetting situations	PROMIS
Global QoL	• Contentment with QoL despite the illness condition	FACT-G (item Gf7)
Psychosocial illness impact	• Trust in one's unique being, ability to handle problems and adjust to things that cannot be changed, and appreciate fully each day	PROMIS (positive 8a) [44]
Psychological well-being	• Sense of whether one's life has purpose • Realizing one's given potential • Quality of ties to others • Feeling in charge of one's own life • Overall well-being • Overall functioning	Interview [17–41]
Individual factors	• Life goals • Personal beliefs • Early life experiences/adversity	Interview [46]
Contextual factors		
Temporal factor	• Strategy in response to crisis is not created instantly but develops over time	
Support from others	• Trusting relationship	NIH TOOLBOX [48]
Warning conditions	• Preexisting psychiatric history • Prolonged symptoms • Absence of hope • Altered subjective experiences	Interview [33]

Abbreviations: FACT-G, the Functional Assessment of Cancer Therapy-General; PROMIS, Patient-Reported Outcomes Measurement Information System [44].

• Absence of hope
• Altered subjective experiences [33].

Intervention toward facilitating adaptation

Basic to the concept of adaptation is the assumption that there is an inherent predisposition toward adaptative functioning in human beings [49]. And as clinical observations and quotations from our case examples above illustrated, people do arrive at their own decisions to take charge of their lives and that they figure out for themselves what they can do to manage symptoms and exert control, even in mentally affected individuals [19]. Strauss [50], for example, concluded from first-hand clinical observations and research work that people play an important role in controlling their own symptoms and in selecting and using the kinds of help available. What appears to be a setback may turn out to be adaptive in the long run [43,51].

It has been the argument in the previous theoretic work concerning mental health [35,52] to view a person *not* from the perspective of normality but as having varying potentialities and limitations under varying conditions. In very many cases, affirmation of personally important values is of utmost importance, which will allow cognitive reorganization or new perspectives possible [46,52,53]. Self-concept or self-esteem is recognized as the most significant determinant of response to the environment as it governs the perceptions or meanings attributed to the environment. Experiences which are inconsistent with self-concept may be perceived as threatening, and may be rejected, denied, or distorted; the self-concept is defended [54]. Thus, self-esteem must be maintained at all costs and enhanced if at all possible [55]. Recent research work [12] designed to help patients adjust to the psychological impact of cancer diagnosis by affirming personally important values or beliefs has provided some preliminary support for the approach of adaptation efforts. Of note, the median age in this sample is 63 years old and intervention effect did not find age differences across individuals. In fact, although research work devoted to the older adults cancer survivors is growing [56,57], still more attention is to be paid to the noteworthy and unique issues that separate older individuals from their younger cancer-survivor counterparts [58].

SALIENCE OF OLD AGE AND CANCER ADAPTATION

Although old age has generally been considered a phase of life in which the person's capacities for adaptation are diminishing due to decreased cognitive functions [47], research revealed an opposite view in that older adults were found to have less severe and more short-lived emotional reactions to detrimental life events than younger adults [59]. Moreover, older adults tend to be motivated to allocate attention on obtaining personally meaningful goals [60,61], thereby likely remember positive memories [60,62] and report positive outcomes [63].

On the other hand, literature supporting a positive link between age and QoL outcomes following cancer diagnosis [64,65] is with mixed results [66] and likely context dependent [60,67]. Given the methodological issues including lack of control of clinical factors (such as stage, comorbidity, and treatment modality) and contextual variables (such as time since diagnosis and social support), it is possible that individual differences other than demographic or clinical factors may more likely account for the divergent patterns of adaptation to cancer diagnosis [68]. The individual-level factors that could influence the outcomes include personality, defense mechanisms, prior life experience, meaning assigned to event, cultural background, roles in the family, etc. [14].

Interestingly, distress symptoms not only can result in no disorders, but also a certain amount of anxiety in a given situation can improve alertness and efficiency for coping [47]. On the other hand, distress may not always be experienced overtly in older adults and may give rise to a variety of other symptoms or defenses [47]. Furthermore, response to an anxiety-producing stimulus in older adults is often delayed and may be increased or decreased depending on which manifestation of anxiety is being measured, for instance, physiologic or psychosocial aspects [69].

CLINICAL IMPLICATIONS

A little help, rationally directed and purposefully focused at a time of need is more effective than more extensive help, given at a period less sensitive to outside influence [18]. It is important for direct care staff members and other caregivers to recognize that coping and adaptation can take different forms, and that what appears to be symptoms may be adaptive in nature [19]. Key to this discussion is that mental disorder may be best identified not from presence of distress but absence of adequate adaptation efforts or resources. It is even more important to recognize that the strength in each individual that can be reinforced by sensitive caregivers to facilitate improvement or recovery [19], and they are not acting as a single resource, but within a social system as part of a network of relationships [18,70].

Clinical professionals including nurses and physicians, not necessarily psychologists, psychiatrists or mental health professionals, may assess the extent to which successful psychological adaptation was reached as well as its associated contextual factors. Unlike mental disorders, assessment and evaluation for adaptation should not require the same training of psychologists, psychiatrists, or mental health professionals, which enables addressing patient's adaptation issues in a timely manner without having to wait until a disorder is established. Focusing on assessing adaptation outcomes to maximize potential for QoL and overall well-being in the context of cancer may be one promising innovative approach to optimize patient outcomes for older adults newly diagnosed with cancer and awaits future investigations to verify.

Moreover, it becomes critical from this review what caregivers say or do to help people in crisis shift from a feeling of powerlessness to one of efficacy and self-direction [19]. What is needed, then, are new ways of thinking that provide a significant shift from focus on limited and negative characteristics of patient and/or families to a more comprehensive and dynamic understanding of individuals and a preventative approach by strengthening the individual's inner resources for adaptation.

SUMMARY

Cancer and its treatment create chronic and severe stress situations in which the limits of patients' coping abilities are constantly challenged, and which may often lead to difficulties in maintaining an optimal adjustment. Adaptation is a concept where psychological, sociologic, and philosophic literature converge. The principle practical significance of adaptation is that the individual is understood not as completely determined by outside forces but to a considerable extent as self-determined, or *autonomy* [71]. Human being has a characteristic tendency toward self-determination, that is, a tendency to resist external influences and to subordinate the heteronomous forces of the physical and social environment to it. Such a perspective is particularly relevant to older adults with a dogged determination toward freedom and optimism, so important in enabling the expected change. Nonetheless, current evidence remains limited to make conclusive remarks about age differences in terms of cancer adaptation and adjustment, awaiting future research to verify.

CLINICS CARE POINTS

- Literature supported the universal efforts of individuals striving to overcome crisis as well as considerable variability.
- Rather than questioning whether one is normal, it is more fruitful to assess one's adaptation resources.
- New ways of thinking are needed to allow of a preventative approach by strengthening inner resources for adaptation, an approach that differs from assessing symptoms and dysfunctions.

DISCLOSURE

The authors declare that no conflict of interest exists.

FUNDING

Preparation of this work was not associated with any funding support.

References

[1] Siegel RL, Giaquinto AN, Jemal A. Cancer statistics, 2024. CA: A Cancer J Clin 2024;74(1):12–49.

[2] Baum A, Posluszny DM. Traumatic stress as a target for intervention with cancer patients. In: Baum A, Andersen BL, editors. Psychosocial interventions for cancer. Washington, DC: American Psychological Association; 2001. p. 143–73.

[3] Weisman AD. A model for psychosocial phasing in cancer. In: Moos RH, editor. Coping with physical illness. New York: Plenum Publishing; 1984. p. 107–22.

[4] Lazarus RS. Coping theory and research: past, present and future. Psychosom Med 1993;55: 234–47.

[5] Krouse HJ, Krouse JH. Cancer as crisis: the critical elements of adjustment. Nurs Res 1982;31:96–101.

[6] McCorkle R, Quint-Benoliel J. Symptom distress current concerns and mood disturbance after diagnosis of life-threatening disease. Soc Sci Med 1983;17:431–8.

[7] Weisman AD, Worden JW. The existential plight in cancer: significance of the first 100 days. Int J Psychiatr Med 1976;7(1):1–15.

[8] Worden JW, Sobel HJ. Ego strength and psychosocial adaptation to cancer. Psychosom Med 1978;40:585–92.

[9] Goncalves V, Jayson G, Tarrier N. A longitudinal investigation of posttraumatic stress disorder in patients with ovarian cancer. J Psychosom Res 2011;70(5):422–31.

[10] Lee LJ, Chung CW, Chang YY, et al. Comparison of the quality of life between patients with non-small-cell lung cancer and healthy controls. Qual Life Res 2011;20(3):415–23.

[11] Mystakidou K, Parpa E, Tsilika E, et al. Traumatic experiences of patients with advanced cancer. J Loss Trauma 2012;17(2):125–36.

[12] Bai M. Self-affirmation intervention for people newly diagnosed with advanced cancer. 2024. Available at: https://clinicaltrials.gov/study/NCT05235750?a=1. Accessed September 5, 2024.

[13] Hartmann H. Psycho-analysis and the concept of health. Int J Psychoanal 1939;20:308–21.

[14] Hatfield AB. Coping and adaptation: a conceptual framework for understanding families. In: Hatfield AB, Lefley HP, editors. Families of mentally ill coping and adaptation. New York: Guilford Press; 1987. p. 60–84.

[15] Caplan G. Principles of preventative psychiatry. New York: Basic Books; 1964.

[16] Roy C. The roy adaptation model. 3rd edition. New Jersey: Pearson Education, Inc; 2009.

[17] Parad HJ, Caplan G. A framework for study families in crisis. In: Parad HJ, editor. Crisis intervention: selected readings. Family Service Association of America; 1965. p. 53–74.

[18] Rapoport L. Crisis intervention. In: Parad HJ, editor. Crisis intervention: selected readings. New York, NY: Family Service Association of America; 1965. p. 22–31.

[19] Hartfield AB, Lefley HP. Surviving mental illness: stress, coping, and adaptation. The Guilford Press; 1993.

[20] Linden W, Vodermaier A, Mackenzie R, et al. Anxiety and depression after cancer diagnosis: prevalence rates by cancer type, gender, and age. J Affect Disord 2012;141(2–3): 343–51.

[21] Waraich P, Goldner EM, Somers JM, et al. Prevalence and incidence studies of mood disorders: a systematic review of the literature. Can J Psychiatr 2004;49(2):124–38.

[22] Mitchell AJ, Chan M, Bhatti H, et al. Prevalence of depression, anxiety, and adjustment disorder in oncological, haematological, and palliative-care settings: a meta-analysis of 94 interview-based studies. Lancet Oncol 2011;12(2):160–74.

[23] Stafford L, Judd F, Gibson P, et al. Screening for depression and anxiety in women with breast and gynaecologic cancer: course and prevalence of morbidity over 12 months. Psycho Oncol 2013;22(9):2071–8.

[24] Néron S, Correa JA, Dajczman E, et al. Screening for depressive symptoms in patients with unresectable lung cancer. Support Care Cancer 2007;15(10):1207–12.

[25] Rayner L, Lee W, Price A, et al. The clinical epidemiology of depression in palliative care and the predictive value of somatic symptoms: cross-sectional survey with four-week follow-up. Palliat Med 2011;25(3):229–41.

[26] Serfaty M, King M, Nazareth I, et al. Manualised cognitive-behavioural therapy in treating depression in advanced cancer: the CanTalk RCT. Health Technol Assess 2019;23(19): 1–106.

[27] National Comprehensive Cancer Network. NCCN guidelines version 1. 2024 distress management. 2024. Available at: https://www.nccn.org/docs/default-source/patient-resources/nccn_distress_thermometer.pdf.

[28] Vodermaier A, Millman RD. Accuracy of the Hospital Anxiety and Depression Scale as a screening tool in cancer patients: a systematic review and meta-analysis. Support Care Cancer 2011;19(12):1899–908.

[29] Zigmond AS, Snaith RP. The hospital anxiety and depression scale. Acta Psychiatr Scand 1983;67(6):361–70.

[30] Dekker J, Braamse A, Schuurhuizen C, et al. Distress in patients with cancer – on the need to distinguish between adaptive and maladaptive emotional responses. Acta oncologica (Stockholm, Sweden) 2017;56(7):1026–9.

[31] Massie MJ. Prevalence of depression in patients with cancer. J Natl Cancer Inst Monogr 2004;32:57–71.

[32] American Psychiatric Association. Diagnostic and statistical manual of mental disorders. 5th edition 2013; https://doi.org/10.1176/appi.books.9780890425596.

[33] Seddon CF, Schnipper HH. Assessing and intervening with the spectrum of depression and anxiety in cancer. In: Christ G, Messner C, Behar L, editors. Handbook of oncology social work : psychosocial care for people with cancer. Oxford University Press; 2015. p. 339–44.

[34] Spitzer RL, Endicott J. Medical and mental disorder: proposed definition and criteria. In: Spitzer RL, Klein DF, editors. Critical issues in psychiatric diagnosis. New York: Raven Press; 1978. p. 15–39.

[35] Wakefield JC. Disorder as harmful dysfunction: a conceptual critique of DSM-III-R's definition of mental disorder. Psychol Rev 1992;99(2):232–47.

[36] Spitzer RL, Wakefield JC. DSM-IV diagnostic criterion for clinical significance: does it help solve the false positives problem? Am J Psychiatr 1999;156(12):1856–64.

[37] Baumeister H, Maercker A, Casey P. Adjustment disorder with depressed mood: a critique of its DSM-IV and ICD-10 conceptualisations and recommendations for the future. Psychopathology 2009;42(3):139–47.

[38] Parry C, Padgett LS, Zebrack B. Now what? Toward an integrated research and practice agenda in distress screening. J Psychosoc Oncol 2012;30(6):715–27.

[39] Watson M, Greer S, Young J, et al. Development of a questionnaire measure of adjustment to cancer: the MAC scale. Psychol Med 1988;18(1):203–9.

[40] Watson M, Homewood J. Mental Adjustment to Cancer Scale: psychometric properties in a large cancer cohort. Psycho Oncol 2008;17(11):1146–51.

[41] Ryff CD, Keyes CL. The structure of psychological well-being revisited. J Pers Soc Psychol 1995;69(4):719–27.

[42] Scott WA. Definitions of mental health and illness. Psychol Bull 1958;55:29–45.

[43] White RW. Strategies of adaptation: an attempt at systematic description. In: Moos RH, editor. Human adaptation: coping with life crises. D.C. Health and Company; 1976. p. 17–32.

[44] PROMIS short form v1.0 - psychosocial illness impact-positive 8a. 2020. Available at: https://www.healthmeasures.net/index.php?option=com_instruments&view=measure&id=173&Itemid=992.

[45] Hinton J. The influence of previous personality on reactions to having terminal cancer. Omega J Death Dying 1975;6(2):95–111.

[46] Adler A. Problems of neurosis: a book of case histories. New York: Harper Torchbooks; 1964.

[47] Busse EW, Pfeiffer E. Behavior and adaptation in late life. Boston, MA: Little, Brown and Company; 1977.

[48] NIH toolbox item bank v3.0 - emotional support (ages 18 plus)(2023). Accessed July 2024.

[49] Pearlin LI, Schooler C. The structure of coping. J Health Soc Behav 1978;19(1):2–21.

[50] Strauss JS. Discussion: what does rehabilitation accomplish? Schizophr Bull 1986;12(4):720–3.

[51] Strauss JS. Mediating processes in schizophrenia: towards a new dynamic psychiatry. Br J Psychiatr 1989;155(Suppl 5):22–8.

[52] Freides D. Toward the elimination of the concept of normality. Journal of Consultation and Psychology 1960;24:128–33.

[53] Tillich P. Courage to be. New Haven & London: Yale University Press; 1952.

[54] Patterson CH. The self in recent Rogerian Theory. Psychologia 1961;4:156–62.

[55] White RW. Strategies of adaptation: an attempt at systematic description. In: Coelho GV, Hamburg DA, Adams JE, editors. Human adaptation: coping and adaptation. New York: Basic Books; 1974. p. 47–68.

[56] Gagliese L, Jovellanos M, Zimmermann C, et al. Age-related patterns in adaptation to cancer pain: a mixed-method study. Pain Med 2009;10(6):1050–61.

[57] Köhler N, Mehnert A, Götze H. Psychological distress, chronic conditions and quality of life in elderly hematologic cancer patients: study protocol of a prospective study. BMC Cancer 2017;17(1):700.

[58] Trask PC, Blank TO, Jacobsen PB. Future perspectives on the treatment issues associated with cancer and aging. Cancer 2008;113(12 Suppl):3512–8.

[59] Hansen T, Blekesaune M. The age and well-being "paradox": a longitudinal and multidimensional reconsideration. Eur J Ageing 2022;19(4):1277–86.

[60] Carstensen LL, Mikels JA. At the intersection of emotion and cognition: aging and the positivity effect. Curr Dir Psychol Sci 2005;14(3):117–21.

[61] Sardella A, Lenzo V, Basile G, et al. Emotion regulation strategies and difficulties in older adults: a systematic review. Clin Gerontol 2023;46(3):280–301.

[62] Fernandes M, Ross M, Wiegand M, et al. Are the memories of older adults positively biased? Psychol Aging 2008;23(2):297–306.

[63] Gurera JW, Isaacowitz DM. Emotion regulation and emotion perception in aging: a perspective on age-related differences and similarities. Prog Brain Res 2019;247:329–51.

[64] Rose JH, Kypriotakis G, Bowman KF, et al. Patterns of adaptation in patients living long term with advanced cancer. Cancer 2009;115(18 Suppl):4298–310.

[65] Yan H, Sellick K. Symptoms, psychological distress, social support, and quality of life of Chinese patients newly diagnosed with gastrointestinal cancer. Cancer Nurs 2004;27: 389–99.

[66] Sehlen S, Hollenhorst H, Schymura B, et al. Psychosocial stress in cancer patients during and after radiotherapy. Strahlenther Onkol 2003;179:175–80.

[67] Schirda B, Valentine TR, Aldao A, et al. Age related differences in emotion regulation strategies: examining the role of contextual factors. Dev Psychol 2016;52(9):1370–80.

[68] Bai M, Cella D. Quality of life outcomes in people newly diagnosed with advanced cancer: a case for individual differences. Poster presentation. ISOQOL 30th annual conference. 2023. Calgary, Alberta, Canada.

[69] Shmavonian BM, Busse EW. Psychophysiologic techniques in the study of the aged. In: Willams R, Tibbitts C, Donahue W, editors. Processes of agingvol. 1. New York: Atherton; 1963. p. 168–83.

[70] Schnipper HH, Varner A. Interventions and ongoing assessment with people living with cancer. In: Christ G, Messner C, Behar L, editors. Handbook of oncology social work : psychosocial care for people with cancer. Oxford University Press; 2015. p. 313–20.

[71] Angyal A. Foundations for a science of personality. New York: The Commonwealth Fund; 1941.

Advances in Family Practice Nursing 7 (2025) 49–65

ADVANCES IN FAMILY PRACTICE NURSING

Depression and Older Adults
A Guide for Assessment, Diagnosis, and Management

Christie Keller, DNP, APRN, PMHNP-BC

College of Nursing, University of Arkansas for Medical Sciences, Little Rock/Fayetteville, 1125 North College Avenue, Fayetteville, AR 72703, USA

Keywords

• Depression • Antidepressants • Older adults • Geriatric psychiatry

Key points

- Primary care providers are the first point-of-care providers for older adults seeking treatment of depression.
- Improved understanding of differential diagnosis and treatment strategies for depression leads to more effective treatments and more efficient care coordination across disciplines.
- Identifying proper treatment strategies leads to earlier remission of symptoms and improves patient outcomes.

DEPRESSION AND OLDER ADULTS: A GUIDE FOR ASSESSMENT, DIAGNOSIS, AND MANAGEMENT

Depression is a prevalent and debilitating mental health condition that often presents in primary care settings. Health care professionals are critical in accurately identifying, assessing, and managing patients with depressive symptoms [1]. Nearly 60% of patients treated for depression in the United States are managed in the primary care setting [1]. Primary care providers are responsible for nearly 78% of antidepressant prescriptions [1]. Less than half of these patients are accurately diagnosed, and more than half are undertreated. Older adults often remain untreated or undertreated due to cognitive decline, inadequate diagnostic tools, and the belief that depression may be a normal part of aging [2].

Research on the use of antidepressants among older adults, particularly in recent years, suggests a significant prevalence of both depression and antidepressant

E-mail address: clkeller@uams.edu

https://doi.org/10.1016/j.yfpn.2025.01.001

Abbreviations

BDNF   brain-derived neurotrophic factor
DASH   dietary approaches to stop hypertension
MAOIs   monoamine oxidase inhibitors
MDD   major depressive disorder
SNRIs   serotonin norepinephrine reuptake inhibitors
SSRIs   serotonin reuptake inhibitors
TCAs   tricyclic antidepressants

usage among this population [3,4]. The geriatric population is especially vulnerable to depression, but prevalence rates are challenging to determine due to methodological differences [3]. One systematic review and meta-analysis [3] found that worldwide, 28.4% of older adults suffer from depression. Antidepressant use in the United States increases with age, particularly among women. The prevalence rate of adults aged 60 years and older is 19% and 24.3% among older adult women [4].

Challenges to appropriate treatment and diagnosis of depression in older adult persons include underreporting of symptoms, cultural stigma, lack of provider awareness, time limitations, scarcity of mental health providers, and lack of access to evidence-based interventions [1,2]. However, regular interactions with primary care providers may facilitate early detection, continuous monitoring, and timely intervention for mental health conditions, contributing significantly to the overall well-being of older adults.

PSYCHIATRIC HISTORY

Accurate psychiatric evaluation relies on strong assessment skills to elicit subjective data from older adults with symptoms of depression [5,6]. Key factors of an older adult's psychiatric history include ascertaining frequency and duration of symptoms, medication history, response to previous medication trials, family psychiatric history, and efficacy of treatment of family members are key elements of a thorough psychiatric history. Questions to consider are as follows:

- Is this the first occurrence, or is this a recurrent episode?
- Any previous antidepressant trials?
- If so, which medication(s) and dose? What was the response for each medication? Was it effective? Were there any side effects? Why did the patient stop this medication?

Additionally, gathering a family psychiatric history is essential, but may be unavailable for older adults. Genetics plays a role in complete psychiatric assessment. It is helpful to know the diagnoses and treatments for immediate family members of each generation, going back to maternal and paternal grandparents, parents, siblings, children, and grandchildren [5,7]. It is important to keep in mind that psychiatric treatment was much less prevalent in previous generations, so parents and grandparents may not have been diagnosed or treated, and any mental health conditions may have gone unrecognized. In these cases, inquire about personality traits, tendencies, eccentricities, and family lore. For example, the patient's mother may not have a diagnosis, but everyone in the family knew that she was highly anxious. Finally, and critically, examine suicide risk factors, such as family attempts and completed suicides, previous and current personal attempts or ideation, and other known risk factors. If the patient is imminently suicidal, refer to a crisis stabilization unit or inpatient treatment if necessary.

ASSESSMENT OF DEPRESSION IN OLDER ADULTS

The American Psychiatric Association [8] lists the diagnostic criteria for major depressive disorder (MDD) as the presence of a depressed mood or loss of pleasure or interest in most activities, along with 5 or more additional symptoms over a 2 week period that represent a change in previous functioning and cause clinically significant distress or functional impairment. Characteristic symptoms of depression include

- Depressed mood by report or observation
- Diminished interest or pleasure in almost all activities
- Significant change in appetite or weight without intent
- Sleep disturbances
- Fatigue or lack of energy
- Psychomotor agitation or retardation
- Feelings of worthlessness or excessive and inappropriate guilt
- Difficulty concentrating or cognitive difficulties
- Recurrent thoughts of death or suicidal ideation

The presentation of depressive disorders in older adults often differs from the clinical diagnostic criteria listed earlier, making it challenging to diagnose with certainty. In addition to a personal or family history of depression, risk factors for depression in older adults include medications, medical conditions, stress, insomnia, socioeconomic status, substance use or abuse, and hearing or vision impairment [7]. Other factors that must be considered when assessing depression in older adults include the association with other psychiatric disorders or degenerative neurologic diseases of the central nervous system. Therefore, the diagnostic process should involve a comprehensive clinical history, a detailed diagnostic interview, and the appropriate use of screening and assessment tools. Accurate assessment of depression in older adults requires a multifaceted approach that considers the unique clinical presentation, risk factors, and the potential comorbidities associated with this condition.

Depressed older adults often exhibit a range of symptoms, including low mood, lack of motivation, loss of physical strength, difficulty sleeping, lack of concentration, and feelings of helplessness, hopelessness, and lack of self-worth [9,10]. However, rather than expressing sadness or a depressed mood, older adults are more likely to focus on somatic complaints, fatigue, anhedonia, poor appetite, insomnia, pain, anxiety, and memory impairments [8,9]. In addition to reported symptoms, observable signs may include social withdrawal, apathy, low energy, cognitive impairment, problems with self-care, and weight loss [9,10]. Older adults may also refuse to eat, drink, or use medications, or they may engage in new or increasing use of substances such as alcohol, pain medications, or sedatives. By addressing these assessment challenges, health care professionals can provide appropriate interventions and support to improve the well-being and quality of life of older adults affected by depression (Table 1).

PATHOGENESIS

Depression can develop for a variety of reasons throughout a person's life. Reactive depression occurs in response to psychosocial stressors or an identifiable precipitating event, such as a recent change, grief, loss of independence, or relationship issues [10,11]. Biologic depression arises from conditions that alter one's neurobiology and may appear to emerge spontaneously [11]. These include medical conditions, medications or substances, hormonal fluctuations, endocrine dysregulation, or biological and genetic vulnerability [10–12]. While medication management may be utilized in both types of depression, it is most useful in treating biologic depression (Table 2).

There is no consensus as to one specific cause for depression, but there are several theories regarding the pathophysiology of the disease process [12,13]. The focus of research into the physiologic mechanisms leading to depression include stress-induced dysregulation of the hypothalamus-pituitary-adrenal axis, neuroprogression, circadian rhythm disorders, neuroinflammation, and the monoamine hypothesis of depression. Realistically, the etiology is multifactorial and any of these models can lead to depressive symptoms. The leading hypothesis upon which most antidepressant drugs have been developed is the monoamine hypothesis, which proposes that a deficiency in any of the

Table 1
Differences in presentation of depression in older adults

Impaired cognition	Social withdrawal
Somatic preoccupation	Obsessive ruminations
Fatigue	Delusions
Pain	Anxiety or panic
Chronic medical comorbidities	Apathy
Poor appetite	Anhedonia
Weight loss	Irritability
Psychomotor agitation	—

Data from American Psychiatric Association. (2022). Diagnostic and statistical manual of mental disorders, Fifth Edition, Text Revision (DSM-5-TR). Washington, DC: Author; Ismail, Z., Fischer, C., & McCall, W. V. (2013). What characterizes late-life depression? Psychiatric Clinics of North America, 36(4), 483-496. https://doi.org/10.1016/j.psc.2013.08.010; Pocklington, C. (2017). Depression in older adults. British Journal of Medical Practitioners, 10(1), a1007.

Table 2
Risk factors for depression in older adults

Psychosocial	Biologic
Personality characteristics	Genetics
Socioeconomic status or change	Female
Stressful life events, such as moving	Endocrine dysregulation
Loneliness	Hormonal fluctuations
Social withdrawal	Medical illness
Inadequate support system	Cerebrovascular changes
Bereavement	Inflammation
Loss of independence	Neurodegenerative illnesses
Elder abuse	

Data from Aziz, R., & Steffens, D. C. (2013). What are the causes of late-life depression? Psychiatric Clinics of North America, 36(4), 497–51 6. https://doi.org/10.1016/j.psc.2013.08.001; Pocklington, C. (2017). Depression in older adults. British Journal of Medical Practitioners, 10(1), a1007; Preston, J. D., O'Neal, J. H., Talaga, M. C., & Moore, B. A. (2021). Handbook of clinical psychopharmacology for therapists (9th ed.). New Harbinger Publications.

monoamines (serotonin, norepinephrine, and dopamine) can lead to depression. This monoamine hypothesis has been extended to include deficient activity in monoamine receptors and dysregulation of brain networks involving these neurotransmitters.

DIFFERENTIAL DIAGNOSIS
Older adults may report a history of previous depressive episodes. However, first-episode depression is not uncommon [7,10]. There is a myriad of causes for depression, including psychosocial factors, medical etiology, and the result of prescribed medications. See Table 3 for list of differential diagnoses to consider [7,8].

Table 3
Differential diagnosis of major depressive disorder in older adults

Differential diagnosis	
MDD (add severity and specifier)	F32.0–F33.9
Adjustment disorder with depressed mood	F43.21
Prolonged grief disorder (bereavement)	F43.8
Depressive disorder due to another medical condition	F06.31, F06.32
Substance/medication-induced depressive disorder	*See specific substances for codes*
Bipolar I disorder/bipolar II disorder	F31.0–F31.9
Depressive episode with insufficient symptoms	F32.89
Persistent depressive disorder	F34.1

Data from American Psychiatric Association. (2022). Diagnostic and statistical manual of mental disorders, Fifth Edition, Text Revision (DSM-5-TR). Washington, DC: Author; Steffens, D. & Zdanys, K. (2023). The American Psychiatric Association Publishing textbook of geriatric psychiatry (6th ed.). American Psychiatric Publishing. ISBN: 9781615373406

Psychosocial factors

Older adults face a variety of psychosocial stressors that can lead to adjustment issues, particularly surrounding loss and changing roles. Challenges facing older adults include life changes such as retirement or loss of occupation, grief involving the loss of a life partner or friend, loss of independence such as no longer driving or moving into an assisted living facility, a serious medical diagnosis, relationship issues, and loneliness [9,10,12]. When stressful events and life changes lead to depressive symptoms that interfere with daily functioning, adjustment disorder may be diagnosed if all criteria for MDD are not met [8]. Time is an essential component of this diagnosis, as the symptom onset must begin within 3 months of an identifiable stressor and last no more than 6 months after removal of the stressor. The treatment of choice for adjustment disorder is psychotherapy, although augmentation with antidepressants during treatment may prove helpful [14].

Prolonged bereavement may also lead to depressive symptoms [9]. Grief is a normal response to the loss of a significant person in one's life, and it shares many symptoms with depression [8,11]. However, the intensity of the depressive symptoms that accompany grief should lessen over time. When symptoms persist or intensify, grief can develop into clinical depression. Table 4 outlines some fundamental differences in depressive symptoms related to grief versus clinical depression [8].

Medical etiology

Multiple medical etiologies can be contributing factors to depression in older adults; for example, normal age-related changes and/or dysregulation of the endocrine system can lead to symptoms of depression [13]. As people age, sex hormones like estrogen and testosterone decrease and low levels of these hormones have been linked to depression. Apart from sex hormones, changes in the glucocorticoid receptor and the responsiveness and secretion of corticotrophin-releasing factor can also affect depressive symptoms. Endocrine dysregulation may cause structural changes in the brain that contribute to depressive symptoms, such as atrophy in the hippocampus and loss of brain volume. Additionally, hypothyroidism is common in older adults [15], which can cause depressive symptoms but is treatable with medication.

Medical illness and chronic pain may lead to depressive symptoms and possible misdiagnosis [9]. Unfortunately, misdiagnosis means that the underlying cause may be left untreated while the patient is unnecessarily exposed to additional medications such as serotonin reuptake inhibitors (SSRIs), leading to increased polypharmacy. All medical conditions must be appropriately documented and considered when treating depression, including cognitive decline, dementia, cerebrovascular disease, hormonal disturbances such as menopause, endocrine disorders, insomnia, and sleep apnea [7,13]. A comprehensive physical examination and medical history can assist in identifying these medical conditions. A thorough laboratory panel should also be obtained to rule out deficiencies and imbalances that may be symptomatic, including vitamin D,

Table 4
Depressive symptoms in grief versus major depressive disorder

	Grief	MDD
Shared features	• Intense sadness • Rumination about the loss • Insomnia • Poor appetite • Weight loss	
Mood and emotions	• Dysphoria decreases in intensity over time • May occur in waves • Associated with reminders of the deceased • Feelings of emptiness and loss • May experience positive emotions and humor along with emotional pain of grief	• Persistently depressed mood unrelated to specific thoughts or preoccupations • Persistent depressed mood • Inability to foresee happiness or pleasure • Pervasive feelings of unhappiness and misery
Thought content	• Preoccupation with thoughts and memories of the deceased	• Self-critical thoughts or pessimistic ruminations
Self-esteem	• Self-esteem preserved	• Low self-esteem (worthlessness and self-loathing)
Suicidal ideation	• Suicidal thoughts focused on the deceased and possibly about "joining" this person	• Suicidal thoughts due to feelings of worthlessness and inability to cope with the pain of depression

Data from American Psychiatric Association. (2022). Diagnostic and statistical manual of mental disorders, Fifth Edition, Text Revision (DSM-5-TR). Washington, DC: Author.; Ismail, Z., Fischer, C., & McCall, W. V. (2013). What characterizes late-life depression? Psychiatric Clinics of North America, 36(4), 483-496. https://doi.org/10.1016/j.psc.2013.08.010; Preston, J. D., O'Neal, J. H., Talaga, M. C., & Moore, B. A. (2021). Handbook of clinical psychopharmacology for therapists (9th ed.). New Harbinger Publications.

vitamin B12, thyroid panel, iron, and hormones, if indicated [7,13]. These laboratories are frequently requested or ordered to rule out medical etiology if referred to psychiatry. Performing them in the primary care setting can sometimes eliminate the need for referral and lead to more timely diagnosis and treatment. All identified medical conditions suspected of contributing to depressive symptoms should be treated when possible.

Therefore, a thorough psychiatric history, medical history, physical assessment, and medication reconciliation to rule out other causes of symptoms to accurately diagnose and treat depression is essential. Treatment options differ according to the underlying contributing factors mentioned earlier.

See Table 5 for medical disorders often associated with depression [8–10,16,17].

Medication considerations

Older adults are highly likely to be prescribed multiple prescription medications, many of which can result in depressive symptoms [10] (see Box 1). For example, β-adrenergic blockers, used to treat hypertension, have been associated with

Table 5
Medical disorders associated with depression

Cerebrovascular diseases	• Stroke
	• Tumor
	• Epilepsy
	• White matter hyperintensities
	• Cerebral arteriosclerosis
Cardiovascular diseases	• Myocardial infarction
	• Ischemic heart disease
Neurodegenerative diseases	• Alzheimer's
	• Parkinson's
	• Huntington's
	• Pick's
	• Wilson's disease
	• Multiple sclerosis
Endocrine disorders	• Hypothyroidism
	• Diabetes
	• Cushing's disease
	• Addison's disease
Inflammatory diseases	• Lupus
	• Asthma
	• Inflammatory bowel disease
	• Systemic inflammation
Metabolic disorders	• Uremia
	• Porphyria
	• Vitamin deficiencies (B-12, D)
Sleep disturbances	• Insomnia
	• Sleep apnea
Miscellaneous disorders	• Migraine
	• Chronic pain
	• Cancer
	• Tuberculosis
	• Mononucleosis
	• Sjögren's syndrome
	• Chronic fatigue syndrome
	• Mild traumatic brain injury
	• Chronic obstructive pulmonary disease

Data from Refs [8–10,16,17].

depression, while angiotensin-converting enzyme inhibitors have not [18]. Long-term corticosteroid therapy is also linked to the development of depression [12,18]. Additionally, the combination of certain medications may have cumulative effects with neuropsychiatric consequences; due to these potential unintended effects, complete medication reconciliation is recommended when treating older adults for depression. When feasible, every effort should be made to eliminate or substitute suspected causal agents. Because individual vulnerabilities can lead some patients to respond differently, if depressive symptoms develop after adding a new medication, an elimination trial with reintroduction of the drug may help to clarify causality of depressive symptoms and whether a switch is necessary [18].

Box 1: Medications that may cause depression

Antihypertensives

Anti-Parkinson drugs

Anti-inflammatory agents

Antibiotics and Antivirals

Stimulants

Benzodiazepines

Corticosteroids and other hormones

Anticonvulsants

Metformin

Immunologic agents

Data from Aziz, R., & Steffens, D. C. (2013). What are the causes of late-life depression? Psychiatric Clinics of North America, 36(4), 497–516. https://doi.org/10.1016/j.psc.2013.08.001; Celano, C. M., Freudenreich, O., Fernandez-Robles, C., Stern, T. A., Caro, M. A., & Huffman, J. C. (2011). Depressogenic effects of medications: A review. Dialogues in Clinical Neuroscience, 13(1), 109–125. https://doi.org/10.31887/DCNS.2011.13.1/ccelano; Pocklington, C. (2017). Depression in older adults. British Journal of Medical Practitioners, 10(1), a1007.

Although medications can lead to depression in older adults, it is equally important to rule out substances of abuse in this population. The National Institute on Drug Abuse [19] reports that substance use disorders are a growing yet often unrecognized concern in the older adult population, with substantial increases in high-risk drinking and other substance use disorders over the past two decades. Providers in the outpatient setting can screen patients for harmful practices such as problematic drinking and misuse of prescription medications by using brief screening tools such as the Short Michigan Alcoholic Screening Test-Geriatric Version, which can lead to more in-depth conversations and treatment recommendations.

Bipolar disorder

Bipolar disorder should always be considered in the differential diagnoses during an evaluation for depression [7]. The treatment and disease trajectory will differ considerably based on these diagnoses, and the use of SSRIs and serotonin norepinephrine reuptake inhibitors (SNRIs) is contraindicated in bipolar disorder because the use of these antidepressants can induce mania and worsen the course of the disease [13]. When bipolar disorder is suspected, the patient should be referred to a psychiatric provider for medication management.

Bipolar disorder rarely emerges late in life [7]; while unipolar depression may occur across the lifespan, bipolar disorder typically begins before the mid-30s [9]. Bipolar II disorder is often misdiagnosed as MDD because hypomanic episodes frequently go unrecognized [13]. Instead, patients are more likely to seek treatment due to depression, which can be debilitating. Bipolar episodes may increase in frequency and intensity over time if left untreated. Underlying bipolar disorder may be unmasked in older adults by factors such as illness, medications, or dementia, leading to a full-blown manic episode [13]. Such patients likely have a longstanding history of depressive episodes. Alcohol abuse, panic attacks, anxiety, and insomnia are common psychiatric comorbidities [9].

Atypical features of depression consist of mood reactivity, significant weight gain or increase in appetite, hypersomnia, leaden paralysis or profound fatigue, and interpersonal rejection sensitivity [8]. Leaden paralysis refers to a heavy, leaden feeling in the arms or legs and is generally accompanied by fatigue or lack of energy. Depression with atypical features is suggestive of a higher risk of bipolar disorder [11]; therefore, when these features are present, further investigation into possible manic or hypomanic episodes is warranted. If these are present and antidepressant trials are ineffective or only partially effective, referral to a psychiatric provider is appropriate.

MANAGEMENT

Proper identification of the etiology of depressive symptoms requires a thorough examination of psychosocial, medical, and medication-related causes. A high-quality assessment of psychiatric history, medical history, physical assessment, and medication reconciliation provides a framework for developing a management plan.

If the underlying cause of depressive symptoms is found to be related to a medical condition, then treatment of the condition is the priority. If the medical condition has been fully treated and depressive symptoms persist, then consider the addition of pharmaceutical agents such as selective SSRIs and SNRIs.

If the cause is due to the effects of another medication, consider removing or replacing the causative agent if possible. If there are no alternatives, consider reasonable nonpharmacological interventions and/or the addition of antidepressant medications.

Nonpharmacological interventions can be overlooked by medical providers, who may lack the time to educate the patient on the need for and efficacy of these interventions. Patients and providers may succumb to the ease of a prescription as a quick fix for a patient's symptoms. However, especially for older adults, the cause of depression most likely took time to develop and will likewise take time to remit. When depression is due to psychosocial stressors, therapy is recommended as a first-line treatment option [7]. Cognitive-behavioral therapy (CBT) or interpersonal therapy can be highly beneficial in helping the patient reframe maladaptive thought patterns, process emotions, learn coping mechanisms and develop resilience to deal with unavoidable stressors [20].

Other nonpharmacological interventions for depression include proper nutrition and possible supplementation with L-methylfolate and omega-3 oils; these have been shown to benefit depression by supporting brain function and neuro-transmitter synthesis [21–23]. Exercise has also been shown to improve depression by increasing blood flow and oxygenation to the brain [24]. Additionally, exercise is thought to improve depression by increasing brain-derived neurotrophic factor (BDNF), which increases neurogenesis and synaptic plasticity [25]. Bright light therapy, via natural sunlight or external light therapy lamp, is another nonpharmacologic intervention, which has been shown to improve mood and sleep. Bright light therapy may be beneficial for seasonal affective disorder [14,26].

Antidepressant is a broad term generically used to refer to SSRIs and SNRIs, which are the first-line recommended treatment of depression and are considered the treatment of choice among nonpsychiatric providers [14]. These medications target depression by increasing the availability of one or more of the monoamine neurotransmitters [26]. While these drugs are used extensively in the United States [27], older adults are frequently maintained at subtherapeutic levels for years and are at risk for undertreatment of depression [14]. When the patient fails to have an adequate response, the drug is often switched rather than maximizing the dose. While other medications for depression are available, such as tricyclic antidepressants (TCAs) and monoamine oxidase inhibitors (MAOIs), these come with negative side effect profiles and toxicity risks that make them better suited for psychiatric specialists, particularly in the older adult population.

The goal of treatment is remission of depressive symptoms [14,26]. When caring for older adults, consider following the adage of *start low and go slow.* The reason for this lies in the physiologic changes that accompany aging. Metabolism and excretion of drugs may be prolonged due to age-associated pharmacokinetic changes; therefore, it is considered best practice to initiate antidepressants (SSRIs and SNRIs) at half the usual initial starting dose (start low) for 1 to 2 weeks as tolerated before titrating up to the usual initial dose recommendations for 3 to 4 weeks. Additional titrations can be done more slowly (go slow) before reaching the maximum recommended dose limits; however, this does not imply that the maximum dose levels are not advised. This misconception may be responsible for the undertreatment of many older adults. Titrating too rapidly may increase side effects but is unlikely to speed a response. A reduction in symptoms is considered a response. If the older adult responds, the dose should be incrementally increased every 4 to 6 weeks until remission of symptoms or until the maximum dose is reached before it is necessary to consider switching to another drug [28]. If the drug is well-tolerated and there is a partial response with room for improvement, consider augmenting with another drug such as bupropion or mirtazapine. When benefits are negligible or side effects are intolerable, consider switching to another agent.

It should be noted that intolerable side effects may be related to initiating a medication at a dose that, while safe, may be too high for older adults to tolerate [13]. In such cases, lower the dose and reevaluate. Patient education regarding side effects may increase adherence and reduce the likelihood of prematurely discontinuing the medication trial. Side effects are usually worse when treatment is initiated (1–2 weeks) or the dose is increased and resolve with time as tolerance develops. Common side effects include gastrointestinal disturbance such as nausea, constipation, or diarrhea, along with sedation and dizziness. Side effects unlikely to resolve with time include cardiac rhythm disturbances, orthostasis, and delirium. In general, avoid drugs with a higher anticholinergic burden and increased risk of sedation and orthostasis, such as those found on the Beers List [29]. Neither paroxetine, TCAs, or drugs with a long half-life, such as fluoxetine, are recommended. Longer half-lives can lead to increased side effects, higher serum levels, and toxicity concerns due to reduced clearance.

Polypharmacy is an unfortunate reality for many older adults due to multiple chronic health conditions [29]. Drug interactions are of particular concern due to the increased number of prescriptions as well as age-related reductions in CYP450 enzymes that can reduce systemic drug clearance [14]. Efforts to avoid polypharmacy can include the use of common side effects as a tool for drug selection. Specific drug profiles may be used to target additional symptoms such as anxiety, poor appetite, and sleep disturbances. For example, a patient with trouble sleeping and a poor appetite may benefit from the sedation and appetite stimulation associated with mirtazapine. Similarly, while the long half-life of fluoxetine is not ideal, it may be useful during discontinuation of SSRIs or SNRIs.

Sudden discontinuation of SSRIs and SNRIs can cause uncomfortable side effects known as discontinuation syndrome [14]. It is advisable to discontinue these medications by tapering to the lowest dose over several weeks, with some patients requiring a slower taper. For some, a slow taper is not enough, and they will continue to experience side effect. In those instances, briefly switching to a low dose of fluoxetine (10 mg) may prove helpful, as its long half-life has the effect of self-tapering. This may be done after tapering the first medication to the lowest dose, then switching to 10 mg of fluoxetine every other day for 1 to 2 weeks.

Older adult patients prescribed SSRIs and SNRIs should be monitored for efficacy and adverse effects regularly or at least every 3 months [14]. Similar to common benign side effects, certain adverse effects, such as suicidal ideation and hyponatremia, are more likely to occur during initiation. Regular monitoring should include weight, pulse, blood pressure, and a list of active medications, which may change frequently. It is important to remember that monitoring also includes the use of rating scales to measure the level of depressive symptoms and the presence of suicidal ideation. Concomitant medications should be monitored for drug interactions and the potential risk of serotonin syndrome in the presence of other serotonergic medications. Electrocardiogram monitoring may be indicated in the presence of bradycardia and in patients with a relevant medical history or active medications that may contribute to irregularities. An elevated risk of bleeding may be of concern, especially with the concomitant use of nonsteroidal anti-inflammatory drugs, which increase the risk of upper gastrointestinal bleeding. Older adults are also at an increased risk of syndrome of inappropriate antidiuretic hormone secretion (SIADH) and hyponatremia. Laboratory monitoring should include electrolytes, serum sodium, renal function tests, and liver function tests at least every 6 months [14].

Equally as important as understanding proper selection and dosing of antidepressant agents is knowing when to refer a patient to a specialist such as a psychotherapist or psychiatric provider. When depression is attributable to psychosocial stressors, therapy is more likely to be beneficial than medication [7]. However, if the stress is prolonged, medication treatment may be beneficial as a supportive tool until therapeutic change is achieved. However, in addition to therapy, referral to a psychiatric specialist may be indicated. How do you know when to refer? The short answer is when you as a provider are not comfortable treating the depression or feel the symptom complexity requires more time or competency than you have available. Other indications for referral [11] include

- Antidepressant (SSRIs and SNRIs) doses have been maximized
- Prolonged grief
- Prolonged dysthymic symptoms without remission
- Depressive symptoms are unresponsive to medication trials
- Suspected bipolar disorder
- Suicidal ideation
- Psychotic symptoms
- Marked impairment in daily functioning

HEALTH PROMOTION

Depression is a complex and multifactorial disorder, particularly among older adults, where the prevalence is linked to various physiologic, psychological, and environmental factors [20]. While pharmacologic interventions remain the cornerstone of treatment, the importance of lifestyle interventions, which can reduce inflammation and support brain health, is increasingly recognized [7]. These modifiable lifestyle factors include nutrition, exercise, social engagement, sunlight exposure, sleep hygiene, and stress management, all of which play an important role in improving mood and cognitive function [7,24]. Education focusing on modifiable lifestyle factors is vital for managing depression, particularly in older adults [20]. Many older adults do not receive adequate advice on the importance of nutrition, exercise, hydration, and sleep in medical settings. The following are health promotion recommendations.

Nutrition
Research shows that deficiencies in key nutrients, such as omega-3 fatty acids, vitamin D, and B vitamins, are linked to depression [20,30]. Diets such as the Mediterranean diet, the Dietary Approaches to Stop Hypertension (DASH) diet, or the Mediterranean-DASH Neurodegenerative Delay diet should be encouraged to reduce the risk for chronic diseases [31]. Maintaining proper

nutrition, including sufficient water intake, protein consumption, and healthy eating habits are key elements in supporting metabolic functions, particularly as metabolism changes with age.

Physical activity

Exercise has been shown to reduce depressive symptoms by improving cardiovascular health and increasing the production of BDNF [25]. BDNF is a molecule that is essential in promoting neurogenesis and synaptic plasticity as well as memory and cognitive function [16,25]. Low levels of BDNF are associated with hippocampal atrophy and implicated in both neurodegenerative disorders and depression [32]; therefore, preservation of BDNF may improve depression and impart neuroprotective benefits. In addition to increasing BDNF, regular physical activity also reduces inflammation, a known contributor to depression [7,12].

Social engagement

Older adults who participate in social networks exhibit fewer depressive symptoms [33]. This is likely because social involvement fosters a sense of belonging and purpose, enhancing well-being and serving as a protective factor against psychological distress.

Sunlight exposure and vitamin D supplementation

Sunlight is essential to produce vitamin D, and deficiencies in vitamin D are strongly correlated with depression [30]. Vitamin D impacts depression through its role in inflammation reduction, immunomodulation, and neurotransmitter and neurotrophic factor synthesis. Older adults are at risk for vitamin D deficiency due to metabolic changes with age. In addition to its role in vitamin D synthesis, sunlight also helps to regulate circadian rhythms and sleep patterns, which are critical for mood stabilization [26].

Sleep hygiene

Inadequate sleep is a significant contributor to depression, as it promotes inflammation and impairs cognitive function [26]. Older adults are particularly vulnerable to poor sleep quality, often due to medical comorbidities or polypharmacy [9]. Sleep education should focus on sleep hygiene, such as creating a regular sleep schedule and limiting activities that interfere with sleep before bedtime.

Stress management

Chronic stress disrupts the endocrine system and contributes to inflammation, both of which have been implicated in the development of depression [7]. Interventions such as mindfulness, meditation, and CBT have shown efficacy in reducing depressive symptoms by managing stress [27].

CLINICAL IMPLICATIONS

Early and accurate diagnosis of depression in older adults is essential for improving quality of life and reducing morbidity and mortality [7]. Addressing modifiable factors such as nutrition, physical activity, social engagement, sunlight exposure, sleep hygiene, and stress management can significantly improve depressive symptoms and enhance the quality of life for this vulnerable population. Integrating lifestyle modifications with pharmacologic treatment provides a holistic approach to managing depression. Health care providers should consider evidence-based recommendations to inform clinical practice and guide interventions when developing personalized care plans.

CLINICS CARE POINTS

- Assess older adults for depressive symptoms at every visit using the Geriatric Depression Scale.
- Maintain accurate and up-to-date active medication list from all prescribers.
- Pay attention to nontraditional complaints that may be indicative of underlying depression.
- Rule out medical conditions, medications, and substance use as causal factors in depression.
- Avoid the use of TCAs, MAOIs, and medications on the Beers List
- Select an SSRI/SNRI antidepressant based on tolerability and symptom presentation.
- Start low and go slow when prescribing antidepressants. May titrate up to maximum dose over time.
- Maximize dose as tolerated before switching to a new medication. May augment if partial response.
- Treat to remission.

CLINICAL VIGNETTE

A 68 year old woman was referred for a psychiatric evaluation after the results of her recent neuropsychological testing were not consistent with Alzheimer's disease or other dementias. Her laboratories were within normal limits, and she was quite healthy. During the psychiatric interview, she reported that she and her husband, who was present, had moved to Arkansas from Southern California 3 years prior during the coronavirus disease 2019 pandemic into an investment property they had purchased for retirement. They had no family or friends in the area. While gathering her psychosocial history, her affect dramatically brightened when she spoke of her life in California. Upon further probing, she revealed that she no longer drives and relies on her husband for transportation. The pandemic prevented social contact the first year; however, when social contact resumed, she had little opportunity to socialize and make friends, and her husband "is an introvert" and did not like going out. Because she depended on him to drive, she spent most of her time at home. This contrasted significantly with her previous lifestyle, as she had a longstanding, close circle of friends and engaged in various social activities, a self-described "social butterfly." She was diagnosed with MDD. After discussion and counseling with the couple, they planned to increase their social activities in a mutually acceptable way. Because the cause of her depression was due to psychosocial factors, they agreed to trial these changes before initiating an antidepressant. She left the appointment with a smile but no prescription. Two weeks later, her husband wrote a letter to the office reporting that they had engaged in many more activities outside of the house and that she had a significant change in her mood. This case highlights the importance of determining the causative factors for depressive symptoms and memory impairment before initiating psychotropic medications, which may not be necessary.

Disclosure
The author has nothing to disclose.

References
[1] Barkil-Oteo A. Collaborative care for depression in primary care: how psychiatry could "troubleshoot" current treatments and practices. Yale J Biol Med 2013;86(2):139–46.

[2] Boehlen FH, Freigofas J, Herzog W, et al. Evidence for underuse and overuse of antidepressants in older adults: results of a large population-based study. Int J Geriatr Psychiatr 2019;34:539–47.

[3] Hu T, Zhao X, Wu M, et al. Prevalence of depression in older adults: a systematic review and meta-analysis. Psychiatry Res 2022;311:114511.

[4] Brody DJ, Gu Q. Antidepressant use among adults: United States, 2015-2018. NCHS Data Brief 2020;1–8.

[5] Carlat DJ. The psychiatric interview. 5th edition. Wolters Kluwer; 2023 (ISBN: 1975212975) Available at: https://www.thecarlatreport.com/products/category/125-ebooks.

[6] Nussbaum AM. The pocket guide to the DSM-5-TR diagnostic exam. Washington (DC): American Psychiatric Association Publishing; 2022 ISBN: 978-1-61537-358-1.

[7] Steffens D, Zdanys K. The American Psychiatric Association Publishing textbook of geriatric psychiatry. 6th edition. Washington (DC): American Psychiatric Publishing; 2023 ISBN: 9781615373406.

[8] American Psychiatric Association. Diagnostic and statistical manual of mental disorders. Fifth Edition. Washington, DC: Author; 2022 Text Revision (DSM-5-TR).

[9] Ismail Z, Fischer C, McCall WV. What characterizes late-life depression? Psychiatr Clin 2013;36(4):483–96.

[10] Pocklington C. Depression in older adults. Br J Med Pract 2017;10(1):a1007.

[11] Preston JD, O'Neal JH, Talaga MC, et al. Handbook of clinical psychopharmacology for therapists. 9th edition. Oakland (CA): New Harbinger Publications; 2021.

[12] Aziz R, Steffens DC. What are the causes of late-life depression? Psychiatr Clin 2013;36(4):497–516.

[13] Boland R, Verduin ML, editors. Kaplan & Sadock's synopsis of psychiatry. 12th edition. Wolters Kluwer; 2022 ISBN: 9781975145569.

[14] Jacobson SA. Clinical manual of geriatric psychopharmacology. 2nd edition. Arlington (VA): American Psychiatric Association Publishing; 2014 ISBN: 9781585624546.

[15] American Thyroid Association. Older patients and thyroid disease. 2024. Available at: https://www.thyroid.org/thyroid-disease-older-patient/.

[16] Gannu L, Devine F, Popadic L, et al. Characterizing the treatment patterns, medication burden, and patient demographics of older adults with major depressive disorder treated with antidepressants with or without selected comorbidities. Curr Med Res Opin 2024;40(6):1027–38; https://doi.org/10.1080/03007995.2024.2348603.

[17] Gotlib IH, Hammen CL. Handbook of depression. 3rd edition. New York (NY): Guilford Press; 2015 ISBN 9781462524167.

[18] Celano CM, Freudenreich O, Fernandez-Robles C, et al. Depressogenic effects of medications: a review. Dialogues Clin Neurosci 2011;13(1):109–25.
[19] National Institute on Drug Abuse (NIDA). 2020. Substance Use in Older Adults DrugFacts. Available at: https://nida.nih.gov/publications/drugfacts/substance-use-in-older-adults-drugfacts (Accessed 23 February 2025).
[20] Fiske A, Wetherell JL, Gatz M. Depression in older adults. Annu Rev Clin Psychol 2009;5(1): 363–89.
[21] Liao Y, Xie B, Zhang H, et al. Efficacy of omega-3 PUFAs in depression: a meta-analysis. Transl Psychiatry 2019;9:190; https://doi.org/10.1038/s41398-019-0515-5.
[22] Shelton RC, Sloan Manning J, Barrentine LW, et al. Assessing effects of l-methylfolate in depression management: results of a real-world patient experience trial. Prim Care Companion for CNS Disord 2013;15(4); https://doi.org/10.4088/PCC.13m01520.
[23] Stahl SM. L-methylfolate: a vitamin for your monoamines. J Clin Psychiatry 2008;69(9): 1352–3.
[24] Rosenbaum S, Tiedemann A, Sherrington C, et al. Physical activity interventions for people with mental illness: a systematic review and meta-analysis. J Clin Psychiatry 2014;75(9): 964–74.
[25] Erickson KI, Miller DL, Roecklein KA. The aging hippocampus: interactions between exercise, depression, and BDNF. Neuroscientist 2012;18(1):82–97.
[26] Stahl SM. Essential psychopharmacology: neuroscientific basis and practical applications. 5th edition. New York (NY): Cambridge University Press; 2021.
[27] Crowe M, Inder M, McCall C. Experience of antidepressant use and discontinuation: a qualitative synthesis of the evidence. J Psychiatr Ment Health Nurs 2023;30(1):21–34.
[28] Srifuengfung M, Pennington BRT, Lenze EJ. Optimizing treatment for older adults with depression. Ther Adv Psychopharmacol 2023;13:20451253231212327.
[29] National Institute on Aging. The dangers of polypharmacy and the case for deprescribing in older adults. 2021. Available at: https://www.nia.nih.gov/news/dangers-polypharmacy-and-case-deprescribing-older-adults.
[30] Akpınar Ş, Karadağ MG. Is vitamin D important in anxiety or depression? What is the truth? Curr Nutr Rep 2022;11(4):675–81.
[31] Cena H, Calder PC. Defining a healthy diet: evidence for the role of contemporary dietary patterns in health and disease. Nutrients 2020;12(2):334.
[32] Arévalo JC, Deogracias R. Mechanisms controlling the expression and secretion of BDNF. Biomolecules 2023;13:789; https://doi.org/10.3390/biom13050789.
[33] Min J, Ailshire J, Crimmins EM. Social engagement and depressive symptoms: do baseline depression status and type of social activities make a difference? Age Ageing 2016;45(6): 838–43.

Advances in Family Practice Nursing 7 (2025) 67–85

ADVANCES IN FAMILY PRACTICE NURSING

ELSEVIER
MOSBY

Understanding End-of-Life Care for the Older Adults
Assessment, Management, and Ethical Considerations

Margaret Love, DNP, APRN, FNP-BC, ACHPN

College of Nursing, University of Arkansas for Medical Sciences, 4301 West Markham Street, Slot #529, Little Rock, AR 72205, USA

Keywords

- Palliative communication • Older adults • Multimorbidity • Frailty • End-of-life care
- Holistic assessment • Functional status • Advance directive

Key points

- End-of-life (EOL) care must address physical, cognitive, and emotional challenges while considering patient autonomy and caregiver support.
- Several assessment tools such as the Barthel Index, Montreal Cognitive Assessment, and Edmonton Symptom Assessment System aid in evaluating functional, cognitive, and symptom burdens in EOL care available to assist clinicians with a comprehensive assessment needed to deliver person-centered care for the older adult at EOL.
- EOL care provision should integrate care across sectors and recognize the varying needs across the continuum of living and dying well for older people with multimorbidity.
- By aligning care with documented preferences and providing caregiver resources, patients and families can feel reassured in the decision-making process while ensuring improved comfort and dignity for the patient.
- Addressing the emotional and physical burden of caregivers is essential to achieving holistic care and ensuring patient and family well-being.

INTRODUCTION

As the aging population grows, managing end-of-life (EOL) care for older adults is an increasingly critical aspect of health care. According to recent demographic trends, 16.8% of the US population is now 65 years and older [1]. Older adults often face complex trajectories of illness. Compared to

E-mail address: MLOVE@uams.edu

https://doi.org/10.1016/j.yfpn.2025.01.007

younger populations, older adults may experience a combination of chronic conditions, cognitive decline, and physical impairments. EOL care for older adults is inherently multidimensional, requiring a balanced approach to managing physical symptoms, addressing psychosocial needs, and supporting families through decision-making. This article explores the essential components of EOL care, focusing on assessing older adults, identifying barriers to care, and integrating current research and updated clinical guidelines to provide compassionate, patient-centered care. It highlights the roles and responsibilities of health care providers in ensuring the quality of life and dignity for older adults during their final stages.

A scoping review examining the palliative care needs of community-dwelling older adults living with multimorbidity found the most identified needs across palliative domains that were pain, function, unhappiness, staying socially connected, future planning, having accessible and tailored care, and having meaning and purpose [2]. Similarly, a study of older adults with cancer determined comprehensive palliative care requires an understanding of geriatric syndromes, proper pain and symptom management, performance status assessment, advance care planning, and EOL care considerations [3]. Moreover, a mixed-method study aimed at improving EOL care for people with dementia found 5 areas for improvement, including timely recognition of EOL, conversations about palliative care and EOL, information and support for people with dementia and caregivers (CGs), person-and-CG-centered care, and assessing quality, coordinated care. The study's finding suggests that addressing the many layers of well-being is needed to enhance the overall quality of life for terminally ill older adults [4]. Early integration of palliative care has been shown to improve quality of life, reduce acute care utilization, and, in some cases, extend survival [5].

The setting of EOL care is a key consideration for older adults. Many older adults with prolonged frailty syndrome may reside in long-term care (LTC) facilities, where the availability and quality of palliative and EOL care vary widely depending on the institution's culture and resources. For those living at home with family, the decision of whether EOL care should take place in a hospice, LTC facility, or at home is complex. This decision must balance the patient's expressed wishes, the potential for CG burnout, and the well-being of the remaining partner, who may also be an older adult. A common concern among older adults nearing death is the desire to avoid burdening loved ones, which underscores the need for comprehensive CG support and education throughout the process.

The National Consensus Project 4th Edition Clinical Guidelines for Quality Palliative Care expanded to include 5 key themes to previously established care domains: structure and process, physical, psychological, and psychiatric aspects, and spiritual, religious, and existential aspects of care. The added themes are comprehensive assessment, family CG assessment and support (especially during care transitions), culturally inclusive care, and communication strategies to ensure the delivery of high-quality care [6].

PATHOPHYSIOLOGY
Physical changes
Aging is accompanied by physiologic changes such as reduced muscle mass (sarcopenia), decreased bone density, and impaired cardiovascular function. These changes increase the risk of falls, fractures, and other complications [7]. As individuals age, they experience a wide range of physical and cognitive changes that impact their overall health and ability to manage chronic conditions. Physically, aging is characterized by a decline in organ function, such as reduced cardiovascular efficiency, diminished lung capacity, and decreased renal and hepatic function. These changes affect how the body metabolizes medications and responds to stress or illness, increasing vulnerability to adverse drug reactions, dehydration, and complications from chronic diseases like diabetes or hypertension. Declines in immune function make older adults more susceptible to infections and reduce their ability to recover from illness or surgery. Additionally, sensory changes, such as diminished vision, hearing, and proprioception, can impair daily activities and increase the likelihood of accidents. These changes increase the risk of falls, fractures, and other complications [7].

Cognitive changes
Cognitive decline, including dementia and delirium, is a common challenge in EOL care for older adults. Cognitive aging may involve processing speed, memory, and executive functioning declines. While some cognitive changes are part of normal aging, others, such as those seen in dementia or mild cognitive impairment (MCI), significantly impact an individual's ability to manage medications, adhere to treatment plans, and make informed decisions about their care. Patients with cognitive impairments may struggle with memory, decision-making, and communication [7]. Impairments are compounded when the older adult experiences polypharmacy, depression, or delirium, common conditions in this population and individuals in the dying stage.

Psychosocial changes
At baseline, impairments, either physical or cognitive, faced by older adults with chronic illnesses complicate self-care tasks, which may lead to social isolation, depression, and anxiety, particularly if they lose social connection [8]. These psychosocial factors can exacerbate physical conditions and decrease

the patient's motivation to engage in activities of daily living [8]. Socioeconomic factors such as access to care or social support may already be exacerbated for the older adult before reaching the EOL phase.

End-of-life assessment

Assessing older adults nearing the EOL is an essential first step in creating an effective care plan. The assessment focus areas are summarized in Table 1. Health care providers must conduct comprehensive evaluations that include the patient's functional, cognitive, emotional, and social baseline status.

Symptoms. Assessment tools are available to aid in identifying clinical conditions, signs, and symptoms that may not fit into clear disease categories and are often referred to as geriatric syndromes in older adults. Geriatric syndromes like delirium, dementia, falls, frailty, dizziness, syncope, pressure ulcers, and urinary incontinence are common in older adults and often signal limited life expectancy. Table 2 provides a summary of commonly used tools in geriatrics and palliative care.

Differentials: aging, pathological decline, progression to end-of-life

Determining a baseline level of physical and cognitive functioning is essential to distinguishing among normal aging, chronic disease progression, and the terminal phase of illness. This distinction is critical for guiding care decisions and aligning them with the patient's values and goals. Cognitive decline, common in older adults with advanced illness, can compromise autonomous decision-making, highlighting the importance of early palliative care involvement to support both patients and families.

In managing EOL care for older adults, it is essential to differentiate symptoms related to the primary terminal illness from those arising from comorbid conditions or geriatric syndromes, such as frailty and polypharmacy [7,8]. Physiologic changes in older adults can worsen risk for predictable terminal symptoms and adverse outcomes (Table 3) particularly in frail older adults [14]. This complexity increases risks associated with polypharmacy, including adverse drug events like delirium, sedation, and falls, highlighting the need for careful medication management using tools such as the Beers List and a "start low, go slow" dosing approach [15]. As terminal illness advances, apparent signs of decline include weakness, anorexia, confusion, and greater dependence on the CG.

Table 1
Assessment focus at end-of-life [7–9]

Assessment dimension	Focus areas
Physical Assessment	Mobility limitations, chronic pain, and comorbidities like heart disease or diabetes [7].
Cognitive Assessment	Identifying signs of cognitive impairment, including dementia or delirium [8].
Psychosocial Evaluation	Emotional well-being, sense of isolation, and depression [8,9].

Table 2
Assessment tools used in the elderly [10–13]

	Population focus	Tool description
Symptom Evaluation		
Generalized Anxiety Disorder-7 (GAD-7) [10]	General adult population, including palliative and chronic illness settings	A 7 item self-report scale measuring the severity of anxiety symptoms over the past 2 wk. Total score of 0–21, with thresholds for mild (5), moderate (10), and severe (15) anxiety.
Geriatric Depression Scale (GDS) [11]	Older adults	Differentiates between depression and cognitive impairment. Higher scores indicate greater depressive symptoms.
Holistic Evaluation		
Edmonton Symptom Assessment System (ESAS) [12]	Palliative care, advanced illness, and cancer.	A comprehensive tool that includes a pain scale (0–10) along with other symptom assessments (eg, nausea, dyspnea, depression).
Comprehensive Geriatric Assessment (CGA) [13]	Older adults with multiple comorbidities	Holistic assessment of physical health, functional status, cognition, and social support.

Performance status is often correlated with prognosis, and for frail older adults experiencing long periods of low functional ability, it can be challenging to accurately identify the EOL phase. Non-cancer diagnoses, such as heart failure or chronic obstructive pulmonary disease, often have less predictable trajectories, making timely discussion about EOL care preferences and settings particularly difficult. These challenges can delay essential planning and result in opportunities for meaningful conversations about care priorities.

Screening tools
The *Comprehensive Geriatric Assessment* evaluates functional status, physical health, cognition, and social support (hospital elder life program [HELP] Guidelines) [13,16]. Several standardized tools are available to assess function and cognition in older adults.

The physiologic process of frailty predisposes older adults to diminished reserve. *Fried Frailty Phenotype* and the *Frailty Index* are 2 models that establish criteria for frailty [14,17]. According to the Fried criteria, an individual is considered frail if they meet 3 or more of the following 5 physical criteria: unintentional weight loss, exhaustion, weakness, slow walking speed, and low physical activity [14]. The frailty index assesses accumulated health deficits, including diseases,

Table 3
End-of-life progression in the older adult: aspects of care [7–9,15]

Aspect	Details
Normal aging changes impacting pharmacokinetics	Reduction in lean body mass, decreased blood flow to kidney and liver, and increased body fat lead to altered drug distribution and clearance.
Common adverse drug effects in older adults	Constipation, diarrhea, indigestion, delirium, dizziness, depression, dermatologic effects.
Specific risks increasing adverse drug events (ADEs)	Dehydration, drug cost, malnutrition, poor compliance, renal failure.
Consequences of polypharmacy	Higher risk of adverse drug reactions, including mental status changes, sedation, and falls. Drug interactions and poor adherence due to regimen complexity.
The transition from living with to dying of the condition	As decline becomes terminal, patients transition from managing chronic illness to experiencing progression toward end-of-life, with signs of body systems gradually failing.
Key indicators of disease progression in terminal illness	Indicators: worsening symptoms like weakness, anorexia, dyspnea, confusion, physical changes (eg, temporal wasting, deep eye sockets), reduced social engagement, and increased caregiving.
Management recommendations for older adults	Use tools like the Beers List for potentially inappropriate medications, apply the "start low and go slow" approach, and review drug necessity.

disabilities, cognitive impairment, and other domains; a ratio of 0.2 or higher indicates a state of frailty [17]. Identifying frailty helps in risk stratification, care planning, and targeted interventions to reduce adverse outcomes, like falls, hospitalizations, and mortality, especially in older adults.

Additional tools include the *Montreal Cognitive Assessment (MoCA)* for cognitive evaluation and the *Barthel Index* for assessing activities of daily living [18,19]. The Minimum Data Set part of the Resident Assessment Instrument (RAI) is required by the Centers for Medicare and Medicaid Services for all long-term-care residents designed to improve quality of life [20]. Standardized tools are vital in assessing function and cognition in older adults at the EOL, providing critical insights into their physical, cognitive, and psychosocial needs. These assessments help health care providers tailor interventions to enhance the quality of life, reduce suffering, and guide care planning, particularly in a population where the under-recognition and undertreatment of pain are common. Persistent pain in older adults has been linked to depression, anxiety, decreased socialization, sleep disturbances, cognitive decline, impaired ambulation, and increased health care costs. The tools listed in Table 4 address these multifaceted challenges and improve overall care outcomes.

Table 4
Select the right screening tool to complete a comprehensive assessment [14,19,21–32]

	Population Focus	Description of Items
Cognitive Evaluation Tools		
Mini-Cog	Dementia screening—older adults, including frail and palliative care populations	A 3 item recall test combined with a clock-drawing task to assess memory and executive function. Effective for detecting moderate-to-severe dementia. Scores of 0–2 suggest cognitive impairment.
Neuropsychiatric Inventory (NPI)	Neurodegenerative diseases and cognitive decline	Assesses behavioral and psychological symptoms of dementia, such as agitation, apathy, and delusions. Severity and distress scores are calculated based on symptoms.
Physical Evaluation Tools		
Palliative Performance Status (PPS)	Palliative care and terminal illness population	Assesses 9 symptoms (eg, pain, fatigue, drowsiness, depression, anxiety) rated on a scale of 0–10.
Karnofsky Performance Status (KPS)	Cancer and palliative patients	Measures ability to carry out daily activities, with scores from 0 (dead) to 100 (normal).
Clinical Frailty Scale (CFS)	Frail older adults	Assesses physical frailty with scores ranging from 1 (very fit) to 9 (terminally ill).
Barthel Index	Older adults for activities of daily living (ADL)	Evaluates the ability to perform 10 ADLs, such as feeding, bathing, grooming, and mobility.
Eastern Cooperative Oncology Group Scale (ECOG)	Cancer and palliative care	Grades functional status from fully active (0) to completely disabled (5).

(continued on next page)

Table 4
(*continued*)

	Population Focus	Description of Items
Functional Assessment Staging Test (FAST)	Older adults with progressive cognitive decline.	Focuses on functional abilities (eg, dressing, bathing). Stages dementia severity, particularly in Alzheimer's disease. Ranges from normal functioning (Stage 1) to severe cognitive decline (Stage 7).
Pain Evaluation Tools		
Multidimensional Pain Inventory (MPI)	Adults with chronic pain	Focuses on pain intensity, psychosocial impacts, and coping mechanisms.
Pain Assessment in Advanced Dementia (PAINAD)	Advanced dementia who cannot verbally communicate pain	Rates 5 domains: breathing, negative vocalization, facial expression, body language, and consolability.
Faces Pain Scale-Revised (FPS-R)	Children and adults with communication challenges.	A visual scale with facial expressions ranging from no pain to worst pain.
Abbey Pain Scale	Dementia in aged care and palliative settings	Assesses 6 domains: vocalization, facial expression, body language, behavioral changes, physiologic changes, and physical changes.
Pain Assessment Checklist for Seniors with Limited Ability to Communicate (PACSLAC)	Seniors with limited communication ability, often in dementia care	Assesses pain based on behavioral indicators like facial expressions and activity changes.
Brief Pain Inventory (BPI)	Patients with cancer and chronic pain conditions	Measures pain intensity, interference with daily activities, and relief from treatments.

Diagnostic testing

As patients approach EOL, the utility of extensive diagnostic testing diminishes. Additional imaging or laboratory tests should be pursued only if they enhance comfort or quality of life, prioritizing comfort measures over curative interventions [8].

COMMUNICATION

Once a comprehensive evaluation of the patient's disease trajectory, psychosocial, spiritual, cognitive, functional, nutritional, and CG support is determined, prognostication is the appropriate next step. The older adults' understanding of their prognosis often influences health care decisions as it relates to treatment or eligibility for hospice care. Clinicians are often hesitant to discuss prognosis; when they do, undue optimism is communicated to patients and families.

Unpredictable exacerbations of illness make prognostication difficult; however, the rate of decline has been identified as a key indicator in determining prognosis. Tools such as the Palliative Performance Scale (PPS) and Palliative Prognostic Index are used periodically to help in estimating survival based on evolving physical deterioration [23,33]. A clinician answering no to the surprise question: "Would I be surprised if this patient dies in the next year?" correlates with a greater likelihood of death in the next year [34].

Clear communication about illness helps patients and families engage in decision-making and prepare for future challenges. It is important to assess what they know, what they wish to learn, their concerns, and their preferences for information sharing. Overly optimistic prognoses can delay hospice referrals, though hospice is most effective when provided for months rather than days. Late understanding of prognosis often results in futile care requests and a difficult transition to palliative care, with delayed do-not-resuscitate (DNR) orders. Providers can guide prognosis discussions, offering information that balances hope with reality. Ideally, communication about EOL care is woven into ongoing advance care planning, respecting personal and cultural preferences and supported by interdisciplinary collaboration. EOL prognosis should be communicated in "hours to days," "days to weeks," or "weeks to months" to provide clarity, set realistic expectations, and guide decision-making. This approach helps avoid miscommunication, undue optimism, or delays in transitioning to appropriate levels of care, such as hospice or palliative services. Clear prognostic communication allows patients and families to prioritize goals, make necessary preparations, and allocate their remaining time according to their values and preferences. Timeframes grounded in clinical experience and evidence-based tools promote trust and facilitate a shared understanding among the health care team, patient, and CG [35].

Discussions about goals of care should start with establishing common ground around what is known and understood, ensuring that the older adult is well informed of their illness. The (Setting, Perception, Invitation, Knowledge, Empathy, Strategy & Summary [SPIKES]) protocol and Ask-Tell-Ask are common communication strategies to encourage an interactive dialogue that enhances relayed and received information [36,37]. The clinician should be aware of and acknowledge emotions by responding with empathy.

A provider can effectively guide and inform EOL discussions by exploring the patient's life context—understanding who they are, what they value, their personal definition of quality of life, and their hopes or fears. This information helps patients establish goals that align with their values and aids in making informed decisions about further medical interventions, life-prolonging measures, or hospice care while incorporating their cultural and spiritual beliefs. Summarize the discussion by reviewing the choices made about treatments, such as opting in or out of procedures (eg, percuraneous endosopic gastrostomy [PEG] tube placement, dialysis), care options (eg, LTC), next steps, code status, completion of advance care documents, and referrals to interdisciplinary team members like chaplains or social workers. Allow time for questions, and reassure the older adult and family that symptom control and comfort will be prioritized if desired and they will not be abandoned.

Advance care planning documents are legal and medical tools that allow individuals to express their health care preferences for future medical care, particularly if they cannot communicate their decision due to illness or incapacity. If not completed at the start of the palliative process, it should be reintroduced as the illness progresses. These documents help ensure that EOL care aligns with the patient's wishes, allowing them to maintain autonomy if they lose decision-making capacity. Advance directives can prevent unwanted care transitions and relieve family members from the burden of making uninformed decisions. Key components of advance care planning (Table 5) include advance directives, which specify wishes for care when decision-making capacity is lost. These may involve instructional directives (eg, living wills), DNR orders, and state-specific medical orders (eg, Physician Order for Life-Sustaining Treatment [POLST], Medical Order for Life-sustaining Treatment [MOLST]). Additionally, appointing a health care proxy (Durable Power of Attorney for Healthcare) ensures that a trusted advocate is available to support the patient's preferences if needed.

CASE STUDY

Mrs. Matty is an 82 year old with a history of Alzheimer's dementia. She was diagnosed 12 years ago, and her daughter Lee has been her caregiver (CG) for the last 10 years. Lee has watched her mother decline. Matty is now bedbound, contracted, and incontinent of bowel and bladder and is hand fed at baseline with progressively weight loss over the last year despite Lee's meticulous care. Matty is followed by home health for stage II pressure ulcer to the coccyx—several recent infections, including urinary tract infection (UTI) and pneumonia, twice in the last 6 months. Lee calls the clinic to report her mother who has stopped eating in the last week and is no longer smiling at her and is overall less responsive and running a low-grade temperature. Lee states that her mother likely has another infection and may need a feeding tube as she is not eating enough to maintain her weight. She expressed her mother is not

Table 5
Advanced care planning components [3,6,38]

Component	Description
Advance Care Planning	Voluntary process to discuss and plan future health care with patients to ensure care aligns with values and goals. Revisits discussions as the patient's condition or life goals change. Involves patient, family, and health care professionals.
Completing Advance Directives	Based on the Patient Self-Determination Act (1991). Legal mechanisms allow patients to state health care wishes and designate a surrogate if they lose decision-making capacity.
Directives	"Living wills" or medical directives. Allows patients to specify preferences for life-sustaining treatments and designate a proxy. Supports autonomy by clarifying wishes for specific treatments under certain conditions.
Do-Not-Resuscitate (DNR)	It specifically outlines the refusal of CPR in cases of cardiopulmonary arrest and ensures that no resuscitative efforts are made, as per the patient's preference.
Proxy Directives	Durable Power of Attorney for Healthcare (DPOA-HC) designates a health care proxy to make decisions if the patient is incapacitated. Often paired with an instructional directive.
Special Forms	State-specific forms allow health care preferences to be summarized as medical orders. Examples include POLST, MOLST, and others. These forms are actionable across all facilities and recognized in the health care community.

able to take her medications and is getting dehydrated. Should I call 911? She cannot be transported to the clinic.

ETHICAL CONSIDERATIONS

In the case of Mrs. Matty, the clinician must address several ethical challenges with compassion and clarity to guide her daughter, Lee, in making informed decisions. As Mrs. Matty no longer has the cognitive capacity to make decisions due to advanced Alzheimer's dementia, the responsibility shifts to Lee, who must act in alignment with her mother's previously expressed values and best interests. The clinician should provide Lee with clear, compassionate information about her mother's prognosis and care options, emphasizing that decisions should prioritize comfort and dignity. Lee's suggestion of feeding tube placement and hospitalization introduces concerns of beneficence and non-maleficence, as these interventions may not improve quality of life and could cause harm, such as aspiration or discomfort [39]. Instead, the clinician should explain the limited benefits and risks of artificial nutrition and hydration in advanced dementia.

The uncertain trajectory of advanced dementia complicates prognostication and decision-making, but framing the prognosis in terms of "weeks to months" can help Lee focus on appropriate care goals, such as hospice eligibility and symptom management. Lee's emotional and practical needs as a primary caregiver are also critical, as her suggestion to call 911 reflects feelings of guilt and helplessness. The clinician must provide reassurance, affirm Lee's exemplary caregiving efforts, and guide her toward hospice services for additional support. Finally, discussions should consider justice in resource allocation, avoiding unnecessary interventions like hospitalization that may not align with Matty's condition or goals. By focusing on comfort and quality of life, the clinician can help Lee make compassionate and ethically sound choices while ensuring ethical, patient-centered care (Table 6).

HOW SHOULD THE CLINICIAN RESPOND?

The clinician ensures that decisions align with Mrs. Matty's presumed values and best interests. Use empathetic prompts to clarify her goals, such as "What do you think your mother would want at this stage?" and discuss options for comfort-focused care. Explain that interventions like feeding tubes are not recommended for advanced dementia due to their lack of benefit and potential to cause discomfort [4,39,40]. Instead, suggest alternatives like handfeeding as tolerated and emphasize the overarching goal of maintaining comfort. Collaborate with home health to address symptom management, including hydration alternatives, pressure ulcer care, and judicious use of antibiotics if consistent with comfort goals.

Discuss hospice eligibility, highlighting that Mrs. Matty's recurrent infections, weight loss, and functional decline meet hospice criteria [41]. Initiate hospice services to provide symptom management, caregiver support, and respite care, offering Lee additional resources to alleviate her emotional and physical burden. Commend Lee for her dedication as a caregiver, provide resources such as support groups and respite programs, and emphasize the importance of self-care. Ensure follow-up to monitor Mrs. Matty's condition, adjusting care plans as needed, while reinforcing that her comfort and dignity remain the top priorities.

Case (Matty continued)–The Advance Practice Registered Nurse (APRN) was available to make a home visit that evening to assess Matty and discuss goals of care. Lee states she knows her mother won't live forever but doesn't want to give up on her if she still wants to be here. Lee expresses I know she will die soon without a feeding tube or antibiotics for the infection. It has improved her condition so many times in the past. The APRN explains the process for feeding tube placement and possible complications of tube feeding in people with advanced dementia. When asked if she has an advance directive, Lee locates the document in the back of her mother's bible and explains it was done years ago. In reviewing the document, the nurse practitioner (NP) explained that her mother elected DNR and opted out of life-prolonging measures, including artificial hydration and nutrients via tube feeding. Although reluctant and tearful, Lee agrees that she should honor her mother's wishes. *She asks what do we do next?*

During the APRN's home visit, Lee is reassured that honoring Mrs. Matty's advance directive respects her autonomy and aligns care with her expressed wishes. The APRN emphasizes that Mrs. Matty's decision to prioritize comfort over life-prolonging measures provides clarity for the next

Table 6
Ethical case application [39,40]

Ethical principle	Challenge	Resolution
Autonomy and Decision-Making	Mrs. Matty lacks cognitive capacity due to advanced Alzheimer's dementia. Ethical responsibility shifts to her surrogate decision-maker, Lee, who must align decisions with her mother's previously expressed wishes and best interests.	The clinician should support Lee with clear, compassionate information about Mrs. Matty's prognosis and care options. Guidance should emphasize alignment with Matty's presumed values and goals of care.
Beneficence vs Non-Maleficence	Lee suggests a feeding tube and potential hospitalization, which may not align with best practices for advanced dementia. Feeding tubes pose significant risks, such as aspiration, discomfort, and reduced quality of life, without proven benefit [39,40].	The clinician should explain the limited benefits and potential harms of artificial nutrition and hydration (ANH) in advanced dementia, emphasizing comfort-focused care. Alternatives like hand-feeding as tolerated should be discussed to preserve dignity and minimize harm.
Prognostic Uncertainty	Advanced dementia is a terminal condition, but its trajectory can be unpredictable, complicating decisions about aggressive interventions vs comfort-focused care.	The clinician should frame the prognosis in terms of "weeks to months" to guide decision-making. This approach facilitates appropriate discussions about hospice eligibility and care goals.
Fidelity to Emotional and Practical Needs	As the primary caregiver, Lee experiences emotional stress, guilt, and decision-making burdens. Her suggestion to call 911 reflects a desire to "do the right thing" while managing feelings of helplessness.	The clinician should provide Lee with emotional support, affirm her caregiving efforts, and reassure her that comfort-focused care is compassionate and ethically sound.
Justice and Resource Allocation	Hospitalization and feeding tube placement may strain health care resources without improving outcomes, raising justice concerns regarding appropriate resource use.	The clinician should discuss care options that prioritize Matty's comfort and avoid unnecessary interventions, aligning with hospice and palliative care principles to optimize resource use.

steps. Comfort-focused care will include hand-feeding as tolerated, oral hydration, and medications for pain and fever, with antibiotics considered only if consistent with the goals of care. Hospice services are introduced to provide symptom management, emotional support, and spiritual counseling.

Case (Matty Continued)—Based on Mrs. Matty's FAST and PPS scores, the APRN gently explains to Lee that her mother's prognosis is likely days to weeks. Overwhelmed and tearful, Lee expresses her distress, stating that this feels too sudden and that she struggles to cope. She admits she has not slept for the past three nights, staying by her mother's side out of worry. Acknowledging Lee's emotional and physical exhaustion, the APRN compassionately recommends hospice support to assist with EOL care and respite. *Lee asked what would happen at the time of death and if her mother would be placed in a hospice facility. How will I be able to afford this? What vital information should the clinician tell Lee about what to expect with hospice care?*

The APRN acknowledges Lee's emotional exhaustion, offering resources such as grief counseling, support groups, and respite care to help her cope during this challenging time. A comprehensive symptom management plan is outlined, focusing on maintaining Mrs. Matty's comfort and dignity. Lee is assured of ongoing guidance and support, helping her find peace in honoring her mother's wishes.

The clinician explains that hospice care prioritizes comfort and quality of life while providing holistic support for both patients and caregivers. Hospice services are typically covered by Medicare, Medicaid, and most private insurers, ensuring minimal or no out-of-pocket costs for most families. These services include medications, equipment, and professional care. Care settings are flexible and tailored to the patient's needs, including routine home care, continuous home care during crises, short-term inpatient care for complex symptom management, and respite care to provide temporary relief for caregivers.

The interdisciplinary hospice team delivers personalized support. Nurses and aides focus on symptom management and caregiver education, social workers connect families with resources and assist with planning, and chaplains provide spiritual care. Bereavement counselors offer grief support both before and after the patient's passing, ensuring that families have the emotional resources they need.

At the time of death, hospice staff manage the pronouncement, coordinate the completion of the death certificate, and handle any required communication with the coroner. They prepare Lee for natural physical changes, such as slowed breathing and unresponsiveness, ensuring that these are understood as part of the dying process. Medications are disposed of following national guidelines, typically through take-back programs or safe at-home methods.

By addressing Lee's concerns with clarity and compassion, the clinician empowers her to honor her mother's wishes and assures her that she is not alone in this journey. Hospice care provides comprehensive support, enabling Lee to focus on her mother's comfort and dignity while receiving the help she needs.

SYMPTOM MANAGEMENT: TAILORING CARE TO THE OLDER ADULT AT END OF LIFE

Tailored pain management and caregiver support are central components, alongside proactive communication about care preferences to honor patient autonomy and avoid conflicts, especially when cognitive decline may impair decision-making [38]. Early discussions and the use of advance directives ensure that patient values are respected, even in cases where families and health care providers might have differing perspectives on care [4].

Pain management presents unique challenges for older adults due to polypharmacy and heightened risk for adverse drug reactions. The AGS Beers Criteria (2023) recommends a "start low, go slow" approach to dosing and emphasizes multimodal strategies, including non-opioid therapies, to minimize adverse effects. However, avoid underdosing the elderly population on opioid therapy at baseline [15]. A study in the *Journal of Palliative Medicine* [42] found that initiating palliative care consults within 24 hours of hospital admission significantly reduced length of stay and hospital charges, regardless of underlying disease. Outpatient palliative care also improves symptom control, reduces hospitalizations, and enhances patient satisfaction [43].

Symptom management at EOL includes addressing reversible issues, such as constipation, and monitoring the impact of symptoms on functional ability and quality of life. The use of multipurpose drugs can help reduce pill burden, while benzodiazepines should be avoided in favor of antipsychotics like haloperidol for delirium. Essential hygiene and basic care help maintain patient dignity as death becomes imminent. Family and caregivers should be prepared for typical signs, including changes in appetite, cardiovascular and cognitive decline, and Cheyne–Stokes breathing, as part of the EOL process.

EDUCATION AND SUPPORT

Family education and support are essential for caregivers of older adults at the EOL, as they face emotional stress, physical exhaustion, and grief. Health care providers should equip families with knowledge on recognizing signs of imminent death, managing complications like hemorrhage or seizures, and understanding post-death procedures. Education on the "7Cs" of care, comfort, control, communication, continuity, and closure can help families feel supported and facilitate meaningful interactions, including life tasks such as forgiveness, gratitude, and farewells [44]. Key signs of approaching death, such as reduced oral intake, cardiovascular changes (eg, hypotension, peripheral cooling), cognitive decline, and Cheyne–Stokes breathing, indicate disease progression and reduced organ perfusion. Care guidance includes hydration and nutrition options, eye and skin care, and symptom management tailored to the patient's needs, helping families navigate EOL stages and prepare for what follows.

MEDICAL AID IN DYING

Medical aid in dying (MAID) is governed by state laws and regulations, with its availability varying across regions. The ethical, legal, and social implications of

MAID and euthanasia are highly debated in EOL care. The *Hospice & Palliative Medicine International Journal* (2024) offers a comprehensive review of these issues, analyzing cultural perspectives and legal frameworks that influence attitudes toward MAID, as well as the psychological impacts on both patients and health care professionals [45]. This research contributes to the ongoing discussion about ethically responsible care in the final stages of life.

TELEMEDICINE IN END-OF-LIFE CARE

Telemedicine has reinvented health care delivery. A 2024 Systematic review of its effectiveness and challenges found that it improves access to specialized palliative care for those in remote or underserved areas [46]. The study highlights the role of telemedicine in continuous monitoring, timely interventions, and overall improvement of patient outcomes and satisfaction.

SUMMARY

EOL care for older adults should be compassionate, individualized, and grounded in patient-centered care that addresses the physical, cognitive, and emotional challenges through continuous communication and assessment. Assessment tools such as the Barthel Index, Mini-MoCA, and Edmonton Symptom Assessment System enable clinicians to evaluate functional, cognitive, and symptom burdens, providing the foundation for person-centered care. Effective EOL care must integrate services across various sectors to meet the unique needs of older adults with multimorbidity, recognizing the continuum, and dying well as part of the progression. Aligning care with patients' documented preferences and offering robust caregiver resources fosters confidence in decision-making and enhances the patient's comfort. Addressing caregivers' emotional and physical burdens is essential to achieving holistic care. Successful clinicians are adept at understanding the ethical legal barrier while balancing care goals with comfort, minimizing family stress, and effective communication to guide decision-making. Emerging technologies and telemedicine may offer new avenues to enhance access to personalized care, supporting the health care team in providing effective.

CLINICS CARE POINTS

- *Assessment:* Health care providers should prioritize regular assessments using geriatric tools to evaluate cognitive and physical function, apply minimal and necessary medications cautiously, and incorporate holistic care strategies, including physical, emotional, and spiritual support.
- *Behavioral and motivational strategies:* Encouraging participation in care through behavioral support to decrease social isolation and increase social networks can significantly improve the dying process of life for older adults.
- *Ethical consideration:* Health care providers should integrate evidence-based guidelines, ethical, and legal decision-making, and decision-making at EOL when guiding patients and families.

- *Communication*: Clear communication and advance care planning are essential in helping patients and families navigate the EOL process, and families should be educated on physical changes they can expect, as well as resources for support.

DECLARATION OF ARTIFICIAL INTELLIGENCE (AI) AND AI-ASSISTED TECHNOLOGIES IN THE WRITING PROCESS

During the preparation of this work, the author used OpenAI/ChatGPT to edit the writing for clarity and to find the latest research, articles, and guidelines referenced in the article. After using this tool/service, the author reviewed and edited the content as needed and takes full responsibility for the publication's content. This declaration does not apply to the use of basic tools for checking, grammar, spelling, references, etc.

References

[1] U.S. Census Bureau. 2020 Census: United States older population grew. 2023. Available at:https://www.census.gov/library/stories/2023/05/2020-census-united-states-older-population-grew.html.

[2] Nicholson CJ, Combes S, Mold F, et al. Addressing inequity in palliative care provision for older people living with multimorbidity: perspectives of community-dwelling older people on their palliative care needs—a scoping review. Palliat Med 2022;37(4):475–97.

[3] Huynh L, Moore J. Palliative and end-of-life care for the older adult with cancer. Curr Opin Support Palliat Care 2021;15(1):23–8.

[4] Triandafilidis Z, Carr S, Davis D, et al. Improving end-of-life care for people with dementia: a mixed-methods study. BMC Palliat Care 2024;23(30); https://doi.org/10.1186/s12904-024-01120-1.

[5] Mah SJ, Ramirez CM, Schnarr KS. Timing of palliative care, end-of-life quality indicators and health resource utilization. JAMA Netw Open 2024;7(10):e2440977. Available at: https://jamanetwork.com/journals/jamanetworkopen/fullarticle/2825394.

[6] National Consensus Project for Quality Palliative Care. Clinical practice guidelines for quality palliative care (4th edition). 2018. Available at: https://www.nationalcoalitionhpc.org.

[7] Resnick B. Biology. Geriatric nursing review syllabus: a core curriculum in advanced practice geriatric nursing. 7th edition. New York: America Geriatrics Society; 2022.

[8] Resnick B. Palliative care. Geriatric nursing review syllabus: a core curriculum in advanced practice geriatric nursing. 7th edition. New York: America Geriatrics Society; 2022.

[9] National Academies of Sciences, Engineering, and Medicine, Division of Behavioral and Social Sciences and Education, Health and Medicine Division, Board on Behavioral, Cognitive, and Sensory Sciences, Board on Health Sciences Policy, Committee on the Health and Medical Dimensions of Social Isolation and Loneliness in Older Adults. Social isolation and loneliness in older adults: opportunities for the health care System. Washington, DC: National Academies Press (US); 2020. p. 3, Health Impacts of Social Isolation and Loneliness on Morbidity and Quality of Life. Available at: https://www.ncbi.nlm.nih.gov/books/NBK557983/.

[10] Spitzer RL, Kroenke K, Williams JBW, et al. A brief measure for assessing generalized anxiety disorder: the GAD-7. Arch Intern Med 2006;166(10):1092–7.

[11] Yesavage JA. Geriatric depression scale. Psychopharmacol Bull 1988;24(4):709–11.

[12] Rolfson DB, Majumdar SR, Tsuyuki RT, et al. Validity and reliability of the Edmonton frail scale. Age Ageing 2006;35(5):526–9.

[13] Castagna A, Militano V, Ruberto C, et al. Comprehensive geriatric assessment and palliative care. Aging Med 2024;7(5):645–8.

[14] Fried LP, Tangen CM, Watson J, et al. Frailty in older adults: evidence for a phenotype. J Gerontol A Biol Sci Med Sci 2001;56(3):M146–56.

[15] American Geriatrics Society Beers Criteria® Update Expert Panel. American Geriatrics Society 2023 updated AGS Beers Criteria® for potentially inappropriate medication use in older adults. J Am Geriatr Soc 2023;71(7):2052–81.

[16] Chen P, Dowal S, Schmitt E, et al. Hospital elder life program in the real world: the many uses of the hospital elder life program website. J Am Geriatr Soc 2015;63(4): 797–803.

[17] Mitnitski AB, Mogilner AJ, Rockwood K. Accumulation of deficits as a proxy measure of aging. Sci World J 2001;1:323–36.

[18] Nasreddine ZS, Phillips NA, Bedirian V, et al. The Montreal Cognitive Assessment, MoCA: a brief tool for mild cognitive impairment. American Geriatrics Society 2005;53(4):695–9.

[19] Barros VDS, Bassi-Dibai D, Guedes CLR, et al. Barthel Index is a valid and reliable tool to measure the functional independence of cancer patients in palliative care. BMC Palliat Care 2022;21(1):24.

[20] CMS. Minimum Data set (MDS) 3.0 resident assessment instrument (RAI) manual. Available at: https://www.cms.gov/medicare/quality/nursing-home-improvement/resident-assessment-instrument-manual.

[21] Mini cog. Available at: https://mini-cog.com.

[22] Cummings JL. The Neuropsychiatric Inventory: assessing psychopathology in dementia patients. Neurology 1997;48:S10–6.

[23] Oh JH, Lee YJ, Seo MS, et al. Change in Palliative Performance Scale (PPS) predicts survival in patients with terminal cancer. J Hosp Palliat Care 2017;20(4):235–41.

[24] Buccheri G, Ferrigno D, Tamburini M. Karnofsky and ECOG performance status scoring in lung cancer: a prospective, longitudinal study of 536 patients from a single institution. Eur J Cancer 1996;32(7):1135–41.

[25] ECOG-ACRIN. Available at: https://ecog-acrin.org/resources/ecog-performance-status/.

[26] Functional assessment staging test (FAST). Available at: https://www.capc.org/documents/download/962/.

[27] Kerns RD, Turk DC, Rudy TE. The West haven-yale multidemensional pain inventory (WHYMPI). Pain 1985;23(4):345–56.

[28] Warden V, Hurley AC, Volicer L. Development and psychometric evaluation of the pain assessment in advanced dementia (PAINAD). Scale. J AM Med Dir Assoc 2003;4:9–15.

[29] Ware LJ, Epps CD, Herr K, et al. Evaluation of the revised faces pain scale, verbal descriptor scale, numeric rating scale, and Iowa pain termometer in older minority adults. PMN 2006;7:117–25.

[30] Abbey J, Piller N, De Bellis A, et al. The Abbey pain scale: a 1-minute numerical indicator for people with end-stage dementia. Int J Palliat Nurs 2004;10(1):6–13.

[31] Warden V, Hurley AC, Volicer L. Development and psychometric evaluation of the pain assessment in advanced dementia (PAINAD) scale. J Am Med Dir Assoc 2003;4(1):9–15.

[32] Cleeland CS. Brief pain inventory user guide. 2009. Available at: https://www.mdanderson.org/documents/Departments-and-Divisions/Symptom-Research/BPI_UserGuide.pdf.

[33] Morita T, Tsunoda J, Inoue S, et al. The palliative prognostic index: a scoring system for survival prediction of terminally ill cancer patients. SCC 1999;7:128–33.

[34] Moss AH, Lunney JR, Culp S, et al. Prognostic Significance of the "surprise" question in cancer patients. J Palliat Med 2010;13:837–40.

[35] National Hospice and Palliative Care Organization. Guidelines for prognostication in hospice and palliative care. 2018. Available at: www.nhpco.org.

[36] Baile WF, Buckman R, Lenzi R, et al. SPIKES—a six-step protocol for delivering bad news: Application to the patient with cancer. Oncologist 2000;5(4):302–11.

[37] Back AL, Arnold RM, Baile WF, et al. Approaching difficult communication tasks in oncology. CA Cancer J Clin 2009;55(3):164–77.

[38] Akdeniz M, Yardımcı B, Kavukcu E. Ethical considerations at the end-of-life care. SAGE Open Med 2021;9:20503121211000918.

[39] American Geriatrics Society Ethics Committee and Clinical Practice and Models of Care Committee. American Geriatrics Society feeding tubes in advanced dementia position statement. J Am Geriatr Soc 2014;62(8):1590–3.

[40] Hospice and Palliative Nurses Association. Medically administered nutrition and hydration at the end of life: position statement. J Hospice Pall Nurs 2020;22(3):E12–4. Available at: https://www.advancingexpertcare.org/wp-content/uploads/2023/05/HPNA_Position_ Statement_MedicallyAdministeredNutrition.Hydration.pdf.

[41] Centers for Medicare and Medicaid Services. Hospice determining terminal status. Available at: https://www.cms.gov/medicare-coverage-database/view/lcd.aspx?LCDId= 34538.

[42] Macmillan PJ, Chalfin B, Soleimani Fard A, et al. Earlier palliative care referrals associated with reduced length of stay and hospital charges. J Palliat Med 2019;23(1); https://doi. org/10.1089/jpm.2019.0029.

[43] Rabow M, Kvale E, Barbour L, et al. Moving upstream: a review of the evidence of the impact of outpatient palliative care. J Palliat Med 2013; https://doi.org/10.1089/jpm.2013. 0153.

[44] Shaw KL, Clifford C, Thomas K, et al. Improving end-of-life care: a critical review of the Gold Standards Framework in primary care. Palliat Med 2010;24(3):317–29.

[45] Bouabida K, Chaves B, Anane E, et al. Recent global perspectives and implications of medical-assisted death and euthanasia. Hos Pal Med Int Jnl 2024;7(3):73–6.

[46] Ghazal KY, Singh Beniwal S, Dhingra A. Assessing telehealth in palliative care: a systematic review of the effectiveness and challenges in rural and underserved areas. Cureus 2024;16(8):e68275.

Advances in Family Practice Nursing 7 (2025) 87–94

ADVANCES IN FAMILY PRACTICE NURSING

Resilience in Older Adults
Evaluation and Implications for Poststroke Recovery

Janice Taylor, DNP, APRN, AGPC-BC

University of Arkansas for Medical Sciences, College of Nursing, 4301 West Markham, Slot 529, Little Rock, AR 72205, USA

Keywords
- Resilience in older adults • Stroke rehabilitation
- Community reintegration after stroke • Caregiver support strategies

Key points

- *Resilience is vital* in overcoming physical, emotional, and social challenges during poststroke recovery in older adults.
- *Collaborative care, including family and community support,* fosters adaptation, independence, and improved quality of life for stroke survivors.
- *Targeted interventions, such as rehabilitation and emotional support,* enhance recovery outcomes and strengthen both patient and caregiver resilience.

INTRODUCTION

Stroke continues to be the leading cause of long-term disability among older adults, often resulting in challenges such as motor deficits, cognitive impairments, emotional disturbances, and a diminished quality of life [1]. According to the American Heart Association in 2021, stroke accounted for approximately 1 of every 21 deaths in the United States [2].

Resilience, a multifaceted concept, plays a pivotal role in the recovery and adaptation of elderly patients experiencing poststroke complications. According to *Merriam-Webster*, resilience is defined as *an ability to recover from or adjust easily to misfortune or change.* [3–5] It is derived from the Latin verb *resilire: to jump back* or *recoil.* [6] Synonyms such as *endurance, adaptability, tenacity,* and *fortitude* reflect its dynamic nature, encompassing both psychological and physiologic dimensions

E-mail address: JLTaylor3@uams.edu

https://doi.org/10.1016/j.yfpn.2024.12.003
2589-420X/25/© 2025 Elsevier Inc. All rights are reserved, including those for text and data mining, AI training, and similar technologies.

Abbreviations

BRS   brief resilience scale
RSOA   resilience scale for older adults

[6]. For poststroke patients, resilience is not merely the capacity to withstand adversity but also an active process of adapting to physical, emotional, and social changes that follow a cerebrovascular event [7].

Complications from stroke demand a comprehensive approach to care that fosters resilience in both the patient and their caregivers. The interplay between biological factors, psychosocial resources, and environmental supports creates a framework through which resilience can be understood and enhanced in this population [1].

This article aims to explore the concept of resilience within the context of elderly patients, particularly those managing poststroke complications. By examining factors that influence resilience—such as coping mechanisms, social support, and rehabilitation strategies—this article seeks to inform evidence-based interventions that promote recovery and improve long-term outcomes. Understanding resilience in the context of stroke recovery is critical to advancing holistic care for a population often burdened by complex challenges following a stroke.

CONCEPTUAL UNDERSTANDING OF RESILIENCE IN THE ELDERLY

Aging is often perceived negatively, associated with the loss of health, cognitive functions, and familial support as inevitable outcomes [8]. However, beginning in the 1980s, a shift toward a more optimistic perspective emerged, particularly through the study of individuals who age *successfully*. [8] Successful aging was once defined by the absence of adversity. Now this concept recognizes resilience as a dynamic interplay of gains and losses [8]. This shift highlights the capacity of older adults to adapt and thrive despite chronic stressors.

A systematic review of resilience in the context of aging highlights 3 core features: the presence of a stressor, a positive or relatively adaptive response to the stressor, and the mechanisms enabling that response [6]. These mechanisms include various factors that facilitate resilience [6]. The most widely accepted understanding of resilience emphasizes a response that exceeds expectations in the face of significant stressors [6]. Among older adults, chronic stressors—such as disabilities and long-term illnesses—are prevalent and influence the capacity to demonstrate resilience. The resilience response may manifest as not only recovery to baseline or improved functioning but also as adaptation to a lower, yet still effective, level of functioning [6]. Assisting the stroke patient in recovery then is an attempt to maximize their abilities to the full extent possible.

Evaluating an individual's ability to accommodate and cope with chronic stressors provides insight into their resilience. Crucial to this process is the older adult's belief in their capacity to overcome adversity, which significantly contributes to their ability to achieve resilience [6]. Moreover, the cumulative life experiences and problem-solving skills acquired over time, combined with a determination to persevere, position older adults as an ideal population for studying resilience. Insights gained from understanding resilience in this demographic can assist in formation of strategies to foster resilience in younger populations [6].

A phenomenological study exploring resilience in 24 chronically ill older adults highlighted spiritual faith, active treatment participation, and family support as critical resilience factors [9]. Early life socialization and religious beliefs emerged as significant coping mechanisms, fostering hope and emotional regulation. These findings accentuate the multifaceted nature of resilience and its dependence on personal, social, and spiritual resources. Interventions tailored to a patient's specific needs were shown to improve resilience by fostering an increased ability to overcome health challenges. These interventions could be implemented by family members, health care providers, or other involved entities [9].

This study highlighted that resilience is both an art and a skill, with adaptation in the face of stress as a key element. Participants underscored the importance of spiritual faith and trust in God in shaping their understanding of resilience. Early life experiences, including family socialization and religious beliefs, contributed significantly to developing trust in God as a coping mechanism to counteract anxiety, depression, and to foster hope [9].

Personal factors also emerged as pivotal in helping participants navigate adversities related to chronic illness. These factors included active participation in their treatment plans, striving to maintain independence, receiving and providing love and support within family and social networks, maintaining hope for medical advancements, and achieving contentment with their circumstances [9]. Together, these findings underscore the complex nature of resilience and its dependence on a blend of personal, social, and spiritual resources.

The conceptual understanding of resilience in the elderly highlights its multidimensional nature, encompassing psychological, social, and spiritual resources that enable individuals to adapt and thrive despite chronic stressors and adversities. Resilience is not merely the absence of distress, but a dynamic process influenced by personal beliefs, early life experiences, social support, and adaptive skills. This comprehensive framework provides a foundation for exploring how resilience can be assessed, measured, and ultimately enhanced to improve the quality of life for older adults facing the challenges of aging and chronic illness [1].

A concept analysis regarding resilience in stroke patients was performed in 2022, as research of this topic has been limited [10]. Results showed defining traits of resilience in stroke patients were segmented into internal personality traits and external environmental support. Psychosocial, physical and family influences, and impairments caused by the disease were considered as the antecedents, while the consequences considered included good adaptation, active cooperation with rehabilitation, optimism for goals, and hope for improvement as time goes on [1]. In working with stroke patients, the focus would then be on enhancing their resilience by improving and strengthening these influences and traits that define resilience.

MEASURING THE RESILIENCE OF THE OLDER ADULT

To effectively understand and support resilience in older adults, it is essential to have reliable tools specifically designed to measure resilience in this population. Below are examples of commonly used screening tools for this purpose.

The resilience scale for older adults (RSOA) is specifically designed to measure resilience within the unique context of aging [10]. This tool considers factors such as coping mechanisms, adaptive behaviors, and the ability to maintain purpose and social connections despite the challenges of aging. It highlights the role of life experience, autonomy, and emotional regulation, which are particularly relevant to older populations. The RSOA is tailored to capture resilience dimensions that resonate with the elderly, including their reliance on accumulated wisdom and adaptive responses to chronic stressors and losses [10].

Another tool used to evaluate resilience is the resilience scale for adults developed specifically for the adult population [2,11,12]. It focuses on measuring the presence of protective factors in adults that are important to recover and sustain mental health. Protective resources, rather than absence of risk factors, are evaluated to assess the adult patient's level of reliance. This tool has 45 questions that assess 5 dimensions of protective resources [11].

The brief resilience scale (BRS) is a 6-item scale that measures a patient's ability to *bounce back* or to recover from stress [11]. This description is most closely related to the Latin verb definition as previously mentioned in the introduction. Although there are areas that it may not specifically measure, as do the previous 2 scales, this tool could easily be used in a clinic situation, where time for screening situations is often lacking. The responses are given in a Likert scale format and would give the provider a quick look at how the individual patient copes with health stressors, such as a stroke [11].

The Connor-Davidson resilience scale has received positive ratings in its utilization and has been used in many studies, and among a wide range of populations. Official versions of the tool include 25-, 10- and 2-item questions. The topics involved include personal competence, acceptance of change and secure relationships, trust/tolerance/strengthening effects of stress, control and spiritual influences [11].

These tools are readily accessible for use in both research and clinical practice. Each scale can be obtained through official publishers or academic institutions and is designed for specific contexts, offering robust frameworks for assessing resilience. Their availability ensures that clinicians and researchers can select tools that align with their goals, whether for comprehensive evaluation in studies or for quick, practical screening in busy clinical settings. Proper licensing and adherence to ethical guidelines for administration further enhance their utility and reliability.

RESILIENCE AMONG STROKE PATIENTS

A 2019 cohort study evaluating resilience in stroke patients over 6 months post-stroke identified significant resilience decline 1 month after discharge, followed by stabilization. Key prognosticators of resilience included self-efficacy, coping styles, functional independence, and religious support. These findings underscore the critical need for psychological and social support, particularly in the early recovery phase [7].

Another study explored family resilience and its influence on stroke survivors' coping and functioning. Results highlighted the mediating effects of patient self-efficacy and confrontational coping styles. Strengthening family support systems and targeting individual and familial strengths can enhance resilience and recovery outcomes [13].

Application for practice: case study
Patient background

Mrs B, a 77-year-old female, recently experienced an acute ischemic stroke affecting her right anterior cerebral artery. This stroke resulted in left-sided hemiplegia and mild to moderate speech impairment. Fortunately, her swallowing function remains intact, allowing her to consume soft foods and thin liquids safely.

Her medical history includes hypertension and diabetes, both of which were managed with moderate adherence to prescribed medications before the stroke. Mrs B previously lived independently in a small, wheelchair-inaccessible cottage home with 3 entry steps. A retired piano and music teacher, she was deeply involved in her church community, with most of her students coming from her congregation. Since the stroke, she has been living with one of her 5 children, which has strained family dynamics.

Now 3 months poststroke, Mrs B faces ongoing challenges requiring focused rehabilitation and support.

CLINICAL PRESENTATION

1. Physical
   - Left-sided hemiplegia: Initial total loss of movement, now improving to the point where she can transfer from bed to chair with standby assistance. She can move lightweight objects with her left hand but still struggles with fine motor skills.
   - Mild expressive aphasia persists, although communication has improved.
   - No swallowing difficulties (dysphagia).
2. Cognitive
   - Mild cognitive impairment with challenges in memory and task organization.
   - Montreal Cognitive Assessment (MoCA) score: 23/30.
3. Emotional and Social
   - Disruption in church attendance has caused feelings of isolation and sadness.
   - She is frustrated with her inability to play the piano fully, though she can still sing and play with her right hand.
   - Currently prescribed fluoxetine to support neuroplasticity and manage depression, which is common poststroke.

○ Patient Health Questionnaire-2 (PHQ-2) score: 6/10, indicative of significant depressive symptoms.
4. Living Situation
   ○ Residing with her caregiving daughter, Pam, who is increasingly frustrated with the demands of care and her mother's desire to live independently.
   ○ Mrs B expresses a strong desire to return to her home with daytime assistance.
   ○ Other children visit occasionally but are unable to offer consistent caregiving support.

EVALUATION OF RESILIENCE

Mrs B demonstrates a history of overcoming significant life challenges, indicating strong intrinsic resilience. Her score on the BRS is 4/6, interpreted as *high resilience*.

During a team meeting with Mrs B, her family, social worker, therapists, and her pastor (with permission), clinical objectives and interventions were collaboratively developed.

CLINICAL OBJECTIVES AND INTERVENTIONS

1. Optimize Poststroke management
   ○ *Medical management*: Prioritize control of hypertension and diabetes through lifestyle modifications, medication adherence, and regular monitoring to prevent recurrent strokes.
   ○ *Rehabilitation*: Continue physical and occupational therapy to maximize recovery of motor function, with a focus on fine motor skills and ambulation. Consistent therapy is essential during the critical recovery period.
   ○ *Home evaluation*: Assess her home for safety modifications. Short visits to her home could help determine if independent living is feasible in the future.
   ○ *Cognitive Support*: Implement cognitive rehabilitation to enhance memory and executive function.
2. Enhance quality of life
   ○ *Emotional and Social Support*: Encourage participation in a stroke support group to improve coping skills and self-efficacy. Reconnecting with her church community through virtual services or member visits could alleviate her sense of isolation.
   ○ *Musical Engagement*: Incorporate music therapy into her routine. Guiding her students during brief lessons could restore a sense of purpose and happiness.
3. Caregiver support
   ○ *Education and respite care*: Provide resources and education to Pam, her primary caregiver, and assess for caregiver burnout at each clinic visit.
   ○ *Family involvement*: Create a caregiving schedule among siblings to distribute responsibilities and allow Pam personal time. This unified approach can strengthen family resilience, benefiting both Mrs B and her caregivers.

INTERVENTIONAL OUTCOMES—3 MONTHS LATER

• Mrs B began visiting her home after a therapist-guided safety evaluation. She now spends 60 to 90 minutes alone while her daughter runs errands, providing her a sense of independence.

- Her music students have resumed brief lessons, which has significantly improved her mood and sense of purpose.
- Physical therapy has enabled her to ambulate with a walker and navigate the steps into her home. She has regained enough left-hand strength to begin playing simple piano pieces with both hands.
- Mrs B attended church for the first time in 9 months, walking in unassisted.
- Communication and understanding between Mrs B and her daughter has improved, reducing conflict and fostering mutual respect.
- Her PHQ-2 score dropped to 0/2, indicating a significant improvement in mood and emotional well-being. Sibling involvement has provided Pam with much-needed respite.

SUMMARY

Poststroke recovery is a multifaceted journey that demands resilience not only from the patient but also from their family and support system. In this case, Mrs B's progress highlights the critical role of resilience in overcoming physical, cognitive, and emotional challenges. The combination of her high personal resilience, supported by therapeutic interventions, community engagement, and tailored caregiver strategies, facilitated a trajectory of meaningful recovery and improved quality of life.

The integration of resilience-building strategies, such as fostering her sense of independence, leveraging her strong faith and musical passion, and addressing caregiver strain, proved instrumental in achieving her recovery goals. Equally important was the recognition of family dynamics and the implementation of supports for her caregiving daughter, which reinforced the family unit's ability to adapt and thrive despite the stressors imposed by her stroke.

This case underscores the importance of systematically evaluating resilience in both patients and their families as part of poststroke care. Resilience serves as a foundation for coping with adversity and regaining function, even in the face of chronic stressors. By focusing on resilience, health care providers can help optimize recovery potential, improve patient and family well-being, and foster a more sustainable and positive caregiving experience. These findings suggest that resilience-building approaches, tailored to the unique needs of each patient and their family, should be an integral part of poststroke rehabilitation programs.

DECLARATION OF AI AND AI-ASSISTED TECHNOLOGIES IN THE WRITING PROCESS

During the preparation of this work the author used OPEN AI/Chat GPT/ November 2024 version, in order to create a case study addressing resilience in older adults. after using this tool/service, the author reviewed and edited the content as needed and takes full responsiblity for ht econtent of the publication.

CLINICS CARE POINTS

- Incorporating psychological and social support early in recovery is vital, as resilience often declines sharply one month after discharge before stabilizing.
- Utilizing proven screening tools for resilience in the primary setting can provide insights into a patient's resilience levels, guiding personalized intervention strategies.
- Inadequate support and education for caregivers can lead to burnout and decreased quality of care, affecting patient resilience and recovery trajectory.

References

[1] Yan HY, Lin HR. Resilience in stroke patients: a concept analysis. Healthcare (Basel) 2022;10(11):2281.

[2] Tsao CW, Aday AW, Almarzooq ZI, et al. Heart disease and stroke statistics—2023 update: a report from the American Heart Association. Circulation 2023;147(8):e93–621.

[3] Merriam-Webster. (n.d.). Resilience. In Merriam-Webster.com dictionary. 2024. Available at: https://www.merriam-webster.com/dictionary/resilience.

[4] Sampedro-Piquero P, Alvarez-Suarez P, Begega A. Coping with stress during aging: the importance of a resilient brain. Curr Neuropharmacol 2018;16(3):284–96.

[5] Taylor MG, Carr D. Psychological resilience and health among older adults: a comparison of personal resources. J Gerontol 2021;76(6):1241–50.

[6] Angevaare MJ, Roberts J, van Hout HPJ, et al. Resilience in older persons: a systematic review of the conceptual literature. Ageing Res Rev 2020;63:101144.

[7] Zhang W, Liu Z, Zhou X, et al. Resilience among stroke survivors: a cohort study of the first 6 months. J Adv Nurs 2020;76(2):504–13.

[8] Borras C, Ingles M, Mas-Bargues C, et al. Centenarians: an excellent example of resilience for successful ageing. Mech Ageing Dev 2020;186:111199.

[9] Hassani P, Izadi-Avanji FS, Rakhshan M, et al. A phenomenological study on resilience of the elderly suffering from chronic disease: a qualitative study. Psychol Res Behav Manag 2017;10:59–67.

[10] Wilson CA, Plouffe RA, Saklofske DH. Assessing resilience in older adulthood: development and validation of the resilience scale for older adults. Can J Aging 2022;41(2):214–29.

[11] PositivePsychology.com. (n.d.). The Connor-davidson brief resilience scale (BRS): an overview. 2024. Available at: https://positivepsychology.com/connor-davidson-brief-resilience-scale/.

[12] Whitson HE, Duan-Porter W, Schmader KE, et al. Physical resilience in older adults: systematic review and development of an emerging construct. J Gerontol A Biol Sci Med Sci 2016;71(4):489–95.

[13] Zhang W, Gao YJ, Ye MM, et al. Post-stroke family resilience is correlated with family functioning among stroke survivors: the mediating role of patient's coping and self-efficacy. Nurs Open 2024;11(7):e223.

Advances in Family Practice Nursing 7 (2025) 95–107

ADVANCES IN FAMILY PRACTICE NURSING

ELSEVIER
MOSBY

Battling Frailty in Older Adults
The Critical Role of Advanced Practice Registered Nurses in Assessment, Management, and Prevention

Pam LaBorde, DNP, APRN, TTS*,
Melodee Harris, PhD, APRN, GNP-BC, AGPCNP-BC

University of Arkansas for Medical Sciences, College of Nursing, 4301 West Markham Street, Mail Slot #529, Little Rock, AR 72205, USA

Keywords
• Frailty • Frailty phenotype • Sarcopenia • Geriatric syndrome

Key points

- Frailty is a geriatric syndrome.
- There is no global definition of frailty.
- Gerontological nurses view frailty from a holistic perspective.
- Gerontological nurses are leaders in the management of frailty.

FRAILTY

The word evokes different meanings and images for many people. Frailty is a geriatric syndrome and vulnerability to decreased function, loss of physiologic reserve, overall poor health, disability, and mortality [1,2]. Frailty in older adults is an emerging global health burden with profound implications for both clinical practice and public health [1,2]. Higher frailty scores are associated with higher health care costs, increased use of health care resources, related cost of hospitalizations, and more use of skilled facilities [2–4]. The overarching impact of frailty is expected to mirror the growth of the aging population [2]. Limited longitudinal frailty studies have reported the paths associated with older population levels of frailty [2]. However, frailty research has heightened health care providers' awareness and sparked more research studies.

*Corresponding author. E-mail address: labordepamelaj@uams.edu

https://doi.org/10.1016/j.yfpn.2024.12.004

Abbreviations
APRN   advanced practice registered nurses
COPD   chronic obstructive pulmonary disease

The impact of frailty on the well-being of older individuals and the substantial strain on health care systems stems from the increasing prevalence and association with adverse health outcomes often seen with frailty [2,3,5]. Advanced practice registered nurses (APRNs) are vital in assessing, managing, and preventing frailty in older adults. This article will define frailty, explore its risk factors and adverse outcomes, and discuss assessment methods and validated tools. The APRN's role will be highlighted through a case study demonstrating their critical contributions to addressing frailty.

FRAILTY DEFINITIONS

There are many definitions of frailty in older adults; however, no *gold standard* definition exists [6,7]. Currently, frailty in older adults is better explained as a concept than limited to a single definition [6,7]. Considering this, the various definitions have some commonalities that have led to defining frailty as a syndrome *marked by loss of function, strength, and physiologic reserve, and by increased vulnerability to sickness and death* [1][(p1106)]. This syndrome can be described as a dynamic state causing losses in human functioning domains (social, physical, psychological), which is attributed to risk factors and leads to adverse outcomes [1,6,8].

Furthermore, frailty has been linked to an increased risk of mortality, falls, worsening disability, hospitalization, and admission to nursing home care among older adults [1,2,4]. Frailty prevalence increases with age, but it is not limited to older people. Frailty can occur at any age, especially in individuals with chronic illnesses, and can potentially be prevented [2,9].

RISK FACTORS

Frailty is a common condition among adults over the age of 65 and is compounded due to pathophysiologic changes that occur with aging, medical comorbidities, and high-risk medication use [2,9,10]. Various risk factors have been identified to contribute to frailty and encompass factors related to public health, lifestyle behaviors, socioeconomic conditions, and physical performance [2,4,7]. These risk factors include but are not limited to, advancing age, decreased physical activity, vitamin D deficiency, sarcopenia, disability, poor health, dietary problems, smoking, and alcohol intake [2,4,6,7]. All older individuals are at risk for developing frailty [9,11]. However, this risk is significantly increased for those with coexisting health conditions, limited financial resources, inactive lifestyles, and inadequate nutrition [2,9,10].

Frailty serves as an indicator of mortality risk in older adults [12]. Individuals with 2 or more conditions face a heightened risk of developing frailty, primarily due to their reduced ability to tolerate the stress associated with their medical conditions [1,13,14]. A meta-analysis of 9 studies involving greater than 14,000 community-dwelling facilities reported that frailty was present in 16% of individuals with comorbidities and had a prevalence of 18% among those with 4 or more diseases [14].

ADVERSE OUTCOMES

The significance of frailty extends beyond medical outcomes. Frailty in the geriatric population can impact their quality of life and functional independence, creating psychological, social, and financial hardships [2,9,10,15,16]. Frailty is associated with increased use of health care resources and adverse health outcomes [2]. These adverse health outcomes are linked to the challenges posed by medical complexity, a higher symptom burden, and more significant social needs [1,9,16–19].

Health care resource utilization

Due to increased comorbidities and medical complexities, frail older individuals use more health care resources [2]. Health care resources commonly used by frail individuals include increased emergency department visits, hospitalizations, consultations, and admission to nursing homes [3]. Garcia- Nogueras (2017) reported that total health care costs comprised *67% associated with hospital admission costs, 29% with specialist visit costs, and 4% with emergency admission costs. Mean hospitalization costs and emergency visit costs increased as frailty status progressed* [3][p209].

Adverse health outcomes

As outlined in the definitions and risk factors, frailty is common and independently linked to notable adverse health outcomes. The progressive nature of frailty facilitates a loss of function and physical reserve, increases vulnerability to diseases, and intensifies the predisposition to falls, fractures, acute illness, disability, and death [1,2,5]. Weakness and fatigue are commonalities in frailty, often attributed to sarcopenia (loss of muscle mass) [13]. Frailty is associated with inflammation [1]. Elevated inflammatory markers, such as C-reactive protein and interleukins, are noted in frail individuals [1]. These elevated levels contribute to feebleness and fatigue due to muscle weakness and decreased physical function. The inflammatory response exacerbating other comorbid medical conditions increases the risk of frailty in the health problems often seen with frailty [1].

Frailty adverse health outcomes can be prevented and managed by addressing 4 areas: nutritional status, physical activity, social activity, and mental activity [8,11]. Nutrition should focus on increasing protein intake and addressing vitamin D deficiency. Increasing balance and strength helps to address physical activity. Staying socially active by engaging and maintaining social connections and attending community events and social gatherings helps to stay mentally active. Keeping the mind active and engaged can be achieved using puzzles, meditation, mindfulness, memory, and physical exercise. Identifying, managing, and preventing adverse health outcomes related to frailty is a crucial priority for the APRN and begins with a comprehensive assessment [8].

ADVANCED PRACTICE REGISTERED NURSES ROLE IN FRAILTY ASSESSMENT

Assessment

Frailty is the heart of gerontology. A clear knowledge of normal age-related changes and frailty is essential to the assessment of older adults. Nurses are uniquely positioned to assess frailty in older adults [8]. Nursing models of assessment view older adults from a holistic standpoint [8]. Because frailty is a geriatric syndrome, there are multiple dimensions [11]. Frailty has a progressive trajectory. An early diagnosis of frailty can prevent or delay adverse outcomes [8]. Nursing assessment orchestrates domains of frailty including, physical, psychological, and social, with adverse outcomes and life-course determinants unique to the older adult [8,11].

Frailty can be primary or secondary [11]. Primary frailty involves multisystem dysregulation [11]. Therefore, frailty syndrome is complex and is not due to a single physiologic system [11]. Sarcopenia or loss of muscle mass is the factor and the main predictor of clinical symptoms of primary frailty in older adults [11,13]. Secondary frailty can accompany major illnesses [11].

Differential diagnoses

It is important to distinguish symptoms of multiple chronic conditions and isolated instances from the criteria for frailty. In addition, the diagnosis is primary or secondary frailty. Differential diagnoses include any chronic conditions such as heart failure, chronic obstructive pulmonary with a cardiovascular, immunologic, respiratory, or any condition that links frailty to another independent factor [11].

APRN in the primary care setting perform a comprehensive geriatric assessment that includes the 5 criteria of frailty: weight loss, exhaustion, slowness, low activity level, and weakness [11,13]. Older adults with 3 of the 5 criteria have a diagnosis of frailty [13].

The importance of frailty in the comprehensive assessment is considered in terms of physical function and symptoms. Unintentional weight loss of more than 10 pounds in the past year is a finding that often includes consideration for swallowing disorders cancer, or other disorders but may also be significant for frailty [17–19]. Exhaustion can be a transient complaint but should not be overlooked in the frailty diagnoses [11,13]. Slowness is assessed by the time to walk 15 feet and is often evaluated due to arthritis or neurologic disorders. While frailty is a critical but frequently overlooked component of the diagnosis, slowness is an important indicator. Low activity levels are often attributed solely to a sedentary lifestyle, but may be due to frailty [1]. Weakness is a common complaint that is confounded by other physical diagnoses [11,13]. The comprehensive geriatric assessment identifies the missing puzzle pieces in diagnosing frailty in older adults.

Frailty screening tools

Similar to the differing definitions of frailty, screening tools vary, with no universally accepted global standard for assessing frailty [2]. There are no clinical guidelines to support routine assessment and screening for frailty in the general population [10,20]. Screening is initiated when there is a suspicion for the diagnosis of frailty syndrome [10]. Because there is no consensus on how to standardize screening for frailty, a case finding approach is useful to identify warning signs of frailty [10,20]. Tools differ in their capability to evaluate frailty's physical, nutritional, and psychosocial dimensions, ensuring comprehensive care for older adults (Table 1). Symptoms vary; so, every tool may not be appropriate for all patients [10]. Frailty scales predict outcomes such as complications, mortality, and health care costs. The scales can be used to correlate the frailty assessment with adverse outcomes [10,24–26].

Some frailty tools include the frailty index, trauma specific frailty index , frail scale, clinical frailty scale, physical frail phenotype, Tilburg frailty indicator, and the Edmonton frail scale [10,13,27–32]. Regardless of the chosen tool, its primary goals are to screen individuals, identify those at risk for frailty, and create a patient-centered plan that includes interventions to prevent and manage frailty progression [10,11]. Overall, the physical frail phenotype is the most widely validated and used tool [13,33].

The selection of a specific scale is determined by the institution and clinical practice venues and how well it aligns with their practice and workflow. However, the chosen scale should enhance medical decision-making, resource allocation, and care planning [10,11]. Identifying frailty can inform health care providers to provide specialized care and direct interventions specific to the frailty level to help mitigate risks and improve outcomes [10,11,24–26].

MANAGEMENT STRATEGIES FOR FRAILTY

The management of frailty is no different than other geriatric syndromes requiring an interprofessional approach [2,11]. Consideration must be given to the person's capability to carry out specific interventions and whether the risk of the intervention outweighs the benefit of the intervention. Either way, the end goal is to align the intervention and management to the individual's goals. The key to meeting this goal is to have a plan in place that reviews the goals of care periodically to monitor for any change in frailty status [11].

APRN play an integral role as the leader of the interprofessional team. Autonomy and independence are the overarching goals for older adults with frailty [11]. Person-centered care promotes individualized interventions to prevent polypharmacy, falls, hospital readmissions, nursing home placement, and to reduce mortality [11].

Prevention is critical to the management of frailty. Physical therapy that includes resistance and strengthening exercises, nutritional support, and reducing

Table 1
Frailty tools

Frailty assessment tools	Time (minutes)	Mobility/ balance	Strength	Physical activity	Endurance	Nutrition	Cognition	Mood	Disability	Medical history	Social
Frail Questionnaire	3	●	●		●	●				●	
Study of Osteoporotic Fractures (SOF Index)	3		●		●	●					
Clinical Frailty Scale	3	●		●	●				●	●	
Preferred Reporting Items for Systematic Reviews and Meta-Analyses (PRISMA-7)	3	●		●			●		●	●	●
Vulnerable Elder Survey-13	5	●	●								
Frailty Phenotype	5	●	●	●	●	●			●		
Tilburg Frailty Indicator	5	●	●		●	●	●	●		●	●
Groningen Frailty Indicator	5	●		●		●	●			●	●
Edmonton Frail Scale	10	●				●	●	●	●	●	●
Comprehensive geriatric assessment (CGA-FI)	30	●	●	●		●	●	●	●	●	

polypharmacy are 3 essential interventions to prevent frailty syndrome [11]. Regardless of the type, physical activity is beneficial when it enhances the individual's mobility, cognition, quality of life, and ability to perform activities of daily living. When the severity of frailty progresses, the focus of management shifts to quality of life [11].

There is a potential synergistic effect of combining physical activity with nutritional interventions in preventing and managing frailty [34]. Protein supplements combined with exercise including resistance training may improve frailty and especially benefit older adults with weight loss and poor nutritional intake [11,35,36]. One longitudinal study showed no improvement in frailty with low dose vitamin D supplements [37]. However, the study did not consider serum baseline vitamin D deficiency [37]. For those who are deficient, vitamin D supplementation may improve physical function and subsequently reduce frailty. The Mediterranean diet is an intervention associated with decreased frailty [38]. Overall, research on nutritional supplementation and frailty is inconsistent and more research is needed [35].

The comorbid conditions, often seen with frail older adults, may require treatment with multiple medications. Health care providers need to include a medication review in frailty assessments and interactions with older adults to optimize their medications and align the care plan with their personal goals and preferences to prevent frailty [10,11].

There are specific recommendations regarding interventions based on the degree of frailty. Kim (2024) thoroughly discusses these recommendations to which providers can refer [7]. The solution to prevent and manage the complex syndrome of frailty is to implement interventions that address the complexities of the domains of physical activity, cognitive stimulation, promotion of healthy nutritional habits, and medication optimization. Doing so positively impacts the frail older adult's physical and mental capacities.

CHALLENGES TO ADVANCED PRACTICE REGISTERED NURSES PRACTICE IN FRAILTY MANAGEMENT

The main challenge for APRN in managing frailty is the need for a standardized, operational definition of frailty. While the assessment, diagnosis, and management of frailty are the strengths of gerontological nursing, the lack of a qualified workforce is a barrier to meeting the needs of older adults with frailty. The management of frailty in older adults has primarily focused on the physiologic domains. The nursing perspective is unique and a valuable contribution to caring for older adults with frailty syndrome [8]. Because of their holistic approach to the care of older adults, nurses are highly in tune with the psychological aspects of frailty syndrome and are leaders in the specialized care of older adults with frailty syndrome [8]. Further, a complete geriatric assessment is time-consuming, especially in primary care [10]. Referral to gerontological nurses is ideal, but often there is a lack of access to nurses with expert knowledge. Nevertheless, more education is needed across disciplines to improve outcomes, decrease use of health care resources, and enhance the quality of life for older adults.

SUMMARY

As individuals continue to age and are at risk of developing frailty, there is a pressing need to heighten the public's awareness of this subject, focusing on frailty prevention. Health care providers and researchers should base their collective efforts on a deeper understanding of frailty prevention and management, with particularly concerning individuals with comorbidities. *To fully realize the benefits of frailty guided clinical care, additional research is needed to narrow the gaps in our knowledge of measurement, new treatments, clinical management, and training for clinicians across diverse settings* [7](po547-8). APRN must navigate the challenge of applying research to clinical practice in managing frailty among the older population. This approach will ultimately improve the well-being of older adults experiencing frailty.

CASE STUDY: ADDRESSING FRAILTY IN OLDER ADULTS

Patient presentation

Mr George Thompson, a 79-year-old male with a history of hypertension, chronic obstructive pulmonary disease (COPD), diabetes, congestive heart failure, osteoarthritis, mild depression, and previous hospitalization for pneumonia, presented to the clinic. His daughter expressed concerns after noticing a significant decline in his physical abilities and overall health during her last visit. Mr Thompson reported frequent fatigue, muscle weakness, difficulty walking in his house, and loss of appetite. He also mentioned difficulty climbing stairs, getting dressed, and preparing meals. Over the past 6 months, he has experienced a noticeable weight loss of 12 pounds and had 2 falls, 1 resulting in a minor wrist sprain.

Assessment

- *Demographics:*
  - Age: 79 years
  - Gender: Male
  - Living Situation: Lives alone in his family home; limited social interaction. Daughter visits monthly
- *Physical examination findings:*
  - Reduced grip strength
  - Difficulty ambulating with mild unsteadiness
  - Body mass index: 19 (previously 22)
- *Frailty assessment* (Table 2)
  - *Fried frailty criteria:* Positive for weight loss, exhaustion, weakness, and low physical activity.
- *Diagnostics:*
  - Comprehensive metabolic panel: Normal.
  - Vitamin D: Deficient (15 ng/mL).
  - Pulmonary function tests: Stable COPD.

| Table 2 |
| Frail scale risk assessment |

Frail scale risk assessment	Score
F Fatigue In the last 4 weeks, did you feel tired all or most of the time?	Yes
R Resistance In the last 4 weeks, by yourself and not using aids, did you have any difficulty walking up 10 steps without resting?	Yes
A Ambulation In the last 4 weeks, by yourself and not using aids, did you have any difficulty walking 300 m (eg, around the block)?	Yes
I Illness Do you have 5 or more illnesses, such as • Hypertension • Diabetes • Cancer (not minor skin cancer) • Chronic lung disease • Have had a heart attack • Congestive heart failure • Angina • Asthma • Arthritis • Kidney disease • Other? Osteoarthritis, mild depression, previous hospitalization For pneumonia	Yes
L Loss of weight In the past year, have you lost more than 5 kg or 5% of your body weight?	Yes
Interpretation score: 0 = robust 1–2 = prefrail‖ ≥ 3 = frail	<ADD UP SCORES>

Recommendations:
1.
  See below write-up
Referrals/Follow-Up:
1.
  Physical therapy
2.
  Nutritional consult
3.
  a. Social worker/case manager consult to discuss possible need of transition to an assisted care facility vs home care options
  b. Support for family
  c. Refer to community resources/senior groups/centers for socialization engagement

Diagnosis

Mr Thompson was diagnosed with frailty, placing him at high risk for adverse outcomes such as falls, hospitalization, and further functional decline.

Table 3
Summary of frailty assessment and interventions

Category	Details
Patient Demographics	79-year-old male; lives alone; limited social interaction.
Presenting Complaint	Fatigue, weight loss, falls, difficulty with daily activities.
Frailty Assessment	Frail scale score indicates frailty
Interventions	Exercise therapy, nutritional support, vitamin D supplementation, social engagement, and care coordination.
Outcomes	Improved strength, confidence, and mobility; no new falls in 3 months.

OpenAI. Response to questions regarding creating a case study addressing frailty in older adults. (Nov 2024 version) [AI language model]. 2024. https://platform.openai.com/ [39].

Management and intervention
- *Physical therapy:*
  - Initiated a tailored exercise program focused on improving strength, balance, and mobility.
- *Nutritional support:*
  - Recommended high-calorie, protein-rich nutritional shakes, and referral to a dietitian.
  - Prescribed vitamin D supplementation.
- *Psychosocial interventions:*
  - Connected with a local senior support group to enhance social engagement.
  - Arranged for weekly visits from a community care worker to assist with daily activities and provide companionship.
- *Care coordination:*
  - Collaborated with his primary care provider and pulmonologist to optimize COPD management.
  - Scheduled follow-ups with physical therapy and dietary services.

Outcomes
After 3 months of intervention:

- Mr Thompson reported improved energy and better ability to manage daily tasks.
- Grip strength increased by 20%.
- No new falls occurred.
- Gait steadiness and confidence improved, and he began attending weekly senior group meetings.

DISCUSSION
This case underscores the APRN's pivotal role in managing frailty by identifying risk factors and implementing comprehensive, interdisciplinary interventions. Early recognition of frailty and proactive care improved Mr Thompson's quality of life and reduced his risk of adverse outcomes.

Key insights for advanced practice registered nurses
- Early identification of frailty using validated tools is essential (Table 3).

- Addressing both physical and psychosocial aspects enhances overall patient outcomes.
- Interdisciplinary collaboration is key to effective frailty management.
- Ongoing monitoring and tailored interventions support long-term improvement.

CLINICS CARE POINTS

- Clinical Care Pearls: Conduct regular Comprehensive Geriatric Assessments (CGA) for early detection of issues.
- Tailor exercise programs to individuals to improve muscle strength and prevent falls.
- Screen for malnutrition and optimize nutrition.
- Perform regular medication reviews to address polypharmacy.
- Combat social isolation by encouraging social engagement.
- Clinical Care Pitfalls: Failure to conduct frailty screenings can delay interventions and can facilitate rapi deterioration.
- Failty to align goals with the individual older adult's preferences can lead to disengagement.
- Insufficient communication among healthcare providers can lead to fragmented care and poor outcomes.

DECLARATION OF GENERATIVE AI

During the preparation of this work, the author used OpenAI (2024) in order to create a case study addressing frailty in older adults. (Nov 2024 version) [AI language model] https://platform.openai.com/. After using this tool/service, the author reviewed and edited the content as needed and takes full responsibility for the content of the publication.

Disclosures

The authors have no disclosures.

References
[1] Espinoza S, Walston JD. Frailty in older adults: insights and interventions. Cleve Clin J Med 2005;72(12):1105–12, PMID: 16392724.
[2] Hoogendijik EO, Afilalo J, Ensrud KE, et al. Frailty: implications for clinical practice and public health. Lancet 2019;394:1365–75.
[3] Garcia-Nogueras I, Aranda-Reneo I, Pena-Longobardo LM, et al. Use of health resource and healthcare costs associated with frailty: the Fradea Study. J Nutr Health Aging 2017;21(2): 207–15.
[4] Kim DH, Glynn RJ, Avorn J, et al. Validation of a claims-based frailty index against physical performance and adverse health outcomes in the health and retirement study. J Gerontol A Biol Sci Med Sci 2019;74(8):1271–6.
[5] Kojima G. Frailty as a predictor of fractures among community dwelling older people: a systematic review and meta-analysis. Bone 2016;90:116–22, Epub 2016 Jun 15. PMID: 27321894.

[6] Sobhani A, Fadayevatan R, Sharifi F, et al. The conceptual and practical definitions of frailty in older adults: a systematic review. J Diabetes Metab Disord 2021;20(2):1975–2013, PMID: 34900836; PMCID: PMC8630240.

[7] Kim DH, Rockwood K. Frailty in older adults. NEJM 2024;391(6):538–48.

[8] Gobbens RJJ, Uchmanowicz I. Frailty viewed from a nursing perspective. SAGE Open Nurs 2023;9:23779608221150598:PMID: 36636626; PMCID: PMC9829991.

[9] Hanlon P, Nicholl B, Dinesh B, et al. Frailty and pre-frailty in middle-aged and older adults and its association with multimorbidity and mortality: a prospective analysis of 493,737 UK Biobank participants. Lancet 2018;3:e323–32.

[10] BC Guidelines. Frailty in older adults: early identification and management. 2023. Available at: https://www2.gov.bc.ca/gov/content/health/practitioner-professional-resources/bc-guidelines/frailty.

[11] Resnick B. Frailty. In: Geriatric nursing review syllabus: a core curriculum in advanced practice geriatric nursing. 7th edition. New York: America Geriatrics Society; 2022.

[12] Breij S, Rijnhart JJM, Schuster NA, et al. Explaining the association between frailty and mortality in older adults: the mediating role of lifestyle, social, psychological, cognitive, and physical factors. Prev Med Rep 2021;24:1–7.

[13] Fried LP, Tangen CM, Watson J, et al. Frailty in older adults: evidence for a phenotype. J Gerontol A Biol Sci Med Sci 2001;56(3):M146–56.

[14] Vetrano DL, Palmer K, Marengoni A, et al. Frailty and multimorbidity: a systematic review and meta-analysis. J Gerontol A Biol Sci Med Sci 2019;74(5):659–66, PMID: 2972 6918.

[15] Kojima G, Iliffe S, Jivraj S, et al. Association between frailty and quality of life among community-dwelling older people: a systematic review and meta-analysis. J Epidemiol Community Health 2016;70(7):716–21, Epub 2016 Jan 18. PMID: 26783304.

[16] Hanlon P, Wightman H, Politis M, et al. The relationship between frailty and social vulnerability: a systematic review. Lancet Healthy Longevity 2024;5(3):e214–26.

[17] Nixon AC, Wilkinson TJ, Young H, et al. Symptom-burden in people living with frailty and chronic kidney disease. BMC Nephrol 2020;21:411.

[18] Verduri A, Clini E, Carter B, et al. Impact of frailty on symptom burden in chronic obstructive pulmonary disease. J Clin Med 2024;13(4):984.

[19] De Biasio JC, Mittel AM, Mueller Ariel L, et al. Frailty in critical care medicine: a review. Anesth Analg 2020;130(6):1462–73.

[20] Allison R, Assadzandi S, Adelman M. Frailty: evaluation and management. Am Fam Physician 2021;103(4):219–26, PMID: 33587574.

[21] eFrailty.org. Available at: https://efrailty.hsl.harvard.edu/. Accessed September 12, 2024.

[22] Kim DH, Cheslock M, Sison Sm, et al. eFrailty: making frailty assessment accessible to clinicians and researchers. J Am Geriatr Soc 2024;1–5; https://doi.org/10.1111/jgs.19138.

[23] Sison ST, Shi SM, Kim KM, et al. A crosswalk of commonly used frailty scales. J Am Geriatr Soc 2023;1–10; https://doi.org/10.1111/jgs.18453.

[24] Curtis E, Romanowski K, Sen S, et al. Frailty score on admission predicts mortality and discharge disposition in elderly trauma patients over the age of 65 y. J Surg Res 2018;230: 13–9.

[25] Hamidi M, Haddadin Z, Zeeshan M, et al. Prospective evaluation and comparison of the predictive ability of different frailty scores to predict outcomes in geriatric trauma patients. J Trauma Acute Care Surg 2018;87(5):1172–80.

[26] Oviedo-Briones M, Rodriguez-Laso A, Carnicero JA, et al. The ability of eight frailty instruments to identify adverse outcomes across different settings: the FRAILTOOLS project. J Cachexia Sarcopenia Muscle 2022;13(3):1487–501, PMID:35429109; PCID: PMC91 78160.

[27] Dalhousie University. Frailty index. Available at: https://www.dal.ca/sites/gmr/our-tools/the-frailty-index.html.

[28] Bellal J, Tawab AT, Amos JD, et al. Prospective validation and application of the trauma specific frailty index: results of an American association for the surgery of trauma multi-institutional observational trial. J Trauma Acute Care Surg 2023;94(1):36–44.

[29] Morley JE, Malmstrom TK, Miller DK. A simple frailty questionnaire (FRAIL) predicts outcomes in middle aged African Americans. J Nutr Health Aging 2012;16(7):601–8.

[30] Rockwood K, Song X, MacKnight C, et al. A global clinical measure of fitness and frailty in elderly people. CMAJ (Can Med Assoc J) 2005;173(5):489–95.

[31] Gobbens RJ, van Assen MA, Luijkx KG, et al. The Tilburg frailty indicator: psychometric properties. J Am Med Dir Assoc 2010;11(5):344–55.

[32] Rolfson DB, Majumdar SR, Tsuyuki RT, et al. Validity and reliability of the Edmonton frail scale. Age Ageing 2006;35(5):526–9.

[33] Lee H, Lee E, Jang I. Frailty and comprehensive geriatric assessment. J Korean Med Sci 2020;35(3):e16.

[34] Woolford SJ, Sohan O, Dennison EM, et al. Approaches to the diagnosis and prevention of frailty. Aging Clin Exp Res 2020;32(9):1629–37.

[35] Dent E, Hanlon P, Sim M, et al. Recent developments in frailty identification management, risk factors and prevention: a narrative review of leading journals in geriatrics and gerontology. Ageing Res Rev 2023;92:1–15.

[36] Kang L, Gao Y, Liu X, et al. Effects of whey protein nutritional supplement on muscle function among community-dwelling frail older people: a multicenter study in China. Arch Gerontol Geriatr 2019;83:7–12.

[37] Bolzetta F, Stubbs B, Noale M, et al. Low-dose vitamin D supplementation and incident frailty in older people: an eight year longitudinal study. Exp Gerontol 2018;101:1–6.

[38] Ntanasi E, Charisis S, Yannakoulia M, et al. Adherence to the Mediterranean diet and incident frailty: results from a longitudinal study. Maturitas 2022;162:44–51.

[39] OpenAI. Response to questions regarding creating a case study addressing frailty in older adults. (Nov 2024 version) [AI language model]. 2024. Available at: https://platform.openai.com/.

Women's Health

Advances in Family Practice Nursing 7 (2025) 109–124

ADVANCES IN FAMILY PRACTICE NURSING

Fragmented Care
Midwifery in a Landscape of Variable Accessibility to Pregnancy Care

Stephanie Mitchell, DNP, CNM, CPM[a,*],
Laila Shad, DNP, CNM[b], Catherine O'Brien, DNP, CNM[c],
Elizabeth G. Muñoz, DNP, CNM, FACNM[d,e]

[a]Birth Sanctuary, PO Box 40, Gainesville, AL 35464, USA; [b]California State University, Fullerton School of Nursing, 800 State College Boulevard, EC-190, Fullerton, CA 92832, USA; [c]Tri-Cities Community Health, 515 W. Cort Street, Pasco, WA 99301, USA; [d]Nurse-Midwifery Pathway, School of Nursing, University of Alabama at Birmingham, 1720 2nd Avenue South, Birmingham, AL 35294-1210, USA; [e]Carle Foundation Hospital, 611 West Park Street, Urbana, IL 81801, USA

Keywords
- Midwifery • Social determinants of health • Collaborative care
- Maternity care deserts

Key points
- The United States does not offer uniform pregnancy care.
- Where a midwife practices, will determine the efficiency and reliability of care.
- Variations in healthcare accessibility highlight the potential of missed and late diagnoses.
- Poor outcomes may be traced to obstacles midwives face in providing prenatal care and to the varying social determinants of health disparities in their surrounding communities.

INTRODUCTION/HISTORY/DEFINITIONS/BACKGROUND

The contiguous United States occupies an area of 3,119,884.69 square miles. In January of 2024, the population was estimated at 335,893,238. According to the latest 2022 reported US census, at any time the fecundability of the population shows a general fertility rate of 54.5 births per 100 people of reproductive ability ages 15 to 44, with birth occurring approximately every 9 seconds [1]. Pregnancy is not generally considered a condition of illness. It would be misguided

*Corresponding author. E-mail address: Stephthemidwife@gmail.com

https://doi.org/10.1016/j.yfpn.2025.01.002

Abbreviations

AFI	amniotic fluid index
BMI	body mass index
BPP	biophysical profile
EFW	estimated fetal weight
EGA	estimated gestational age
GDM A1	diet controlled gestational diabetes
GDM A2	insulin dependent gestational diabetes
GTT	glucose tolerance test
IUGR	Intrauterine growth restriction
LMP	last menstrual cycle
SDH	Social Determinants of Health
SMFM	Society for Maternal-Fetal Medicine
US	ultrasound

to believe that pregnancy care is classified and carried out the same systematic way as in illness, as stark variation in the healthcare system creates a wide range of pathways to pregnancy care. These variations in care are not based on variations in the accepted standards of care, but rather are based on factors that are inconsistent depending on where someone receives prenatal care. It may come as a surprise that the healthcare system will vary so widely based on the geographic location of the pregnant individual. In addition to nuances of the healthcare system, the resources the pregnant person has access to may drive the follow-up care they receive, as opposed to established and accepted standards for particular pregnancy conditions.

More than half (53%) of pregnancy-related deaths happen up to 1 year after delivery, and 80% of pregnancy-related deaths are classified as preventable [2]. Prevention of maternal mortality could be as simple as receiving follow-up testing for a diagnosed condition or returning to the clinic environment to have their blood pressure checked again by a nurse. Depending on the patient's ability to access health care, these follow-up visits may not be easily obtained. Therefore, not all pregnant patients in the United States will have access to basic prenatal care touch-points recommended by professional guidelines. To examine what this means on a micro level, we must understand that standards of care are established by professional organizations, which use the best evidence to increase the likelihood of identification of disease processes and circumvent the sequela leading to morbidity and mortality. The nuances of care are then influenced by a variety of factors, such as a provider's ability to stay up to date on best practices, and then further, by what resources may be available within a practice setting. The 2 case studies that follow will consider the variable nature of the nuances in care across different healthcare settings in the United States for 2 complications in pregnancy, Intrauterine Growth Restriction (IUGR) and Gestational Diabetes Mellitus (GDM).

INTRAUTERINE GROWTH RESTRICTION

IUGR is a complication of pregnancy that has been associated with a variety of adverse perinatal outcomes [3]. The etiology of IUGR can be categorized into issues relating to the person carrying the pregnancy, the fetus, or placental insufficiency. Experts offer recommendations for the identification and management of this diagnosis, which include ultrasound (US) growth, Doppler studies, and recommendation for delivery at a certain gestational age via induction of labor or cesarean section. Initially, the signs of IUGR are detected through prenatal care via a discrepancy in measurements of the uterine fundal height in centimeters and its correlation to the gestational age of the fetus. This primary screening leads to the initiation of diagnostic imaging, which will provide the diagnosis and subsequent management. Current professional recommendations for practice are provided in a bulleted format below:

Society for Maternal-Fetal Medicine (SMFM) recommendations for IUGR:

- Growth US every 3 to 4 weeks if risk factors for IUGR are present [4].
- Delivery between 38.0 and 39.0 weeks Estimated Gestational Age (EGA) if between 3rd and 10th percentile and normal umbilical artery Doppler [4].
- Delivery at 37.0 weeks EGA or earlier if estimated fetal weight (EFW) is less than 3rd percentile or if elevated umbilical artery Doppler discovered on US [4].
- Earlier delivery is required for absent or reversed umbilical artery flow [4].

American College of Obstetricians and Gynecologists (ACOG) recommendations for IUGR:

- Growth US every 3 to 4 weeks if risk factors for IUGR are present [3].
- Delivery between 38.0 and 38.6 weeks EGA if no other complications present [3].
- Delivery between 34.0 and 37.6 weeks EGA if other complications present [3].
- Earlier delivery is required for absent or reversed umbilical artery flow [3].

CASE STUDY

The following case study and chart will illuminate how providing the patient with evidence-based care may vary based on location, resources, and practice environment.

Sonya is a 27-year-old G3P2002 at 37 weeks dated by a certain LMP and confirmed by an 8-week US with a 2-day difference. She presents to care for a routine prenatal visit with a midwife. On examination, she is found to be vertex by Leopold and a fundal height was found to be 33 cm from the symphysis. Table 1 discusses the variations in care for patients with IUGR in various regions of the US.

GESTATIONAL DIABETES MELLITUS

ACOG recommends a 2-step approach to diagnosing gestational diabetes mellitus (GDM) [5]. In circumstances where economic or social barriers exist, a 2-h glucose test may also be used. Studies have correlated use of a fasting 3-h glucose tolerance test captures approximately 2% to 10.5% more cases of

Table 1
Midwifery care for intrauterine growth restriction in various regions

Location/Practice type	Steps to care for IUGR
Urban California Private nonprofit health plan and hospital system 420 beds	• Stat US order, the patient goes directly to radiology. If overall growth or AC measures <10%ile, Doppler studies will also be done. If IUGR is noted, the patient is sent to labor and delivery (L&D) for a fetal non-stress test (NST). • If <36 wk MFM message is sent to request a detailed MFM US. • In L&D based on findings of overall measurements, Dopplers and NST evaluation delivery timing will be organized. If any concerns, the patient will be directly admitted for delivery.
Rural Illinois Rural nonprofit trauma I and level III perinatal teaching hospital 453 beds	• MFM US and consultation were ordered. • <34 wk, transfer to MFM. • >34 wk, remain in CNM care and delivery at 39.0 wk EGA. • If elevated Dopplers are present, transfer to MFM care and most likely scheduled for Induction of Labor.
Rural Alabama Private homebirth practice, 1:1 care under the only legal midwifery credential (CPM) accepted for independant midwifery practice in Alabama	• Create an US order. • Fax US order to local private US office (45 miles away). • Patients will need to call to schedule an appointment on their own and will advise the midwife of the appointment date. • Results will be faxed to the provider. Results are not automatically uploaded into EMR. • For diagnosis of IUGR, the client is risked out of care and will need to transfer to OB practice. • Records will be faxed to the accepting provider.

Rural Reservation
Located in Pine Ridge South Dakota at an IHS hospital the primary federal health service provider for enrolled tribe members of American Indian and Alaska Native people. 45 beds

- Place a referral for the patient to schedule the patient for an US at the nearest diagnostic radiology department (90 miles away).
- If the referral is accepted, the patient can make an appointment.
- If a patient has their own transportation, they can drive to the appointment; otherwise, provisions must be made for the patient to get a shuttle ride from the clinic to the radiology center, which leaves the clinic at 9 AM daily.
- Patients must have an active state medicare card and an appointment verification letter to access the van.
- Results will be faxed to the provider in about 1–2 wk. Provider may request stat results on the requisition or may call the radiology office for results.
- If the results show the fetal growth is at or <10%tile and an MFM consult is needed, the process for referral is repeated, this time to an MFM specialist who accepts medicare patients. MFM appointments are on Wednesdays only unless the patient can make a 5.5-h drive to another area of the state for another day of the week.
- If fetal surveillance is indicated NST can be done at the L + D on site, as can AFI/BPP (if there is a provider available that can perform US; this is not always the case).
- The radiology department does not perform fetal US with an exception made for viability.

diabetes than a 2-h test. Diagnosis of GDM is made with 2 out of 3 elevated values in the 3-h glucose tolerance test (GTT) or values greater than 200 mg/dL in the 1-h GTT.

ACOG updated guidance on GDM:

- Offers guidance on the diagnosis and management of GDM A1 and A2 [5].
- Recommends universal screening for GDM in pregnancy [5].
- Recommends nutrition consultation for those diagnosed [5].
- Blood glucose levels must be monitored in clients with GDM A1 to diagnose GDM A2 [5].
- Insulin considered first-line treatment for GDM A2 [5].
- Metformin is a reasonable alternative to insulin if the patient cannot access insulin treatment [5].
- In patients with well-controlled GDM A1, delivery should not be recommended before 39.0 weeks [5].
- Pregnancies with well-controlled GDM A1 could go as long as 40.6 weeks EGA before delivery, as long as fetal testing is performed [5].
- In patients whose blood glucose levels are not well-controlled, delivery between 39.0 and 39.6 weeks EGA is recommended [5].
- Clients with GDM and an estimated fetal weight of greater than 4500 g should be counseled on electing for a cesarean-section (C-section) versus attempting a vaginal birth [5].

SMFM guidelines on GDM:

- Insulin considered first-line treatment for GDM A2 [5].
- Metformin is an appropriate alternative to begin treatment if there are concerns about adherence to the plan-of-care [5].
- SMFM does not have recommendations on the diagnosis of GDM.

GESTATIONAL DIABETES MELLITUS CASE STUDY

Debra is a 30-year-old G2P1001 at 30 weeks dated by a 26-week US with a Body Mass Index (BMI) of 40, who had a 3 h glucose value of 144 (fasting), 182 (1 h), 160 (2 h), and 145 (3 h) today. She did not have GDM with her first pregnancy 2.5 years ago, but she did have a macrosomic baby who weighed 4700 g and was delivered by primary C-section after a diagnosis of "failure to descend" in the second stage following 4 h of active maternal bearing efforts. She presents to care for a routine prenatal visit. Table 2 will illuminate the steps when providing Debra with evidence-based care.

SOCIAL DETERMINANTS OF HEALTH

Social Determinants of Health (SDH) are non-medical conditions that affect the health outcomes, quality-of-life, and functioning of individuals [6]. Pre-existing environments where one lives, works, grows, and receives healthcare, all contribute to factors that impact long-term and short-term outcomes for any given health scenario [6]. In situations where access to nutritious foods and opportunities for physical exercise are abundant, the less often we run into the development of health conditions. The environmental landscape

Table 2
Midwifery care for GDM in various regions in the United States

Location	Steps to care for GDM
Urban California	This patient, based on a previous OB history of fetal macrosomia and BMI >/ = 30, would have qualified for early diabetes screening by way of early 1 h, and hemoglobin A1C (HA1C). If elevated, move to 3-h testing as above. If early 1-h screening is normal, repeat 1-h screening would be ordered 26–28 w. If an early 1-h elevated with normal 3-h a repeat 3-h GTT would then be ordered at 26–28 w.

Supplies:

Testing supplies will be ordered for glucose monitoring, and patients can pick them up at onsite pharmacies. Chart routed to designated GDM case managers.

Education:

Online GDM class will be scheduled for the patient through case management with a plan of a telemedicine visit with the diabetes nurse 1 w later for a review of values. Patient glucometer values are uploaded and synched into the patient portal where the GDM case manager, as well as providers are able to retrieve and review values. The patient is advised to sync values for all clinic visits and GDM case manager appointments.

Monitoring:

Glucose values and medication management are managed by case managers through an MFM-dictated protocol and routed to the provider for signing of insulin/metformin dosing. If medication is indicated it can be picked up in the pharmacy at the clinic/hospital.

Patients will be offered TOLAC or repeat cesarean delivery and counseled on risks/benefits.

Growth US will be ordered to be done around 36-w gestation for the EFW for A1 GDM, if A2 GDM will have every 4-w growth US from 28-w or time of A2 GDM diagnosis until delivery. If extrapolated, EFM >4500g patients will be counseled for repeat cesarean delivery in the presence of GDM. If <4500g, will proceed with delivery per patient preference.

If the A1 GDM patient will be scheduled for delivery by 40w0d-40w6d A2GDM patient will be scheduled for delivery by 39w0d-39w6d or sooner depending on BG control, in collaboration with the MFM/OB generalist and midwife. If A2GDM, the patient will also be scheduled for twice weekly NST in the designated NST clinic along with an Amniotic Fluid Index (AFI). If any abnormalities in testing, patient sent to L&D for further evaluation.

(continued on next page)

Table 2
(continued)

Location	Steps to care for GDM
Rural Illinois	This patient meets the criteria for an early glucose screening test due to her pre-pregnancy BMI >40. The type of early glucose screening would be up to the CNM but would be either 1-h GTT or HA1C. If the patient had elevated glucose screening before 20 w EGA, would be presumed Type 2 DM instead of GDM. This patient would then transfer to MFM care. If early screening was normal, patients would remain in CNM care, and repeat GTT would be performed between 24.0–28.6 wk EGA. If the patient had an elevated GTT between 24–28 wk EGA, they move to the 3-h OGTT if the value is over 140 and considered GDM A2 if the result is over 200. If the patient meets the criteria for a 3-h OGTT and they have two or more elevated values, they receive the diagnosis of GDM A1. Supplies: Glucose testing supplies will be ordered by the midwifery clinic nurse. Education: Chart routed to MFM office to schedule an MFM consult visit and education with the APRN in the MFM department. Each patient receives the same teaching on glucose monitoring and dietary modifications. Monitoring: Fasting and postprandial blood glucose values are reviewed by the CNM office during the initial 2 wk of testing blood glucose levels. If >20% (or 6 of 28 values) are elevated, the patient is diagnosed with A1GDM and continues testing glucose levels throughout the remainder of pregnancy. If >20% of values in any week are elevated, the patient is diagnosed with A2GDM and insulin is initiated. The CNM co-manages the patient with MFM. at this point and the patient would be transferred to MFM if blood glucose levels were not controlled with insulin or *additional problems were present.* The patient's MFM consult would also address the history of cesarean section and the patient would be offered at TOLAC as long as fetal weight was estimated to be <4500 g. If the estimated fetal weight is >4500 g, a repeat cesarean section would be recommended. These recommendations would be communicated at the MFM consult and the patient would be co-managed along with the CNM service. Timing of delivery would depend on the glucose control during the pregnancy and the US reports on fetal growth, which would be performed every 4 wk from diagnosis of GDM until delivery. Patients with GDM would begin twice-weekly antenatal testing at 32 wk and continue through the week of delivery. Delivery would be recommended before 40.0 wk EGA for patients with A1 GDM and before 39.0 wk EGA for clients with A2 GDM. All clients are offered informed consent for all decision points along the way from diagnosis of GDM through delivery. The patient understands they can decline recommendations and the CNM would document their decision to do so in their electronic health record.

Rural Alabama

Important note for this particular case study: A trial of labor after a cesarean section (TOLAC) in an out-of-hospital setting, according to Alabama state regulations, constitutes an illegal practice of midwifery. A midwife could care for a person who had a previous c-section for prenatal care, but the patient would need to present for intrapartum care at a hospital. Out-of-hospital care is not an option

Early screening would be offered in this case due to the history of fetal macrosomia. In cases of HA1C >5.7 would offer early 1-h testing as well.

Supplies:

The client will have to obtain testing supplies over the counter.

The patient has an option of attempting to record and control blood sugars using diet only.

Education:

Clients will meet with the midwife once a week for 2 w for education on testing, recording values, and reinforcement of dietary and lifestyle modifications. The clients have 2 w to collect and record results and present to care with the blood glucose values to determine if the patient needs insulin control or if dietary control is sufficient.

Monitoring:

Each homebirth midwifery practice may vary on their parameters of glucose control. Two fasting elevations in a week, or 4 postprandial elevated values >140 during the week without clear identifiable causation will risk the client out of care. The midwife will make contact with the OB physician of the patient's choosing, and request a 1:1 provider-to-provider warm handoff to transfer care for management of A2 GDM. Shared decision-making will dictate if the patient will continue with co-care with a plan to birth at the hospital.

No routine growth US for A1 GDM unless S>D on clinical examination.

No induction of labor for A1 GDM. The patient will risk out of care routinely at 41 w.

(continued on next page)

Table 2
(continued)

Location	Steps to care for GDM
Rural Reservation	All patients receive initial screening by HA1C to differentiate gestational diabetes from Type II diabetes. This patient would qualify for early diabetes screening based on OB history of macrosomia by 2-step glucose testing. Supplies: The clinic nurse will provide testing supplies. Education: The clinic nurse provides 1:1 education on how to use the glucometer and record results. The patient is given a glucose log to record values for 2 w. Monitoring: At the next scheduled visit (usually 2 w from diagnosis) elevations in 20% of values (or 6 of 28 values) OR 3 instances of fasting elevations >95 OR any 2 postprandial values >140 a referral is made to Maternal Fetal Medicine if there is not an OB physician on-site to manage insulin. The referral process is similar to any other high-risk perinatal conditions requiring care outside of IHS. A purchased Referral Care order is placed in the computer. A hospital committee meets weekly to approve or deny referrals to outside IHS facilities. Upon approval, an appointment will be scheduled. If a patient has their own transportation, they can drive to the appointment. Otherwise, provisions must be made for the patient to get a shuttle ride from the clinic to the radiology center, which leaves the clinic at 9 AM daily. Patients must have an active state medicare card and an appointment verification letter to access the van. Appointments are on Wednesdays only for a provider who is onsite once weekly and must be scheduled after 11:00 AM to account for travel time. The van returns to IHS in the afternoon. Fetal testing would start at 32 wk and consist of twice weekly NST, and a weekly AFI. As there is no OB US available on site, 1 NST would be on-site at the IHS hospital, and patients would have to commute to the largest closest city for MFM care once weekly for testing and NST. Induction of labor is electively scheduled after 39 w.

Table 3
Social determinants of health in various regions of the United States

	Urban California	Rural Illinois	Rural Alabama	Rural Indian Reservation
Economic Stability	27.3% live below the poverty level. in 2023 The median income for a household in the city was $45,782. [10]	18.7% live below the poverty level. Median income- $61,090 [10]	30.4% live below the poverty level. Median income- $31,726 [10]	47.7% of the population live below the poverty level. 61% of residents <age 18 live below the poverty level. Oglala Lakota County, per-capita income makes it the second poorest county in the United States, at $6286 [7,8] 80% of residents are unemployed.
Access to Healthcare	85.3% have health coverage 53 hospitals in Southern California offer OB services 1483:1 primary care provider/person [10]	996:1 primary care provider/person	Defined as a Maternity Care Desert 1746:1 primary care provider/person No Obstetric hospital services in Sumter County. No US services in Sumter County	Defined as a Maternity Care Desert; low-access to care. 100% of enrolled tribal members have access to IHS health services. Availability of obstetricians varies anywhere from 0-31 d a month contingent on contractual staffing arrangements, which fluctuate throughout the year. 300% higher incidence of infant mortality 800% increase incidence of diabetes. Suicide rates are among the highest in the northern hemisphere and are 4 times higher than the national rate for persons aged 15–25.

(continued on next page)

Table 3
(continued)

	Urban California	Rural Illinois	Rural Alabama	Rural Indian Reservation
Neighborhood Context	In 2023 32% of the population had housing instability Median Property value in 2022 was $722,200 Walk score of 37/100 [11] some public transportation and does not have many bike lanes. [10]	19% with housing instability The median property value in 2022 was $189,700 Walk score of 52/100 [11] Some public transportation is available and is somewhat bikeable.	Sumter County, Alabama is 903.8 square miles of land area and is the 14th largest county in Alabama with 13.8% housing instability. The median property value in 2023 was $88,000 No public transportation Walk score of 11/100 [11] The location is car-dependent. Most errands require a car.	2.8 million acres in South Dakota that held Indigenous prisoners of war in 1889. The median property value in 2022 was $55,000 No public transportation Walk Score of 26/100. [11] The location is car-dependent. Most errands require a car.
Environmental	Multiple hospitals with obstetric services. Not a food desert [14] Multiple grocery stores are located throughout the location.	1 hospital with obstetric services Not a food desert [14] Multiple grocery stores throughout the general location	45 miles to the closest hospital with obstetric US services and Maternal-fetal Medicine services 1 day out of the week by referral. Defines as a food desert. [14] 3 grocery stores in Sumter County.	90 miles to the closest access to a hospital with obstetric services. Maternal Fetal Medicine access 1 d out the week by referral. Defined as food desert. [14] 2 grocery stores within a 90-mile radius of the reservation.

| Social/community context | The largest ethnic populations are Hispanic (61.4%) white Hispanic, (19%) white non-Hispanic, (10.7%) Black (12.3%) Chinese including Mandarin and Cantonese (3.54%) Korean (3.48%) American Indian or Alaskan Native (<1%) Culturally congruent maternity care is available. [12,13] | The largest ethnic populations are white (67.4%), Black (12.1%), Asian (10.2%), Hispanic - all types (5.83%). Multiracial (3.76%) Culturally congruent maternity care is available. [12,13] | The largest ethnic populations are Black (72.3%), white (25.2%), multiracial (<2%), Asian (<1%), American Indian/Alaskan Native (<1%), Hispanic (<1%) Culturally congruent maternity care is not available for the majority of the population. [12,13] | The largest ethnic populations in Pine Ridge, SD are American Indian & Alaska Native (Non-Hispanic) [79.9%), American Indian & Alaska Native (Hispanic) (12.8%), White (Non-Hispanic) [7.29%), White (Hispanic) (0%), and Black or African American (Non-Hispanic) (0%). Culturally congruent pregnancy care is not available. Of all racial and ethnic groups in America, members of the Lakota nation have the lowest life expectancy. The average life expectancy for men is 47 y. Women's average life expectancy has been described as 52–55 y [7,8] Culturally congruent maternity care is not available for the majority of the population. [12,13] |

for the aforementioned case studies not only illuminates the differences in care that one might experience but also shows that though people may be receiving midwifery-led care, the outcomes could be negatively impacted by the key differences of highlighted SDH across geographic regions in the United States [7–17]. Cultural congruence discussed in Table 3 is defined as the ability to access primary health care resources in the context of one's cultural lived experience [12,13]. Table 3 describes and compares some specific indicators of the SDH with the area where the client/patient is receiving perinatal care. According to the United States Department of Agriculture, a food desert is an area that has either a poverty rate greater than or equal to 20% or a median family income, not exceeding 80% of the median family income in urban areas or 80% of the statewide median family income in nonurban areas [14]. Proximity to living in a food desert has been correlated to chronic disease and illness [15].

DISCUSSION

Experts in perinatal care offer recommendations on the management of conditions that arise in pregnancy. These recommendations are based on evidence that lends to uniform screening and management of these conditions. We also know that midwifery care, and specifically access to collaborative perinatal care has been shown to improve perinatal and fetal outcomes [18,19]. As we have highlighted, factors that contribute to care outside of the context of these recommendations can be directly linked to SDH. Based on where geographically a pregnancy occurs in the United States and whether you have robust access to collaborative care, or if you are in a low-resource setting will inversely and inevitably affect the streamlining of these processes. For some conditions, hospital or facility policy does not dictate the precise timeline for early screening for some conditions. There is leeway, and Midwives have guidance that they may refer to, but may choose early screening such as Hemoglobin A1C, or an early 1-h glucose tolerance testing. Education on the disease process varies by location as well. In larger, high-resource settings, there are staffs available to provide education and teaching to increase compliance and dietary changes, which lend to optimal glucose management.

Midwifery care in a high volume, high acuity, and high resource setting such as in Urban California the turnaround time from possible concern, as in laboratories outside of reference range for gestational diabetes, or US diagnostics may take a few minutes. Streamlined and specific coordinators are tasked with tracking and coordinating care. From possible concerns, diagnostics for conditions such as IUGR can be identified in a few minutes to a few hours. Conversely, when we look at lower resource settings and maternity care deserts such as in rural Alabama diagnostics may occur within a few days, and on a rural reservation, diagnosis may take up to a few weeks, and follow-up may be disjointed or delayed due to transportation issues, issues related to inability to take leave from work, or related to reliable childcare.

SUMMARY

Variations in perinatal care, in addition to SDH impact perinatal and fetal outcomes. Disparities in outcomes can be traced to barriers to receiving evidence-based care. Care recommendations are difficult to meet in places such as Pine Ridge Reservation and rural Alabama because there simply is not enough access of infrastructure to support best practices. Research is not lacking on how poor access leads to detrimental outcomes; however, the focus should be on supporting midwives to meet the established care criteria for those who experience elevated risk in pregnancy. The location should not dictate best practice.

CLINICS CARE POINTS

- The United States does not offer uniform pregnancy care.
- Access to a collaborative care model increases efficiency of pregnancy care and improved outcomes.
- Uniform independent practice of Midwives will increase access to pregnancy care.

Disclosures

The authors have nothing to disclose.

References

[1] Census (2024). Fertility of women in the United States: 2022. Available at: https://www.census.gov/data/tables/2022/demo/fertility/women-fertility.html. Accessed November 8, 2024.

[2] CDC (2022). Four in 5 pregnancy-related deaths in the U.S. are preventable. Available at: https://www.cdc.gov/media/releases/2022/p0919-pregnancy-related-deaths.html#:~:text=Four%20in%205%20pregnancy%2Drelated,preventable%20%7C%20CDC%20Online%20Newsroom%20%7C%20CDC. Accessed November 8, 2024.

[3] ACOG Practice Bulletin No. 227 fetal growth restriction. Obstet Gynecol 2021;137(2):e16–28.

[4] Abuhamad A, Martins JG, Biggio JR. Diagnosis and management of fetal growth restriction: the SMFM guideline and comparison with the ISUOG guideline. Ultrasound Obstet Gynecol 2021;57:880–3.

[5] ACOG Practice Bulletin No. 190: gestational diabetes mellitus. Obstet Gynecol 2018;131(2):e49–64.

[6] CDC. Social determinants of health. date unknown. Available at: https://www.cdc.gov/health-disparities-hiv-std-tb-hepatitis/about/social-determinants-of-health.html#:~:text=Social%20determinants%20of%20health%20(SDOH,the%20conditions%20of%20daily%20life. Accessed November 8, 2024.

[7] Strickland P. Life on the Pine Ridge Native American Reservation. Available at: https://www.aljazeera.com/features/2016/11/2/life-on-the-pine-ridge-native-american-reservation. Accessed November 8, 2024.

[8] Ulmer KK. Disparities in healthcare: a focus on Native American Women's health and the system that is failing them. Proceedings in Obstetrics and Gynecology 2020;9(3):1–10.

[9] March of dimes. Peristats maternity care deserts. Available at: https://www.marchofdimes.org/peristats/data?top=23. Accessed November 6, 2024.

[10] Datausa.io website. Available at: https://datausa.io/profile/geo/sumter-county-al?redirect=true#:~:text=Poverty%20%26%20Diversity&text=30.4%25%20of%20the%20

population%20for,the%20national%20average%20of%2012.5%25. Accessed November 8, 2024.

[11] Walkscore.com website. Available at: https://www.walkscore.com/. Accessed July 12, 2024.

[12] Schim SM, Doorenbos A, Benkert R, et al. Culturally congruent care: putting the Puzzle together. J Transcult Nurs 2007;18(2):103–10.

[13] Schim SM, Doorenbos AZ. A three-dimensional model of cultural congruence: framework for intervention. J Soc Work End Life Palliat Care 2010;6(3–4):256–70.

[14] Dutko P, Ver Ploeg M, Farrigan T. United States department of agriculture: characteristics and influential factors of food deserts. Available at: https://www.ers.usda.gov/webdocs/publications/45014/30940_err140.pdf. Accessed November 8, 2024.

[15] Ghazaryan A, Carlson A, Rhone AY, et al. Association between the nutritional quality of household at-home food purchases and chronic diseases and risk factors in the United States. Nutrients 2015;13(9):3260.

[16] Ginsbach KF. The Oglala Lakota and the right to health: the forgotten Americans. Quinnipiac Health LJ 2021;24:237. Available at: https://racism.org/articles/citizenship-rights/-rights-of/9727-the-oglala. Accessed November 8, 2024.

[17] Healthy people 2030, U.S. Department of health and human services, office of disease prevention and health promotion. Available at: https://health.gov/healthypeople/objectives-and-data/social-determinants-health. Accessed November 8, 2024.

[18] Carlson NS, Breman R, Neal JL, et al. Preventing cesarean birth in women with obesity: influence of unit-level midwifery presence on use of cesarean among women in the consortium on safe labor data set. J Midwifery Wom Health 2020;65:22–32.

[19] Sandall J, Fernandez Turienzo C, Devane D, et al. Midwife continuity of care models versus other models of care for childbearing women. Cochrane Database Syst Rev 2024;4(4):CD004667.

Advances in Family Practice Nursing 7 (2025) 125–138

ADVANCES IN FAMILY PRACTICE NURSING

Interpreting Bone Density Screenings and Treatment for Osteopenia and Osteoporosis

Mary Lauren Pfieffer, DNP, FNP-BC*,
Queen Henry-Okafor, PhD, FNP-BC, PMHNP-BC,
Shannon Cole, DNP, APRN-BC, Jannyse Tapp, DNP, FNP-BC

Vanderbilt University School of Nursing, 461 21st Avenue South, Nashville, TN 37240, USA

Keywords

• Osteoporosis • Osteopenia • Bone mineral density • Fracture risk assessment tool
• Osteopenia treatment • Osteoporosis treatment

Key points

- Osteopenia and osteoporosis prevalence is increasing as the aging population in the United States is increasing.
- Patients most at risk are postmenopausal women. Bone denisty tests are re-ccomended for postmenopausal women, men over 70 and those with increased risk factors.
- Dual-energy X-ray absorptiometry helps classify bone health status and guide clinical decision-making regarding prevention and treatment strategies.
- Treatment is aimed at reducing bone loss and improving bone mineral density. Pharmacologic treatment options include bisphosphonates, selective estrogen receptor modulators, and monoclonal antibodies.
- Health promotion is imperative to prevent progression of bone loss. Interventions include dietary modifications, physical activity, lifestyle modification, and fall prevention strategies.

INTRODUCTION

Osteopenia and osteoporosis are progressive skeletal disorders characterized by decreased bone mineral density (BMD) and compromised bone strength, predisposing individuals to an increased risk of fracture. These conditions represent significant public health challenges due to their prevalence and associated morbidity, impacting millions worldwide [1]. Menopause is a

*Corresponding author. E-mail address: mary.pfieffer@vanderbilt.edu

https://doi.org/10.1016/j.yfpn.2025.01.003
2589-420X/25/© 2025 Elsevier Inc. All rights are reserved, including those for text and data mining, AI training, and similar technologies.

Abbreviations

BMD	bone mineral density
DXA	dual-energy X-ray absorptiometry
FRAX	Fracture Risk Assessment Tool
WHO	World Health Organization

significant risk factor for bone loss in women during late adulthood. After the onset of menopause, women typically lose about 2% of cortical bone and 5% of trabecular bone per year for the first 5 to 8 years. Additionally, Caucasian women aged 50 years have a lifetime risk of osteoporotic fracture of around 40%. In addition to gender and age, a family history of osteoporosis or broken bones can increase the risk. Certain medications, such as corticosteroids, thyroid hormone replacement, and blood thinners, can also increase the risk of osteoporosis. Other risk factors include smoking, heavy alcohol use, low vitamin D or calcium levels, lack of physical activity, and certain medical conditions. White and Asian women aged 50 and over, as well as men with low testosterone levels, are at a higher risk of developing osteoporosis.

Approximately 10 million people are affected by osteoporosis or osteopenia [2]. This condition leads to nearly 1.5 million fractures each year [2]. The impact of a fracture is significant, affecting both physical and emotional health and often leading to a decline in overall health. Additionally, a fracture places a substantial economic burden on our country. As the aging population in the United States continues to grow, there will likely be an increase in the prevalence of fractures [2].

The U.S. Centers for Disease Control and Prevention (CDC) states that osteoporosis can significantly reduce the quality of life by limiting activities due to the fear of fractures. Fractures can be painful and lead to long-term disability and complications such as pneumonia and pressure sores. Osteoporosis-related fractures cost the US $17.9 billion per year, primarily due to acute and rehabilitative care [2]. Each year in the United States, there are 1.5 million osteoporotic fractures [2]. These fractures result in over half a million hospitalizations, more than 800,000 emergency room visits, over 2.6 million physician office visits, and lead to almost 180,000 individuals being placed into nursing homes [2].

PATHOPHYSIOLOGY OF OSTEOPENIA AND OSTEOPOROSIS

The pathophysiology of osteopenia and osteoporosis is rooted in an imbalance between bone formation and bone resorption processes. Under normal physiologic conditions, bone remodeling–a dynamic process involving the coordinated actions of osteoblasts (bone-forming cells) and osteoclasts (bone-resorbing cells)–ensures skeletal integrity and maintains BMD [3]. However, this equilibrium is disrupted in osteopenia and osteoporosis, leading to net bone loss over time.

Key factors contributing to bone loss include hormonal changes, particularly estrogen deficiency in postmenopausal women, which accelerates bone turnover and resorption [4]. Chronic inflammatory conditions, such as rheumatoid arthritis, and prolonged use of glucocorticoids can also exacerbate bone loss by affecting osteoblast and osteoclast function [1]. Additionally, inadequate calcium and vitamin D intake, sedentary lifestyle, and genetic predisposition further contribute to the development and progression of these bone disorders. Understanding the pathophysiology of osteopenia and osteoporosis is essential for developing effective diagnostic, preventive, and therapeutic strategies to preserve bone health and reduce fracture risk.

DIAGNOSTIC TESTS, SCREENING, AND INTERPRETATION FOR OSTEOPENIA AND OSTEOPOROSIS

Accurate diagnosis and early detection of osteopenia and osteoporosis are crucial for implementing timely interventions to prevent fractures and mitigate bone loss. The frequency of bone density screening tests depends on a person's risk of bone fractures. In general, the recommendations are as follows: high-risk individuals should have screenings every 2 years; moderate-risk individuals should be screened every 3 to 5 years; low-risk individuals should undergo screenings every 10 to 15 years.

Several diagnostic tools and screening modalities are employed to assess bone health, evaluate fracture risk, and guide therapeutic decisions. Regular bone density tests are recommended for postmenopausal women, men over 70, and individuals with risk factors such as a family history of osteoporosis, low body weight, or previous fractures [5,6]. The guidelines for getting a BMD and the frequency of repeat scans vary. Medicare typically covers dual-energy X-ray absorptiometry (DXA or DEXA) scans every other year for women over 65 and men over 70 [5,6]. However, other medical organizations and the Bone Health and Osteoporosis Foundation suggest that scans can start as early as age 50 for individuals with risk factors for fractures, including both women and men [2].

METHODOLOGY USED FOR BONE DENSITY SCREENINGS

Bone density screenings primarily involve the use of noninvasive imaging technologies to measure BMD. The most common method is DXA or DEXA, which uses low-level X-rays to assess bone density at various sites in the body, usually the hip and spine [1]. The procedure is quick, painless, and involves minimal radiation exposure. The resulting images provide detailed information about bone density, which is compared against standard reference values to determine bone health status [7].

BMD via DXA remains the gold standard for diagnosing osteoporosis and osteopenia. DXA assesses BMD at the hip and lumbar spine, providing T-scores that compare an individual's BMD to that of a young adult reference population [1].

DIAGNOSTIC CRITERIA AND CLASSIFICATIONS

The World Health Organization (WHO) has established diagnostic criteria for osteopenia and osteoporosis based on BMD measurements. These criteria use T-scores, which compare an individual's BMD to the average peak BMD of a healthy young adult. A T-score of −1.0 to −2.5 indicates osteopenia, while a T-score of −2.5 or lower indicates osteoporosis [3]. Additionally, the Fracture Risk Assessment Tool (FRAX) can be used in conjunction with BMD measurements to estimate an individual's 10-year probability of hip and other major osteoporotic fractures, aiding in risk stratification and management decisions [8].

TOOLS COMMONLY USED FOR BONE DENSITY MEASUREMENTS

Fracture Risk Assessment Tools

Various fracture risk assessment tools (Fig. 1) integrate clinical risk factors with BMD measurements to predict the likelihood of future fractures. The FRAX tool, endorsed by the WHO, incorporates age, sex, body mass index , prior fracture history, parental history of hip fracture, glucocorticoid use, smoking status, alcohol intake, and BMD to estimate 10-year fracture probabilities [1]. Clinicians use FRAX scores to guide treatment decisions, such as initiating pharmacotherapy for osteoporosis.

Laboratory Tests and Biomarkers

Laboratory tests, such as serum calcium, phosphate, alkaline phosphatase, and vitamin D levels, may be utilized to identify secondary causes of osteoporosis

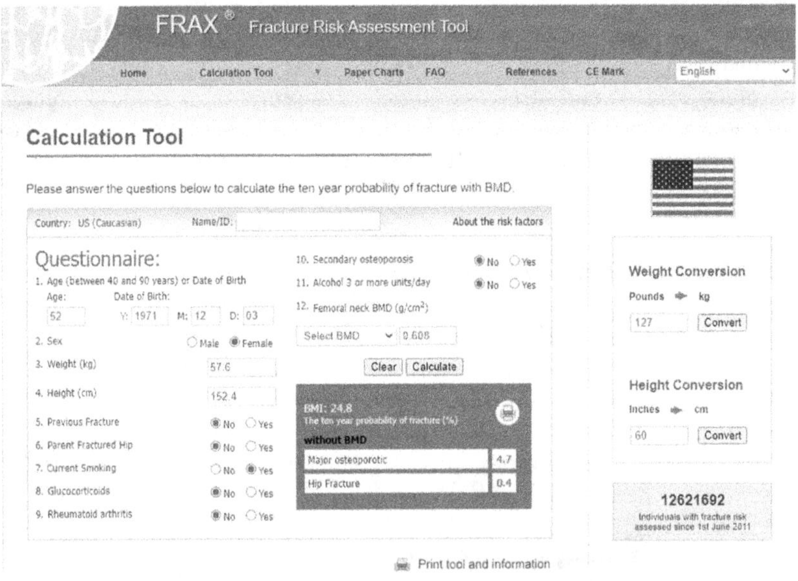

Fig. 1. Fracture risk assessment tool. (University of Sheffield [26]).

[9]. Markers of bone turnover, including serum C-terminal telopeptide and procollagen type I N-terminal propeptide, reflect bone resorption and formation rates, aiding in disease monitoring and treatment response assessment [4].

Imaging Modalities
The gold standard for measuring bone density is DXA, renowned for its accuracy, speed, and low radiation dose. DXA scans provide detailed images of the hip, spine, and sometimes the forearm, allowing for precise assessment of bone health. In addition to DXA, quantitative computed tomography provides a 3-dimensional assessment of BMD at the spine and hip, offering insights into bone geometry and trabecular bone density [3]. High-resolution peripheral quantitative computed tomography evaluates microarchitecture at peripheral skeletal sites, enhancing fracture risk prediction beyond BMD alone. Peripheral devices like peripheral dual-energy x-ray absorptiometry and quantitative ultrasound are also used, particularly in settings where DXA is unavailable. These methods measure bone density at peripheral sites such as the wrist, heel, or finger, providing valuable screening information, though they are less comprehensive than central DXA scans [5].

Interpreting and Classifying Bone Density Results
The interpretation of bone density results involves analyzing the BMD measurements obtained from diagnostic tests such as DXA. These results are compared to reference values to determine the relative bone health of the patient. The primary metrics used for this comparison are T-scores and Z-scores [10]. These scores help classify bone health status and guide clinical decision-making regarding prevention and treatment strategies.

Interpreting DXA results involves considering T-scores, fracture risk assessment, and clinical context. Treatment thresholds for initiating pharmacotherapy are influenced by fracture risk, BMD status, and the presence of significant clinical factors [4]. Integrated assessment with FRAX scores helps tailor interventions to individual risk profiles, optimizing fracture prevention strategies in clinical practice.

T-score and Z-score Significance
The T-score is a critical metric in assessing bone health. It compares an individual's bone density to the average peak bone density of a healthy young adult of the same sex. The T-score is expressed in standard deviations from this reference point.

- A T-score of -1.0 or above is considered normal bone density.
- A T-score between -1.0 and -2.5 indicates osteopenia, signifying lower than normal bone density and an increased risk of developing osteoporosis.
- A T-score of -2.5 or below is diagnostic of osteoporosis, indicating significantly reduced bone density and a higher risk of fractures.

Conversely, the Z-score compares an individual's bone density to the average bone density of people of the same age, sex, and size. It is particularly useful in evaluating bone health in premenopausal women, men under 50, and children. A Z-score of −2.0 or lower may suggest an underlying condition contributing to bone loss and warrants further investigation.

Differences Between Osteopenia and Osteoporosis

The key difference between osteopenia and osteoporosis lies in the severity of bone density reduction, as indicated by T-scores. A T-score between −1.0 and −2.5 characterizes osteopenia. It reflects a stage of bone loss that is not severe enough to be classified as osteoporosis but indicates a higher risk of progressing to osteoporosis without intervention. Osteopenia is considered a warning sign, highlighting the need for lifestyle modifications and possible pharmacologic treatment to prevent further bone loss.

Osteoporosis, defined by a T-score of −2.5 or lower, represents a more advanced stage of bone loss. It is associated with a significantly higher risk of fractures, even with minimal trauma. Osteoporosis involves decreased bone density and changes in bone microarchitecture, further compromising bone strength. The management of osteoporosis typically requires a more aggressive approach, including medications to slow bone resorption or stimulate bone formation, alongside lifestyle and dietary interventions [9].

By understanding and accurately interpreting bone density results through T-scores and Z-scores, health care providers can effectively classify bone health status, identify individuals at risk, and implement appropriate measures to prevent and treat osteopenia and osteoporosis. See Table 1.

EVIDENCE-BASED STRATEGIES FOR OSTEOPENIA AND OSTEOPOROSIS MANAGEMENT

Osteopenia and osteoporosis represent a spectrum of BMD disorders characterized by decreased bone mass and microarchitectural deterioration of bone tissue, leading to increased fracture risk. Effective management strategies are crucial to mitigate the progression of bone loss and reduce fracture incidence in affected individuals.

Lifestyle Modifications

1. Nutrition and Diet: Adequate calcium intake is fundamental for bone health. The National Osteoporosis Foundation recommends 1000 mg/day for adults aged 19 to 50 years and 1200 mg/day for adults over 50 years through diet and supplements if necessary [8]. Vitamin D supplementation is essential as it facilitates calcium absorption. The Endocrine Society recommends 800 to 1000 IU/day for adults at risk of osteoporosis [11].
2. Physical Activity: Weight-bearing exercises (eg, walking, jogging, resistance training) and muscle-strengthening activities help maintain bone density and reduce fracture risk [1]. Balance and posture exercises are also beneficial in preventing falls, particularly in older adults [12].

Pharmacologic Interventions

Medication therapy is typically initiated based on BMD and fracture risk. There are differences regarding mechanism of action; however, the aim for

Table 1
Diagnostic tests and interpretation of results

Diagnostic test	Methodology	Measurement site	Interpretation Metric	Normal Range	Osteopenia Range	Osteoporosis Range
Dual-energy x-ray absorptiometry	Uses low-dose x-rays to measure bone density	Hip, spine, forearm	T-score	≥ -1.0	-1.0 to -2.5	≤ -2.5
Quantitative Computed Tomography	Uses CT scans to measure volumetric bone density	Spine	T-score	≥ -1.0	-1.0 to -2.5	≤ -2.5
Peripheral DXA	Uses low-dose x-rays to measure bone density at peripheral sites	Wrist, heel, finger	T-score	≥ -1.0	-1.0 to -2.5	≤ -2.5
Quantitative ultrasound	Uses sound waves to assess bone density and structure	Heel, tibia	Z-score	≥ -1.0	-1.0 to -2.5	≤ -2.5

Interpretation of T-scores and Z-scores: T-score compares an individual's bone density to the average peak bone density of a healthy young adult of the same sex. Score compares an individual's bone density to the average peak bone density of a healthy young adult of the same age, sex, and body size.

all is reducing bone loss and improving BMD. It has also been suggested that medication therapy offers analgesia for alleviating pain [13].

1. Bisphosphonates: Bisphosphonates (eg, alendronate, risedronate) inhibit bone resorption and are first-line treatments for osteoporosis [1]. They reduce fracture risk significantly and are generally well-tolerated with long-term use [2].
2. Selective Estrogen Receptor Modulators (SERMs): SERMs like raloxifene mimic estrogen's effects on bone without affecting the uterus and breast. They reduce vertebral fracture risk but may increase thromboembolic events [2].
3. Monoclonal Antibodies: Denosumab, a monoclonal antibody targeting receptor activator of nuclear factor kappa-B ligand (RANKL), decreases bone resorption and fracture risk. It is effective in postmenopausal women and men with osteoporosis [2].

Emerging Therapies
1. Romosozumab: Romosozumab, a sclerostin inhibitor, promotes bone formation and inhibits bone resorption. It reduces fracture risk significantly and is approved for postmenopausal women at high risk of fracture.
2. Teriparatide: Teriparatide, a recombinant parathyroid hormone, stimulates bone formation. It is indicated for severe osteoporosis in individuals at high fracture risk [2].

Multidisciplinary Approach
Effective management of osteopenia and osteoporosis requires a multidisciplinary approach involving health care providers, nutritionists, physical therapists, and pharmacists. Regular monitoring of BMD and adherence to treatment guidelines are crucial to optimize outcomes and reduce fracture risk in affected individuals. See Table 2.

In conclusion, the management of osteopenia and osteoporosis is evolving with advancements in pharmacotherapy and a greater emphasis on lifestyle modifications. Tailored interventions based on individual risk profiles and regular assessment are crucial to preventing fractures and improving the quality of life in patients with these bone disorders.

Health Promotion
Health promotion for osteoporosis focuses on preventing bone loss and fractures through a combination of lifestyle changes, dietary adjustments, and medical interventions. Key strategies for promoting bone health and preventing osteoporosis include dietary modifications, physical activity, lifestyle modification, and fall prevention strategies [14–18].

Dietary Modifications
Proper nutrition is essential for the prevention and treatment of osteoporosis. A balanced diet, rich in key nutrients, can greatly enhance bone health and reduce the risk of fractures [14,19]. For individuals over the age of 50, it is recommended to consume 1200 mg of calcium per day. Calcium is crucial for maintaining strong bones and preventing bone loss, significantly impacting

Table 2
Summarizing evidence-based strategies for osteopenia and osteoporosis management

Category	Strategy	Key points
Lifestyle Modifications	Nutrition and diet	Calcium intake: 1000 mg/day (19–50 y), 1200 mg/day (>50 y) Vitamin D supplementation: 800–1000 IU/day
	Physical activity	Weight-bearing exercises and muscle-strengthening activities Balance and posture exercises to prevent falls
Pharmacologic Interventions	Biphosphonates	First-line treatment for osteoporosis Reduce fracture risk and inhibit bone resorption
	Selective estrogen receptor modulators	Raloxifene: reduces vertebral fracture risk, watch for thromboembolic events
	Monoclonal antibodies	Denosumab: Targets receptor activator of nuclear factor kappa-B ligand (RANKL), reduces bone resorption and fracture risk
Emerging Therapies	Romosozumab	Sclerostin inhibitor, promotes bone formation and inhibits resorption
	Teriparatide	Recombinant parathyroid hormone, stimulates bone formation
Multidisciplinary Approach	Regular monitoring and adherence	Multidisciplinary team involvement, monitor bone mineral density regularly Tailored interventions based on individual risk profiles
	Patient education and support	Importance of treatment adherence and lifestyle modifications

bone mineral density [14]. Good sources of calcium include dairy products, leafy green vegetables, and fortified foods [19].

Alongside calcium, vitamin D is vital for bone health as it aids in calcium absorption. Vitamin D deficiency has been shown to increase bone turnover and bone loss [14]. The optimal range for vitamin D intake is 800 to 1000 IU per day to improve bone health [14]. Vitamin D can be obtained from sunlight exposure, fatty fish, fortified dairy products, and supplements [20].

While calcium and vitamin D are critical, other nutrients also play significant roles in bone health. Magnesium is essential for bone formation and affects the concentrations of parathyroid hormone and the active form of vitamin D to maintain bone homeostasis [14,20]. Several studies have found positive associations between magnesium intake and bone mineral density in both men and women [14,20]. Sources of magnesium include nuts, seeds, whole grains, and green leafy vegetables [20].

Vitamin K deficiency is correlated with low BMD and an increased risk of bone fractures caused by osteoporosis [14,20]. Vitamin K can be found in green leafy vegetables such as kale and spinach, as well as in vegetable oils and some fruits [20].

Additionally, increased consumption of potassium has been shown to enhance bone mineral density [20]. Rich sources of potassium include fruits, vegetables, legumes, and potatoes [20].

By following these dietary guidelines, individuals can significantly improve their bone health, reduce the risk of osteoporosis and fractures associated with osteoporosis, and maintain an active and healthy lifestyle.

Physical Activity

It is recommended that those with osteoporosis and those trying to prevent osteoporosis should exercise for at least 30 minutes 3 times per week [17]. This recommendation is widely accepted despite the small effect that physical activity has on bone mineral density [17]. To date, there is no definitive exercise program for individuals with osteoporosis [15,16]. However, evidence increasingly supports a multimodal approach that incorporates various types of exercises and training. Resistance training and weight-bearing impact exercises are considered the most effective for reducing fracture risk by strengthening the musculoskeletal system [15–18].

Balance and mobility exercises are also highly recommended to enhance functionality and minimize the risk of falls [16,17]. Although low-impact aerobic activities like cycling or swimming have a limited effect on bone loss prevention, these aerobic exercises offer significant advantages for cardiovascular health, metabolic function, and body composition in individuals with osteoporosis [16]. Overall, the integration of individualized exercise plans has significant potential to reduce the morbidity and mortality of osteoporosis [18].

Lifestyle Modification

Lifestyle modifications are crucial for managing osteoporosis and improving bone health. Recommendations include smoking cessation, limiting alcohol, and maintaining a healthy weight. Nicotine, which is found in cigarettes, is known to cause peripheral vessel vasoconstriction, which is linked to the development of osteoporosis and delayed fracture healing [21]. Therefore, smoking cessation is recommended to prevent primary and secondary osteoporosis and its associated risks [21,22].

Similarly, it is recommended to avoid excessive alcohol intake. Increased alcohol intake has been associated with reduced calcium absorption and increases the risk of falls [22]. Therefore, LeBoff et al suggest limiting alcohol consumption to 2 drinks per day for women, and 3 drinks per day for men [22].

Fall Prevention Strategies

Fall prevention is crucial for individuals with osteoporosis, as most osteoporosis-related fractures result from falls [17]. Strategies for fall prevention include assessing for visual impairment, gait abnormalities, musculoskeletal impairment, and polypharmacy. Ensuring home safety is essential. The homes of individuals with osteoporosis should be evaluated and modified to reduce fall risk.

Recommended modifications include ensuring proper lighting, removing slippery surfaces, wearing low-heeled, rubber-soled, skid-free shoes, standing up slowly, and using assistive devices for walking as needed [23].

Monitoring and Follow-Up

The recommendations on routine follow-up for patients diagnosed with osteoporosis vary. According to LeBoff et al, clinicians should perform BMD testing 1 to 2 years after initiating or changing medical therapy for osteoporosis, and subsequently at appropriate intervals based on clinical circumstances [22]. They suggest that more frequent BMD testing may be necessary for individuals at higher risk for fractures, such as those with previous fractures, older age, or very low BMD. Conversely, less frequent BMD testing may be appropriate for patients with initial T-scores in the normal range, those with osteopenia, and those who have remained fracture-free while on treatment [22]. Kaiser Permenente has similar guidelines suggesting that those with no previous facture a T-score of -1.5 to -1.9, should repeat BMD testing in 5 years, while those with a -2.0 to -2.4 should repeat testing in 2 years [24].

For patients receiving pharmacologic treatment for osteoporosis, clinicians should routinely reassess the risk of fracture, patient satisfaction, adherence to therapy, and the need for continued or modified treatment [22,25]. Reassessment of the patient's BMD status and overall condition should include consideration of a drug holiday after 5 years of oral bisphosphonates or 3 years of intravenous bisphosphonates in patients who are no longer at high risk of fracture (T-score ≥ -2.5, no new fractures) [22,25]. This decision should be based on a comprehensive evaluation of the patient's fracture risk, including any new fractures, changes in BMD, and overall health status [22,25].

During each health care visit, clinicians should engage patients in discussions about their treatment, including any side effects or concerns. It is crucial to clearly explain the risk-benefit trade-offs, emphasizing that while the risk of adverse events is generally very low, the risk of fractures and their associated negative outcomes is significantly higher without treatment. Additionally, clinicians should provide continuous education on the importance of adhering to the prescribed therapy and adopting lifestyle modifications, such as a balanced diet and regular exercise, to support bone health.

Furthermore, clinicians should monitor patients for any signs of treatment-related complications or adverse effects, adjusting the treatment plan as needed. Regular follow-ups should be scheduled to review the patient's progress, address any issues, and make necessary adjustments to the treatment regimen. By maintaining an active and informed approach to osteoporosis management, clinicians can help optimize patient outcomes and reduce the risk of fractures.

Case study: osteopenia

History of presenting illness (HPI): BA is a 52-year-old white female (WF) with a past medical history of hypertension, depression, and migraines. She presents today for a routine annual physical. She reports that she has not had an annual physical or routine screening in several years. Her last mammogram, colonoscopy, and pap smear was more than 5 years ago, and she has never had a bone density screen. She denies any alcohol or illicit drug use, but does report a 40-year pack history. No history of prior fractures.

Review of systems (ROS): General: Denies fever, headache, fatigue, chills.
Endocrine: Denies intolerance to heat or cold, excessive thirst, or sweating.
Respiratory: Chronic cough. Denies any wheezing and shortness of breath.
Cardiovascular (CV): denies any chest pain, palpatations and edema.
Gastrointestinal/genitourinary (GI/GU): Denies any abdominal pain, nausea/ vomitting/diarrhea (NVD). LMP 10 years ago (status/post [S/P] complete hysterectomy)
Musculoskeletal: Denies any back pain, joint pain, muscle aches. Any previous fractures.
Neuro: Denies any dizziness, fainting, lightheadedness.

Physical exam (PE): Vitals Wt: 129 lbs, Ht: 60 in, BMI: 25.19, Blood Pressure: 124/84, Temp: 97.3, HR: 89, and O2: 98%
Physical examination is normal.

Diagnostics: Mammogram–normal, Pap smear–normal, Colonoscopy–normal
DXA Bone Densitiometry
Lumbar Spine L1: *BMD* 0.766 gm/sq cm, *T-Score*–2.0
Lumbar Spine L2: *BMD* 0.796 gm/sq cm, *T-Score*–2.1
Lumbar Spine L3: *BMD* 0.828 gm/sq cm, *T-Score*–2.3
Lumbar Spine L4: *BMD* 0.865 gm/sq cm, *T-Score*–1.8
Lumbar Spine: *BMD* 0.816 gm/sq cm, *T-Score*–2.1
Left Femoral Neck: *BMD* 0.608 gm/sq cm, *T-Score*–2.2
Left Total Hip: *BMD* 0.744 gm/sq cm, *T-Score*–1.6
Right Femoral Neck: *BMD* 0.608 gm/sq cm, *T-Score*–2.2
Right Total Hip: *BMD* 0.744 gm/sq cm, *T-Score*–1.6

Differentials

Osteopenic bone mineral density
Osteoporotic bone mineral density

Treatment

Based on her FRAX score, BA would have a low to moderate estimated fracture risk. For most patients with a low to moderate chance of a fragility fracture, pharmacologic therapies are not generally recommended to prevent bone loss or fractures. Instead, treatment decisions are based on what each person prefers and considering the benefits and possible risks of the medications.

Patient Education

Lifestyle modifications are imperative to improve bone health and prevent further bone loss.

Calcium and Vitamin D: Consume or supplement with about 1200 mg of calcium with Vitamin D per day.

Healthy Diet: Eat a well-balanced diet with enough calories to avoid malnutrition.

Exercise: Postmenopausal women should do weight-bearing exercises, like walking or jogging, for at least 30 minutes most days of the week. Also, include muscle-strengthening and posture exercises 2 to 3 days a week.

Smoking Cessation: Avoid cigarette smoking as it speeds up bone loss.

Limit Alcohol: Avoid excessive alcohol intake.

Fall prevention: BA should have regular eye examinations; ensure to avoid slippery surfaces and other interventions to prevent falls. Long-term use of glucocorticoids should be avoided, if possible.

SUMMARY

Osteopenia and osteoporosis is a current health challenge facing older adults in the United States. It is important for providers to be up to date on current screening algorithms and management. This equips patients with knowledge to stay on top of bone density screenings. Referral to a specialist may be necessary, but often these conditions can be treated in primary care. Educating patients and promoting health promotion is important in clinical practice as it will decrease further bone mineral demineralization. Together we can improve the overall health promotion of our aging population and decrease fracture risk.

CLINICS CARE POINTS

- Prevalence of osteoporosis and osteopenia is increasing in the United States.
- Providers need to ensure they are adequately screening patients for bone loss.
- Dual-energy X-ray absorptiometry helps classify bone health status and guide clinical decision-making regarding prevention and treatment strategies.
- Pharmacologic treatment options include bisphosphonates, selective estrogen receptor modulators, and monoclonal antibodies.
- Lifestyle changes that can aid in bone loss progression are dietary changes, increased physical activity, and fall prevention.

Disclosure

The authors have nothing to disclose.

References

[1] Cosman F, de Beur SJ, LeBoff MS, et al. Clinician's guide to prevention and treatment of osteoporosis. Osteoporos Int 2020;31(7):1193–208.

[2] Bone health and osteoporosis: a report of the surgeon general. Office of the Surgeon General (US): U.S. Department of Health and Human Services; 2020.

[3] Compston JE, McClung MR, Leslie WD. Osteoporosis. Lancet 2019;393(10169): 364–76.

[4] Eastell R, Rosen CJ, Black DM, et al. Pharmacological management of osteoporosis in postmenopausal women: an Endocrine Society clinical practice guideline. J Clin Endocrinol Metabol 2020;105(3):e1–46.

[5] Harvey NC, Odén A, Orwoll E, et al. Falls predict fractures independently of FRAX probability: a meta-analysis of the osteoporotic fractures in men (MrOS) study. J Bone Miner Res 2018;33(3):510–6.

[6] Sornay-Rendu E, Duboeuf F, Chapurlat RD. Postmenopausal women with normal BMD who have fractures have deteriorated bone microarchitecture: a prospective analysis from the OFELY study. Bone 2024;182:117072:Epub 2024 Mar 15. PMID: 38492712.

[7] Silva BC, Broy SB, Boutroy S, et al. Fracture risk prediction by non-BMD DXA Measures: the 2015 ISCD official positions part trabecular bone score. J Clin Densitom 2017;20(3): 290–307.

[8] National Osteoporosis Foundation. Clinician's guide to prevention and treatment of osteoporosis. 2021. Available at: https://www.nof.org/.

[9] Kanis JA, McCloskey EV, Johansson H, et al. European guidance for the diagnosis and management of osteoporosis in postmenopausal women. Osteoporos Int 2019;30(1):3–44.

[10] Eastell R, Rosen CJ, Black DM, et al. Pharmacological management of osteoporosis in postmenopausal women: an Endocrine Society clinical practice guideline. J Clin Endocrinol Metabol 2019;104(5):1595–622.

[11] Endocrine Society. Endocrine Society clinical practice guideline on vitamin D deficiency. J Clin Endocrinol Metabol 2020;105(5):e42–5.

[12] Hauer K, Lamb SE, Jorstad EC, et al. Systematic review of definitions and methods of balance and falls in older adults. J Am Geriatr Soc 2016;53(5):728–38.

[13] Pickering ME, Javier RM, Malochet S, et al. Osteoporosis treatment and pain relief: a scoping review. Eur J Pain 2024;28(1):3–20.

[14] Hejazi J, Davoodi A, Khosravi M, et al. Nutrition and osteoporosis prevention and treatment. Biomed Res Therapy 2020;7(4):3709–20.

[15] Pinheiro MB, Oliveira J, Bauman A, et al. Evidence on physical activity and osteoporosis prevention for people aged 65+ years: a systematic review to inform the WHO guidelines on physical activity and sedentary behaviour. Int J Behav Nutr Phys Activ 2020;17:150.

[16] Marini S, Barone G, Masini A, et al. The effect of physical activity on bone biomarkers in people with osteoporosis: a systematic review. Front Endocrinol 2020;11; https://doi.org/10.3389/fendo.2020.585689.

[17] Anam AK, Insogna K. Update on osteoporosis screening and management. Med Clin 2021;105(6):1117–34.

[18] Bae S, Lee S, Park H, et al. Position statement: exercise guidelines for osteoporosis management and fall prevention in osteoporosis patients. J Bone Metabol 2023;30(2):149–65.

[19] Healthy Living. Calcium: shopping list. US department of health and human services. Office of disease prevention and health promotion. 2023. Available at: https://health.gov/my healthfinder/healthy-living/nutrition/calcium-shopping-list#:~:text=Onegoodwaytoget, absorb(takein)calcium.

[20] Strengthening Knowledge and Understanding of Dietary Supplements. Vitamin D Fact Sheet for Consumers. National Institutes of Health. Office of Dietary Supplements. 2022. Available at: https://ods.od.nih.gov/factsheets/VitaminD-Consumer/#:~:text=VitaminDisaddedto, smallamountsofvitaminD.

[21] Kiyota Y, Muramatsu H, Sato Y, et al. Smoking cessation increases levels of osteocalcin and uncarboxylated osteocalcin in human sera. Sci Rep 2020;10(1):16845.

[22] LeBoff MS, Greenspan SL, Insogna KL, et al. The clinician's guide to prevention and treatment of osteoporosis. Osteoporos Int 2022;33(10):2049–102.

[23] Bhatnagar A, Kekatpure AL. Postmenopausal osteoporosis: a literature review. Cureus 2022;14(9):e29367.

[24] Osteoporosis Screening, Diagnosis, and Treatment Guideline. Kaiser permanente. 2022. Available at: https://wa.kaiserpermanente.org/static/pdf/public/guidelines/osteoporosis. pdf.

[25] Morin SN, Feldman S, Funnell L, et al, Osteoporosis Canada 2023 Guideline Update Group. Clinical practice guideline for management of osteoporosis and fracture prevention in Canada: 2023 update. Can Med Assoc J 2023;195(39):E1333–48.

[26] The University of Sheffield. Fracture risk assessment tool - FRAX ®- University of Sheffield. 2024. Available at: https://frax.shef.ac.uk/frax/tool.aspx?country=9.

Advances in Family Practice Nursing 7 (2025) 139–157

ADVANCES IN FAMILY PRACTICE NURSING

Episiotomy
Indications, Techniques, and Postpartum Care Considerations

Sharon L. Holley, DNP, CNM[a],*,
Sarah E. Barton, DNP, CNM, C-EFM[b],
Mary Catherine Carpenter, MSN, CNM[c]

[a]Nurse-Midwifery Pathway, School of Nursing, University of Alabama at Birmingham, 1701 University Boulevard, NB 580, Birmingham, AL 35233-1815, USA; [b]Certified Nurse-Midwife (Private Practice), Rutland Women's Health, Rutland, VT, USA; [c]Certified Nurse-Midwife (Private Practice), MaineHealth, 64 Knox Street, Thomaston, ME 04861, USA

Keywords

- Episiotomy • Obstetric anal sphincter injuries • Perineal trauma • Informed consent
- Vaginal tears • Midline episiotomy • Mediolateral episiotomy • Postpartum care

Key points

- *Restrictive use recommended*: Major health organizations recommend against routine episiotomy due to increased severe perineal injury risks, advocating restrictive use based on specific clinical indications.
- *Informed consent and shared decision-making*: Obtain informed consent before episiotomy. Discuss risks and benefits prior to labor to respect patient autonomy and ensure ethical practice.
- *Types of episiotomies*: Midline episiotomies are easier to repair but risk severe lacerations. Mediolateral episiotomies are harder to repair but less likely to cause severe lacerations.
- *Complications and postpartum care*: Episiotomy can cause trauma, blood loss, pain, dyspareunia, infection, and wound breakdown. Proper postpartum care, including inspection and pain management, is crucial for recovery.

INTRODUCTION

Episiotomy is defined as a controlled surgical incision in the perineum performed during the second stage of labor to enlarge the vaginal opening just prior to a vaginal birth of the fetus [1–4]. This increases the size of the vaginal

*Corresponding author. E-mail address: sharonholley@uab.edu

https://doi.org/10.1016/j.yfpn.2025.01.004

Abbreviations

FGM   female genital mutilation
NSAID   nonsteroidal anti-inflammatory drug
OASIS   Obstetric anal sphincter injuries
WHO   World Health Organization

outlet. It has been used in an attempt to decrease second stage pushing efforts and to reduce the incidence of severe perineal trauma, 3rd and 4th degree lacerations, also known as Obstetric anal sphincter injuries (OASIS) [5], There is a belief that uncontrolled lacerations can lead to possible extensions, and be more difficult to repair [6,7]. Incidence of episiotomy varies geographically, and rates range from as low as 1% to as high as 90% [5]. There are 7 types of episiotomies described in the literature; however, the 2 types most commonly described in the literature are the midline, also known as median, and the mediolateral [1]. The technique used most frequently in the United States and Canada is the midline episiotomy whereas the mediolateral is more commonly performed in Europe [2,4].

Episiotomy was used commonly during the 20th century based on the belief that it prevents pelvic floor relaxation, cystoceles, and other pelvic floor injury to the fetal head by reducing the pressure on the perineum and preventing vaginal lacerations as the fetal head and body emerges through the introitus [7–9]. More recent studies have demonstrated that routine use should be avoided as it is associated with an increased risk for severe perineal laceration, is linked to over-medicalization, and the decision to perform is often financially driven rather than by the indications of the patient [2,10,11].

RECOMMENDATION AGAINST ROUTINE USE

In 1996 the World Health Organization (WHO) recommended use of episiotomy should not exceed 10% [5]. Episiotomy has been one of the most frequent interventions during childbirth. It was theorized that the wound created would be easier to repair than one that occurred spontaneously. This has since been refuted, and restrictive use of episiotomy has been shown to lower the risk of severe perineal trauma [12]. A Cochrane Review in 2017 concluded that routine episiotomy is associated with an increased risk of severe perineal lacerations [12]. However, when a policy of selective use was implemented, there was a 30% reduction in severe perineal trauma as compared to a routine episiotomy policy [10]. Episiotomy increases the risk for 3rd and 4th degree lacerations, as well as postpartum hemorrhage and has not been found to protect against OASIS [4]. Routine use of episiotomy is associated with an increase in severe perineal injury, additional morbidity that may impact patient healing, and long-term well-being. Its use is linked to over-medicalization, which drives up cost with an unnecessary intervention.

Consequently, birth providers should not routinely perform an episiotomy, but rather use a restricted policy and consider risk factors when deciding to perform this procedure [4,11,13].

INDICATIONS FOR EPISIOTOMY

The American College of Obstetrics and Gynecology and the International Federation of Gynecology and Obstetrics both recommend restrictive use of episiotomy [4,14]. Indications should be based on the need to expedite delivery such as category III fetal heart rate patterns suggesting the fetus is at risk for newborn acidemia [9]. Other considerations include, but are not limited to, prolonged second stage, rigid perineum, short perineal body, history of advanced perineal tear, preterm birth, intravaginal band, a history of female genital mutilation (FGM), breech vaginal birth, fetal macrosomia, shoulder dystocia, need to facilitate the birth of a compromised fetus, or operative vaginal birth [9,15,16]. Classifications of degree of vaginal tears, or lacerations, are listed in Table 1.

RISK FACTORS

Risk factors for an episiotomy, regardless of parity, include advanced gestational age, regional analgesia, meconium-stained fluid, increased birth weight, and mother or sister with OASIS [4,18]. A meta-analysis published in 2020

Table 1
Classification of vaginal tears

Classification	Definition	Additional information
First degree	Involves the vaginal mucosa and perineal skin with no underlying tissue involvement [6].	
Second degree	Includes underlying subcutaneous tissue and perineal muscles [6].	
Third degree	The anal sphincter musculature is involved in the tear [6].	Can be further broken down based on the total area of anal sphincter involvement: 3a is <50% external anal sphincter involvement 3b is >50% external anal sphincter involvement 3c involves external and internal anal sphincter but is not fully extended through the rectal muscle into rectal mucosa [17].
Fourth degree	The tear extends through the rectal muscle into rectal mucosa [6].	

found additional risk factors included instrument facilitated birth, and persistent occiput posterior presentation of the fetal head [19]. Nulliparae have been found to have additional risk factors including birthing a male fetus and having an induction of labor. Multiparae factors include higher maternal age, and shoulder dystocia. Protective factors include lower maternal age, and previous vaginal birth [8].

COMPLICATIONS FOLLOWING EPISIOTOMY

Immediately following episiotomy potential complications include additional perineal trauma, including OASIS, blood loss, and pain. Postpartum risks include dyspareunia, infection, and wound breakdown. Long-term complications include scarring, increased risk of OASIS in subsequent vaginal births, and possible dyspareunia within the first year or 2 following birth [4,9,10]. The inherent risk of wound complications following OASIS repair is significant and may be exacerbated by factors such as missed diagnoses, improper repair techniques, and the primary surgeon's lack of experience. Therefore, it is crucial for the birth attendant to be proficient in accurately identifying and repairing various types of perineal trauma to ensure optimal short-term and long-term outcomes [20].

INFORMED CONSENT

Ideally, discussing the need for a possible episiotomy should be done prior to labor using shared decision-making, raising awareness of possible indications and risks, should this procedure become necessary. Even if not discussed before labor, informed consent should always be obtained prior to performing an episiotomy in the birth setting to ensure that the basic ethical principle of autonomy is upheld. The discussion about the need for an episiotomy to expedite birth may occur under urgent conditions such as prolonged fetal heart rate decelerations and present limited opportunity for in-depth discussion on the risks and benefits but all efforts to avoid coercive communication should be employed. If the fully informed patient then declines, respectful discussion of alternative options should be reviewed.

Ultimately consent is required for an episiotomy and if refused cannot be performed. In this situation, alternatives should be pursued to assure the best outcome for mother and infant. All conversations regarding episiotomy, including indication, risks, benefits, alternatives, and the patient decision should be thoroughly documented in the medical record. Informed consents as compared to shared decision-making are listed in Table 2.

TIMING OF AN EPISIOTOMY

There is little evidence regarding the best time to perform an episiotomy. Carrying out this procedure too soon may result in unnecessary blood loss. Conversely waiting too long until the perineum is bulging and thinned out may contribute to an abrupt uncontrolled birth with extension of the original episiotomy or additional lacerations. Some obstetric providers recommend

Table 2
Informed consent versus shared decision-making

	Definition	Criteria that must Be met	Responsibility of the healthcare provider
Informed Consent	Informed consent is a principle in medical ethics and medical law that a patient should have sufficient information before making their own free decisions about their medical care [21].	Criteria that must be met: 1. The patient must be competent. 2. The patient must be adequately informed. 3. The patient must not be coerced.	The provider must give enough information about the diagnosis and treatment or procedure including risks, benefits, alternatives, and what might happen by doing nothing in order that the patient may make an informed voluntary decision. This is often given both verbally, as well as in writing [21].
Shared Decision-Making	Shared decision-making occurs when patients and their health care providers work together with key objectives to provide person-centered care and to maximize patient autonomy with regard to making health care decisions [22].		

performing the incision when birth is expected imminently, and the fetal head remains crowning without retracting between contractions. When the fetal head is well-applied to the perineum, this will often tamponade the area and lead to decreased bleeding as compared to if the incision is performed too early.

CLASSIFICATION OF EPISIOTOMY TYPES

The 7 classifications include midline (median and medial), modified median, mediolateral, J-shaped, lateral, radical lateral, and anterior and are listed in Table 3. Currently, 2 are more commonly described in the literature: mediolateral and midline.

PERINEAL ANATOMY

The perineum is comprised of multiple layers of muscles, ligaments, and connective tissue, inferior to which lies the anal sphincter complex and is identified in Fig. 1 below [32]. The pelvic floor, otherwise known as pelvic diaphragm, is a complex muscular structure including the levator ani and coccygeus muscles. Levator ani muscle's function is a key to the support of the pelvic floor; it has multiple different muscles with different origins and insertions. Muscles included in the levator ani group include pubococcygeus, puborectalis, and iliococcygeus muscles. The pubococcygeus muscle is further broken down into 3 separate areas: pubovaginalis, puboperinealis, and puboanalis. Pubovaginalis is u-shaped and wraps around the vaginal introitus; these muscle fibers are responsible for elevating the urethra during vaginal contraction despite no direct connection to it and likely contribute to urinary continence. Puboperinealis attach to the perineal body and pull the complete perineal structure upwards toward the pubic symphysis. Puboanalis's fibers lie between the internal and external anal sphincters; it is a key in elevating the anus and supporting the contraction of the urogenital hiatus. Puborectalis is a u-shaped muscle around the anal rectal junction this muscle is also included in the anal sphincter complex. Iliococcygeus is the most posterior muscle of the levator ani, passing behind the rectum attaching to the coccyx. It is unlikely to be affected in the event of laceration or episiotomy due to its location.

The bulbocavernosus muscle attaches to the central tendinous point and surrounds the vaginal introitus covering the Bartholin glands. When a midline, or median, episiotomy is performed the bulbocavernosus and superficial transverse perineal muscles are separated. If this is a deeper cut, it may additionally separate the deep transverse perineal muscle. When a mediolateral episiotomy is performed, the bulbocavernosus, superficial, deep transverse perineal muscles, and levator ani muscle are separated [33].

PERFORMING AN EPISIOTOMY

Prior to cutting an episiotomy, good management of pain should be obtained. This can be achieved using a variety of options including nitrous oxide at the bedside, an epidural, infiltration of 1% Lidocaine without epinephrine to the

Table 3
Types of episiotomies

Name	How incision is Performed	Angle of Incision	Advantages	Disadvantages
Midline Also *known as* Median or Medial	The incision is performed starting at the posterior fourchette, the vaginal apex, runs anterior to posterior (midline) through the central tendon of the perineal body and then proceeds separating the bulbocavernosus and superficial transverse perineal muscles [2]. Depending on the depth of the cut, the deep transverse perineal muscle may also be cut into 2 sides. The perineal apex is above the anal sphincter, with the incision extending to roughly half the length of the perineum [2].	The pre-birth incision angle from midline should be between 0–25° of the sagittal plane [2].	The primary advantages include ease of repair and better cosmetic results. Postpartum pain may be less than mediolateral episiotomies; however, prospective studies have not found a significant difference. Using this technique also avoids risk of incising the Bartholin's gland and duct [23].	Increased risk of extension into a 3rd or 4th degree laceration as compared to a mediolateral episiotomy. This is due to the inferior apex of the midline episiotomy being created directly above the rectal sphincter [9].

(continued on next page)

Table 3
(continued)

Name	How incision is Performed	Angle of Incision	Advantages	Disadvantages
Mediolateral	The incision starts at or 3 mm laterally from the midline from the midline vaginal apex at the central tendinous point of the perineum and is then cut laterally, right, or left, and downwards away from the rectum cutting through the bulbocavernosus and the superficial and deep transverse perineal muscles, into the pubococcygeus (levator ani) muscle [2]. The points of the scissors directed right or left toward the ischial tuberosity on the same side as the incision [9].	The pre-birth incision angle should be at 60° away from the midline to achieve a post-birth suture angle of 45° [2,4,24].	The primary advantage is fewer extensions into 3rd or 4th degree lacerations occur compared to midline episiotomies. May be protective of OASIS, particularly with use of instrument assisted vaginal births for nulliparous patients [25,26].	Some studies have found mediolateral is associated with more blood loss; others have not. Potential risk of injury to the Bartholin's gland and duct if performed incorrectly. Compared to midline episiotomies, mediolateral episiotomies can be more challenging to repair, and distortion of the site may occur during repair if suturing is done horizontally like is done with repair of a medial episiotomy. Correct repair of a mediolateral episiotomy should follow a diagonal slant along the line of the incision and, the superior side of the incision has a larger area of exposed tissue than the inferior side, requiring larger bites of tissue superiorly when suturing [9].

| Modified median | A median episiotomy that is modified at the end by adding 2 transverse incisions in opposite directions just above the expected location of the anal sphincter so that it creates an inverted "T-shape". | | The diameter of the vaginal outlet is increased by 83% when compared to the median episiotomy due to the separation of the perineal membrane/sphincter attachments, and so allows true posterior displacement of the anus with no risk of any resultant traction injury [2,27,28]. |
| J-shaped | This episiotomy is a modification of the midline but with a J-shape. | The perineum is incised at the apex of the fourchette but then instead of going toward the anus the incision is redirected and curved laterally to avoid the anus. After the 40-degree angle is made the incision is continued another 2–2.5 cm and away from the anus [2,21]. | Using this angle is thought to prevent the development of a 3rd or 4th degree laceration. | Suturing the J-shaped episiotomy is difficult due to the shape of the opposing edges not being straight and this can lead to tissue sheering and a puckered suture line following repair. Therefore it is not commonly used [21]. |

(continued on next page)

Table 3
(continued)

Name	How incision is Performed	Angle of Incision	Advantages	Disadvantages
Lateral	This type of incision is started in the vaginal introitus 1–2 cm lateral to the midline and is directed downwards toward the ischial tuberosity [2]. Lateral episiotomy is rarely described in the obstetric literature and is rarely used except in Finland [2,7,29].	The incision is started laterally 1–2 cm from the midline of the vaginal introitus and goes downward ischial tuberosity [2].		This type of episiotomy has a higher risk of damaging the Bartholin's gland and duct related to the position and angle the incision is made therefore this type is no longer used.
Radical lateral *Also known as* Schuchardt incision	This type of episiotomy is often not considered an obstetric incision.	The incision is a fully extended deep into one vaginal sulcus and is curved downward and laterally to around the side of the rectum.	It may be performed at the beginning of radical vaginal hysterectomy or trachelectomy to allow access to the parametrium, to assist with extraction of a vaginal pessary or, during childbirth in complicated deliveries such as a large fetal head, breech fetal presentation, or assist with correction of shoulder dystocia [2].	

Anterior *Also known as* Deinfibulation	The opening during delivery of the scar associated with some degrees of previously performed female genital mutilation. It should be noted that it is possible that a second type of perineal episiotomy may be required during childbirth.	The practitioner's finger is inserted through the introitus and directed toward the pubis. To free the scar, fused labia minora are incised in the midline until the external urethral meatus can be seen and the anterior flap is completely open. The clitoral remnants should not be incised [30,31].

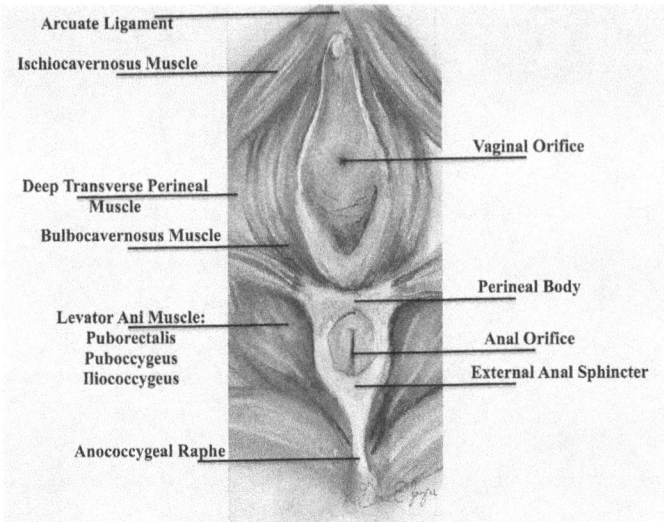

Fig. 1. Perineal anatomy. (*Courtesy of* Grace Elizabeth Joyner, BFA, MS, LPCAT.)

area. Intravenous or intramuscular narcotics may be considered in situations where pain is unmanageable by other means.

When an episiotomy must be cut, evidence indicates that a mediolateral episiotomy cut at a crowning angle of 60° decreases risk of OASIS, particularly when vacuum or forceps are used [10,24]. Previous studies have demonstrated that when an episiotomy is performed during crowning of the fetal head the starting angle of the episiotomy is greater than the angle of the resulting incision due to the perineal degree of distortion. For example, an episiotomy performed starting 40° from the midline of the posterior fourchette will result in an incision angle of 20°, and an episiotomy angle performed at 60° would result in an incision angle of 45° [24]. The angle of the incision following birth is ultimately more important than the angle pre-birth; therefore, it is critical to understand the correct angle to cut each type of episiotomy and perform the smallest necessary episiotomy [34,35].

Once the episiotomy is cut, the clinician should continue to apply gentle pressure to the fetal head to control and direct a slow extension of the head. This will help avoid a rapid birth, sudden pressure on the perineum, and extension of the incision. Pressure on the wound to control bleeding may also be required between maternal pushing efforts.

REPAIR OF EPISIOTOMY

A thorough evaluation of perineal trauma should be conducted following every vaginal birth. Prior to the examination, or repair, it is important to inform the patient about the necessity and purpose of the examination [20]. Repair of an episiotomy is not unlike that of a spontaneous laceration. It is crucial to have the supplies gathered and accessible prior to birth. A prompt thorough assessment of the wound should be made immediately allowing for early consultation with a provider experienced and privileged in repair of 3rd and 4th degree perineal injuries. Repair requires adequate lighting and patient positioning. A digital rectal examination should be performed for significant wounds to allow thorough assessment of OASIS [32]. Patient comfort can also be determined at this point and allow the clinician to assess the need for additional pain management.

Pain management should be achieved if needed prior to repair. 20 mL of 1% Lidocaine without epinephrine should be available for use. Initial injections should be placed at the exterior edge of the wound and continue to the apex, always withdrawing prior to injecting to assure the needle has not entered a vessel. Generally, delays in repair should be avoided to minimize blood loss, decrease discomfort and risk of infection; however, a brief delay of 3 to 5 minutes to allow the best effect from lidocaine is recommended.

Episiotomies with complex lacerations or brisk bleeding may require the help of an assistant to allow good visualization and speed up wound closure [32]. Maternal habitus and comfort level may also necessitate the use of an assistant. Use of a radio-opaque tampon or lap sponge will control uterine blood flow if needed and may allow for improved visualization and quicker repair.

Rapidly absorbing synthetic suture should be used to decrease short-term perineal pain [32]; 2.0 and 3.0 diameter sutures are appropriate for closure of obstetric wounds. The anchoring stitch needs to be 0.5 cm above apex. Closure of the vaginal wall is accomplished with continuous non-locking stitches to the hymnal ring. These should approximate the edges and provide hemostasis while left loose enough to accommodate postpartum edema. This run of suture will end at introitus and ideally the same suture can be passed through the vaginal wall to complete the repair.

The repair of the perineal body including the bulbocavernosus muscle is then begun. Closure of this space starts with a secure crown stitch in the bulbocavernosus muscle and then closure is accomplished with a running barber pole stitch of the perineal tissue. The dead space should then be eliminated, and the superficial closure can begin. Final closure starts at the perineal edge of the wound with subcuticular stitches ending at the introitus. Suture should be securely knotted, and suture left loose enough to accommodate swelling while still approximating the edges. This is often the most uncomfortable part of the repair. It has been suggested that an adhesive may also provide adequate closure of this portion of the repair while decreasing pain and repair time [32]. Most repairs can be completed in 25 minutes.

Patients with episiotomies that extend to 3rd and 4th degree injuries should receive a dose of antibiotics and this can be started while waiting for the consultant to arrive for repair [32]. Repairing a 3rd and 4th degree laceration is beyond the scope of this article and would require additional training beyond Core Competencies to request privileges in most institutional settings.

DOCUMENTATION
Documentation of the procedure should be included within the delivery summary and provide the following information:

1. Informed consent
2. Description of the type of episiotomy performed
3. The classification of the laceration
4. Any additional lacerations or extensions
5. Type of suture used
6. Technique used for repair
7. Any lacerations left unrepaired and if they are bleeding or not
8. Pain management used, and how the patient tolerated the repair

SPECIAL CONSIDERATIONS
Short perineal body
Perineal body is defined as the area between the posterior of the fourchette and the mid-anus. Shortened length of perineum, less than 3 cm, has been suspected to increase risk of perineal trauma, which has led to the suggestion that episiotomy should be used in this circumstance to reduce this risk of OASIS [29]. Komorowski and colleagues (2014) found in their study of 448 births no correlation between length of perineum and degree of perineal trauma [36]. A perineal body length of ≤ 3.0 cm combined with episiotomy resulted in a substantially higher rate of third-degree and fourth-degree lacerations [37]. Given this evidence along with the referenced recommendations of the WHO, an episiotomy is not recommended as a routine intervention for patients with a short perineal body for the purpose of preventing perineal trauma [11].

Female genital mutilation
FGM, also known as female circumcision, is defined by WHO (2020) as the partial or total removal of external female genitalia or other injury to the female genitalia organs for non-medical reasons. WHO (2020) states there are 4 types of FGM. The scope of this article will not go in depth regarding type of FGM; however, it is important to consider that caring for patients with FGM Type III may warrant further training beyond that which is received in education programs. Therefore, it is recommended to refer the patient to a provider who is proficient in anterior episiotomy technique, most likely an obstetrical-gynecological physician, at the beginning of the third trimester. In settings where there is a high incidence of FGM, it may be beneficial to have proficiency in all types of episiotomies to prevent sequelae. There are 4 types of FGM described and are identified in Table 4.

Equity
There is the consideration of equity of care, particularly regarding interventions during the time of labor and birth. One study with 2490 participants, found Black patients reported significantly more nonconsensual perinatal procedures than any other identified minority by race, including episiotomy,

Table 4
Categories of female genital mutilation

Name	Definition	Types	Additional Information
Type I	Partial or total removal of the clitoris and/or the prepuce (clitoridectomy) [38]	Type I a: Removal of the clitoral hood or prepuce only Type I b: Removal of the clitoris with the prepuce [38]	Anterior episiotomy was the most protective against third- and fourth-degree lacerations specific to Type III or infibulation. Anterior episiotomy was compared with posterior lateral and a combination of both posterior lateral and anterior performed together. All types of episiotomies with this type of FGM have been found to be protective against postpartum hemorrhage [39].
Type II	Partial or total removal of the clitoral glans and the labia minora, with or without removal of the labia majora [38]	Type II a: Removal of the labia minora only Type II b: Partial or total removal of the clitoris and the labia minora Type II c: Partial or total removal of the clitoris, the labia minora and the labia majora [38]	
Type III	Infibulation - the narrowing of the vaginal opening through the creation of a covering seal. The seal is formed by cutting and repositioning the labia minora, or labia majora, sometimes through stitching, with or without the addition of Type 1 FGM [38]		
Type IV	Includes all other harmful procedures to the female genitalia for non-medical purposes, for example, pricking, piercing, incising, scraping, and cauterizing the genital area [38].		

artificial rupture of membranes, and prophylactic IV medications [40]. Particular attention should be paid to use of informed care, particularly with those who identify as Black, indigenous, or people of color (BIPOC) to give their consent for perinatal procedures including [10].

Financial

Some providers may be motivated by increased financial reimbursement in their decision to perform an episiotomy [11]. Conversely, an episiotomy should not be avoided based solely on the cost of performing it. In other words, the decision to perform or not perform should be made with the individual clinical situation at hand and not be influenced by financial reimbursement.

Cultural

The WHO document on Positive Birth Experiences notes that some cultures hold the belief that performing an episiotomy will facilitate a shorter labor and birth and is therefore culturally accepted whereas other cultures are more reluctant to accept an episiotomy [11]. This requires an understanding of the expectations of a given population and then having an informed conversation, preferably prior to labor and birth.

POSTPARTUM CARE

During the first 24 to 48 hours the perineum should be visually inspected at least twice daily to ensure there is no excessive bleeding, formation of a hematoma, or improper healing. Pain management can often be accomplished using nonsteroidal anti-inflammatory drugs (NSAID) medication such as Ibuprofen. However, if there is a third-degree or fourth-degree laceration, then use of short-term opiates is often helpful, but then should move toward use of the NSAIDs. Additionally, with third-degree or fourth-degree lacerations use of stool softeners and oral laxatives should be offered on a schedule to avoid constipation, particularly the first week following birth [20].

LONG-TERM EFFECTS OF EPISIOTOMY

The long-term effects of episiotomy are difficult to assess. What information we do have is a product of research into pelvic floor deficits including prolapse, urinary and fecal incontinence, and those have yielded mixed results. Research into the long-term psychologic impact of episiotomy and other birth trauma is in its infancy and primarily qualitative. While there is evidence to demonstrate that patients who have had a routine episiotomy are more likely to have pain with intercourse in the months following giving birth, and are slower to resume sexual intercourse, than those who had restricted use of episiotomy, there is no evidence that episiotomy is associated with long-term impact on dyspareunia or pelvic pain [4].

SUMMARY

The decision to perform an episiotomy should be based on individual circumstances rather than a routine policy and must include documented informed consent. The purpose is to prevent OASIS injury or expedite the second-stage of labor when there is concern for fetal acidemia. While there are 7 types of episiotomies described in the literature, 2 are used more frequently: median and mediolateral. Pain management should be achieved prior to cutting or repairing an episiotomy and suturing should leave good cosmetic results.

Implications for practice
Implications for practice include the following items:

a. Emphasize the importance of informed consent and shared decision-making to respect patient autonomy and ensure ethical practice. Discuss the potential need for an episiotomy with patients prior to labor whenever possible.
b. Adhere to guidelines recommending restrictive use of episiotomy, reserving the procedure for specific clinical indications such as category III fetal heart rate patterns, prolonged second stage, or other risk factors.
c. Ensure that birth attendants are proficient in identifying and repairing various types of perineal trauma. Adequate training in episiotomy techniques and repair is crucial to minimize complications and improve outcomes.
d. Implement thorough postpartum care protocols, including regular inspection of the perineum, effective pain management, and the use of stool softeners for severe lacerations. This helps in early detection and management of complications.
e. Further research into the long-term implications of episiotomy, including the impact on pelvic floor health and sexual function is needed. Educate health care providers on the latest evidence-based practices to improve patient outcomes.

The long-term effects of episiotomy are unknown, largely because they are unstudied. We have found no research on the long-term impact of episiotomy on sexuality. As clinicians, we owe it to ourselves and our patients to undertake the necessary research identifying the evidence-based indications, the safest technique and repair, as well as the short-term and long-term implications of this surgical intervention in childbirth.

CLINICS CARE POINTS

- Selective Indications: Perform episiotomy based on specific clinical indications such as fetal distress, prolonged second stage, or rigid perineum, rather than as a routine procedure.
- Informed Consent: Always obtain informed consent prior to performing an episiotomy. Discuss potential risks, benefits, and alternatives with the patient.
- Optimal Timing: Perform episiotomy when the fetal head is crowning and the perineum is bulging to minimize blood loss and additional lacerations.
- Pain Management: Ensure adequate pain management before performing and repairing an episiotomy. Options include local anesthesia, nitrous oxide, or epidural.
- Postpartum Monitoring: Monitor for complications such as infection, wound breakdown, and dyspareunia. Provide appropriate postpartum care and support to promote healing and comfort.

- Patient Education: Educate patients on postpartum care, including signs of infection, proper wound care, and when to seek medical attention. Encourage open communication about any concerns or symptoms.

Disclosure

The authors have nothing to disclose.

References

[1] Carroli G, Mignini L. Episiotomy for vaginal birth. Cochrane Database Syst Rev 2009;1: CD000081.

[2] Kalis V, Laine K, de Leeuw J, et al. Classification of episiotomy: towards a standardization of terminology. BJOG 2012;119(5):522–6.

[3] Goueslard K, Cottenet J, Roussot A, et al. How did episiotomy rates change from 2007 to 2014? Population-based study in France. BMC Pregnancy Childbirth 2018;18(1):208, PMID: 29866103; PMCID: PMC5987447.

[4] American College of Obstetricians and Gynecologists (ACOG). Practice Bulletin No. 165: prevention and management of obstetrical lacerations at vaginal delivery. Obstet Gynecol 2016;128:e1–15.

[5] Laine K, Yli BM, Cole V, et al. European guidelines on perinatal care- Peripartum care Episiotomy. J Matern Fetal Neonatal Med 2021;12:1–6.

[6] K Barjon, H. Mahdy, Episiotomy. In: StatPearls [Internet]. StatPearls Publishing; Treasure Island (FL), 2022. Available at: https://www.statpearls.com/ArticleLibrary/viewarticle/87999 (Accessed 2 January 2025).

[7] Ghulmiyya L, Sinno S, Mirza F, et al. Episiotomy: history, present and future - a review. J Matern Fetal Neonatal Med 2020;35(7):1386–91.

[8] Thacker SB, Banta HD. Benefits and risks of episiotomy: an interpretative review of the English language literature, 1860-1980. Obstet Gynecol Surv 1983;38(6):322–38.

[9] Hersh SR, Emeis CL. Mediolateral episiotomy: technique, practice, and training. J Midwifery Womens Health 2020;65(3):404–9.

[10] Jiang H, Qian X, Carroli G, et al. Selective versus routine use of episiotomy for vaginal birth. Cochrane Database Syst Rev 2017;2:CD000081.

[11] World Health Organization. WHO recommendations: intrapartum care for a positive childbirth experience. Geneva: World Health Organization; 2018.

[12] Carroli G, Mignini L. Episiotomy for vaginal birth. Cochrane Database Syst Rev 2009;1:CD000081 [Update in: Cochrane Database Syst Rev. 2017 Feb 08;2:CD000081].

[13] Mahgoub S, Piant H, Gaudineau A, et al. Risk factors for obstetric anal sphincter injuries (OASIS) and the role of episiotomy: a retrospective series of 496 cases. J Gynecol Obstet Hum Reprod 2019;48:657–62.

[14] Wright A, Nassar A, Visser G, et al. FIGO Good clinical practice paper: management of second stage labor. Int J Gynaecol Obstet 2021;152:172–81.

[15] Sagi-Dain L, Sagi S. Indications for episiotomy performance – a cross-sectional survey and review of the literature. J Obstet Gynaecol 2016;36(3):361–5.

[16] Saadia Z. Rates and indicators for episiotomy in modern obstetrics - a study from Saudi Arabia. Mater Sociomed 2014;26(3):188–90.

[17] Arnold MJ, Sadler KS, Leli K. Obstetric laceration: prevention and repair. Am Fam Physician 2021;103(12):745–52.

[18] Shmueli A, Gabbay Benziv R, Hiersch L, et al. Episiotomy - risk factors and outcomes. J Matern Fetal Neonatal Med 2017;30(3):251–6, Epub 2016 Apr 19. PMID: 27018243.

[19] Pergialiotis V, Bellos I, Fanaki M, et al. Risk factors for severe perineal trauma during childbirth: an updated meta-analysis. Eur J Obstet Gynecol Reprod Biol 2020;247:94–100, Epub 2020 Feb 14. PMID: 32087423.

[20] Schmidt PC, Fenner DE. Repair of episiotomy and obstetrical perineal lacerations (first-fourth). Am J Obstet Gynecol 2024;230(35):S1005–13.

[21] Cocanour CS. Informed consent- it's more than a signature on a piece of paper. Am J Surg 2017;214:993–7.

[22] Hower EG. Beyond shared decision making. J Clin Ethics 2020;31(4):293–302.

[23] Muhleman MA, Aly I, Walters A, et al. To cut or not to cut, that is the question: a review of the anatomy, the technique, risks, and benefits of an episiotomy. Clin Anat 2017;30(3): 362–72, PMID: 28195378.

[24] Sultan AH, Thakar R, Ismail KM, et al. The role of mediolateral episiotomy during operative vaginal delivery. Eur J Obstet Gynecol Reprod Biol 2019;240:192–6.

[25] Van Bavel J, Hukkelhoven CWPM, de Vries C, et al. The effectiveness of mediolateral episiotomy in preventing obstetric anal sphincter injuries during operative vaginal delivery: a ten-year analysis of a national registry. Int Urogynecol J 2018;29(3):407–13.

[26] Ankarcrona V, Zhao H, Jacobsson B, et al. Obstetric anal sphincter injury after episiotomy in vacuum extraction: an epidemiological study using an emulated randomised trial approach. BJOG 2021; https://doi.org/10.1111/1471-0528.16663.

[27] Hudson CN, Sohaib SA, Shulver HM, et al. The anatomy of the perineal membrane: its relationship to injury in childbirth and episiotomy. Aust N Z J Obstet Gynaecol 2002;42: 193–6.

[28] May JL. Modified median episiotomy minimizes the risk of third degree tears. Obstet Gynecol 1994;83:156–7.

[29] Cunningham FG, editor. Williams Obstetrics. 26th edition. New York, NY: McGraw-Hill Medical; 2022. p. 18–22, Chapter 27.

[30] Husic A, Hammoud MM. Indications for the use of episiotomy in Qatar. Int J Gynecol Obstet 2009;104:240–1.

[31] Shaw E. Medical protocol for delivery of infibulated women in Sudan. Am J Nurs 1985;85: 687.

[32] Committee on Practice Bulletins-Obstetrics. ACOG Practice Bulletin No. 198: prevention and management of obstetric lacerations at vaginal delivery. Obstet Gynecol 2018;132(3):e87–102, PMID: 30134424.

[33] Phillippi J, Kantrowitz-Gordon I. Varney's midwifery. 7th edition. Burlington, MA: Jones & Bartlett Learning; 2024.

[34] Royal College of Obstetricians & Gynaecologists. The management of third-and fourth-degree perineal tears: green-top guideline No. 29. London, UK: RCOG; 2021.

[35] Kalis V, Landsmanova J, Bednarova B, et al. Evaluation of the incision angle of medilateral episiotomy at 60 degrees. Int J Gynaecol Obstet 2011;112:220–4.

[36] Komorowski LK, Leeman LM, Fullilove AM, et al. Does a large infant head or a short perineal body increase the risk of obstetrical perineal trauma? Birth 2014;41(2):147–52.

[37] Djusad S, Purwosunu Y, Hidayat F. Relationship between perineal body length and degree of perineal tears in primigravidas undergoing vaginal delivery with episiotomy. Obstet Gynecol Int 2021;2621872; https://doi.org/10.1155/2021/2621872.

[38] Mishori R, Warren N, Reingold R. Female genital mutilation or cutting. Am Fam Physician 2018;97(1):49–52.

[39] Rodriguez MI, Seuc A, Say L, et al. Episiotomy and obstetric outcomes among women living with type 3 female genital mutilation: a secondary analysis. Reprod Health 2016;13(1): 131.

[40] Logan RG, Vedam S, Declercq E. Giving voice to mothers: a national survey of the experiences of care during and after pregnancy and childbirth among women of color in the United States. Birth 2021;48(3):297–305.

Advances in Family Practice Nursing 7 (2025) 159–171

ADVANCES IN FAMILY PRACTICE NURSING

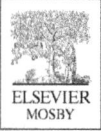

Understanding Intersectionality in African American Breastfeeding
Insights for Health Care Professionals

Alexis L. Woods Barr, MS, PhD[a],*,
Stephanie Devane-Johnson, PhD, CNM[b]

[a]Department of Health and Human Behavior, Gillings School of Public Health, University of North Carolina at Chapel Hill, 116 Orange Mill Avenue, Ruskin, FL 33570, USA; [b]School of Nursing, Vanderbilt University, 461 21st Avenue South, Nashville, TN 37240, USA

Keywords
- Intersectionality • Cultural competence • African American breastfeeding
- Health care disparities • Intergenerational support

Key points
- Intersectionality offers crucial insights into the complex factors influencing breastfeeding among African American women.
- Health care professionals must recognize historic trauma and provide culturally-competent, intersectionally-aware care.
- Engaging family members and community resources is vital for supporting breastfeeding in African American communities.

INTRODUCTION

Breastfeeding provides numerous health benefits for both mothers and infants, yet racial disparities in breastfeeding rates persist in the United States [1,2]. African American women consistently have lower rates of breastfeeding initiation and duration compared to other racial/ethnic groups [3]. Health care professionals play a crucial role in supporting breastfeeding among African American families [4]. To provide culturally sensitive and effective care, it is essential to understand the complex intersecting factors that shape African American women's infant feeding experiences and decisions.

*Corresponding author. University of North Carolina Chapel Hill, 116 Orange Mill Avenue, Ruskin, FL 33570. E-mail address: alexiswoodsbarr@unc.edu

https://doi.org/10.1016/j.yfpn.2025.01.005
2589-420X/25/Published by Elsevier Inc.

Abbreviation

WIC   Women, Infant, and Children

It is important to note that socioeconomic status alone does not shield African American women from health care discrimination or health disparities. This phenomenon, known as *Blacks' diminished returns,* refers to the consistently smaller health benefits that African Americans receive from equivalent socioeconomic resources compared to their white counterparts [5]. Even African American women with higher education levels and incomes continue to face systemic barriers and biases within the health care system [6]. For instance, highly educated African American women may still experience lower quality of care or reduced access to lactation support services compared to white women of similar socioeconomic status [7]. This persistence of disparities across socioeconomic strata underscores the deep-rooted nature of racial inequities in health care and highlights the need for an intersectional approach that considers how race intersects with other social identities to influence health outcomes, including breastfeeding practices and support.

This article explores the concept of intersectionality as it relates to breastfeeding in African American communities. We will examine how interlocking systems of oppression based on race, gender, and class influence infant feeding practices across generations. By understanding these intersectional dynamics, health care professionals can better support African American mothers in their breastfeeding journey.

Understanding Intersectionality and Black Feminist Thought in Breastfeeding

Intersectionality, coined by legal scholar Kimberlé Crenshaw, provides a crucial framework for understanding the complex factors influencing breastfeeding among African American women [8]. In this context, intersectionality illuminates how the overlapping identities of race, gender, and class create unique challenges for African American mothers. An African American woman may face racial discrimination in health care settings, gender-based workplace barriers to pumping, and class-related constraints on accessing quality lactation support—all simultaneously affecting her breastfeeding experience.

Black Feminist Thought, developed by Patricia Hill Collins, complements intersectionality by centering the experiences and knowledge of African American women [9]. Applied to breastfeeding, this theory highlights several key aspects. It considers the historic context, where the legacy of slavery and forced wet-nursing continues to influence perceptions of breastfeeding in African American communities. It also addresses stereotypes and stigma, recognizing how negative stereotypes about Black women's bodies and sexuality can create barriers to breastfeeding support and acceptance. Moreover, it emphasizes resistance and empowerment, acknowledging that many African American women view breastfeeding as an act of reclaiming their bodies and maternal identities. Lastly, it values collective wisdom, recognizing the crucial roles of intergenerational knowledge and community support in breastfeeding decisions and practices.

These theories inform the analysis of breastfeeding disparities by revealing how multiple, interacting forms of oppression create unique barriers for African American women, beyond those explained by race or socioeconomic status alone. They highlight the importance of historic and cultural contexts in shaping current breastfeeding attitudes and practices. Furthermore, they emphasize the need for culturally competent care that recognizes and respects the diverse experiences and knowledge of African American women. These frameworks also help identify points of resilience and empowerment within African American communities that can be leveraged to support breastfeeding. Ultimately, they guide the development of multi-faceted interventions that address the complex, intersecting factors influencing breastfeeding disparities.

By applying these 2 theoretic lenses, we can develop a more nuanced understanding of breastfeeding disparities and create more effective, culturally sensitive strategies to support African American women in their breastfeeding journeys. This approach allows us to move beyond simplistic explanations and develop comprehensive solutions that address the multifaceted nature of breastfeeding challenges faced by African American women.

African American Multi-generational Perspectives on Infant Feeding

Infant feeding practices among African American families are deeply influenced by historic, cultural, and socioeconomic factors that span generations. Recent research has shed light on how intersectionality affects infant feeding practices across multiple generations of African American families, revealing a complex interplay of changing societal norms, persisting structural barriers, and evolving family dynamics [10]. This study found that while some grandmothers had breastfed their children, others had not, reflecting varied infant feeding experiences across generations. Importantly, regardless of their own feeding choices, grandmothers were generally supportive of the mothers' decisions to breastfeed.

The transmission of infant feeding knowledge and attitudes through generations plays a crucial role in shaping new mothers' feeding choices. In many cultures, matriarchs are the maternal grandmothers, aunties or other senior female relatives of women who remain salient figures during childbirth and rearing, wielding considerable influence over women's behavior and decision-making. Black women seek support and advice from their mothers and their grandmothers in parenting and infant care decisions, and in general, Black matriarchs are empowered to provide such infant care and feeding guidance to their daughters of healthy infants [11]. In fact, grandmothers are routinely identified in studies seeking to identify influences over infant feeding decisions among Black women with healthy infants [10–13]. Interventions to increase breastfeeding rates among Black women have called for the direct or indirect involvement or acknowledgment of the role that the Black matriarch plays in the infant feeding decision [11,13].

The intersection of matriarchal influence and race and the impact of this interaction on infant feeding decisions have been described in the literature. Family members, especially grandmothers, often serve as the key influencers in infant feeding decisions, sometimes perpetuating outdated information or personal biases against breastfeeding [14]. However, this intergenerational influence can also be a powerful force for positive change when older family members support and encourage breastfeeding [15]. The intergenerational support, coupled with mothers' increasing access to breastfeeding information and resources, has contributed to a shift toward more positive breastfeeding attitudes among younger generations of African American women [11].

This dynamic underscore the importance of family-centered interventions when promoting breastfeeding in African American communities. Health care providers must recognize and engage with these familial dynamics, addressing concerns and misconceptions while respecting the valuable role that family wisdom and support play in a new mother's breastfeeding journey. However, despite this positive trend, many African American mothers continue to face significant structural barriers to breastfeeding, such as limited access to culturally competent lactation support [16].

Importantly, African American women are beginning to view breastfeeding through a lens of cultural reclamation and resistance against historic oppression [11]. For some, the act of breastfeeding becomes a way to reclaim their bodies and maternal identities in the face of longstanding stereotypes and the historic trauma of forced wet-nursing during slavery [17]. This perspective of resilience and empowerment is a powerful motivator for some mothers and can be a valuable point of discussion in breastfeeding promotion efforts.

However, it is crucial for the health care providers to approach this topic with sensitivity, recognizing that each woman's relationship with breastfeeding is unique and shaped by her individual experiences and the intersecting aspects of her identity. By understanding these multi-generational perspectives and the complex factors that influence them, health care professionals can provide more nuanced, culturally sensitive support to African American mothers, and their families throughout their breastfeeding journey.

CASE STUDIES

To illustrate how intersectionality and Black Feminist Thought manifest in real-world health care settings, we present 2 case studies. These examples demonstrate the practical application of intersectional analysis and highlight the importance of culturally-competent care. Case Study 1 explores multigenerational experiences in a hospital delivery room, while Case Study 2 examines challenges faced by a young mother navigating the Special Supplemental Nutrition Program for Women, Infant, and Children (WIC) program. Through these narratives, we will see how these theoretic concepts translate into lived experiences, informing our subsequent discussion on improving breastfeeding support for African American women.

Case Study 1: The Johnson Family in the Delivery Room

Tanya Johnson, a 28-year-old African American woman, is in labor with her first child. She is accompanied by her mother, Linda (50), and grandmother, Ruth (72). Tanya, a college-educated professional, has researched breastfeeding extensively and is determined to breastfeed. However, she is nervous about potential challenges, having heard stories from family members and colleagues about difficulties with breastfeeding initiation. Linda, who formula-fed Tanya, is supportive of her daughter but harbors concern about breastfeeding. She thinks it might be best for Tanya to formula feed, worried that breastfeeding could hinder Tanya's career growth and opportunities at work. Ruth, who breastfed her children out of necessity in a time when formula was less accessible, offers traditional wisdom but is unfamiliar with modern breastfeeding supports.

The family's interactions with health care professionals illuminate the multi-faceted intersectional challenges they face. As the nurses come in and out of the room, subtle microaggressions and assumptions become apparent. One nurse, while checking Tanya's vitals, casually asks, "Is this your first?" When Tanya confirms, the nurse responds with, "Good for you for choosing breastfeeding. Many young moms in your community don't even try." This comment, while seemingly supportive, carries stereotypical assumptions about African American mothers and breastfeeding rates, and puts unnecessary pressure on Tanya.

The nurse, looking around the room, comments, "It's nice to see such strong family support." She then hesitates briefly before adding, "Will the father be joining us later? It's really best for the baby if he's involved from the start." This comment shows how health care professionals might unknowingly perpetuate harmful stereotypes about African American families, even in what they might consider casual conversation. It puts Tanya in the uncomfortable position of either explaining her personal situation or feeling judged, adding unnecessary stress during an already intense time.

Changing the subject, Tanya mentions her concerns about balancing breastfeeding with her career as a marketing executive. The nurse looks visibly surprised, subtly revealing preconceived notions about Tanya's professional status, and demonstrating how deeply ingrained racial and gender stereotypes can affect patient care, even when health care professionals are not consciously aware of their biases.

Linda, feeling increasingly uncomfortable with the nurse's assumptions, interjects, "Tanya has a demanding career. I'm just concerned that breastfeeding might be too much for her to handle alongside her job." The nurse responds, "Oh, I'm sure she can manage. It's what's best for the baby, after all." This dismissive response makes Linda feel defensive about her own feeding choices and concerns for her daughter, heightening the tension in the room.

Ruth, sensing the growing discomfort, begins to share her own breastfeeding experience, "When I had my children, we didn't have all these fancy pumps and—" the nurse interrupts, "Things have changed a lot since then. We have much better methods now." Feeling dismissed, Ruth becomes hesitant to share more of her experiences, despite the valuable cultural and historic perspective she could offer.

As the labor progresses, a new nurse takes over. This nurse's approach is noticeably different, demonstrating cultural competence and intersectional awareness. She takes the time to listen to Tanya's concerns about balancing breastfeeding and her career, sharing experiences of other working mothers. She acknowledges the challenges but also provides practical strategies for managing breastfeeding in a demanding work environment.

As the labor progresses, a new nurse, Keisha, an African American woman, takes over. Keisha's approach is noticeably different. She takes the time to listen to Tanya's concerns about balancing breastfeeding and her career, sharing her own experiences as a working mother. She acknowledges the challenges but also provides practical strategies for managing breastfeeding in a demanding work environment.

The new nurse also engages Linda and Ruth, recognizing the importance of intergenerational support. She asks Ruth about her breastfeeding experiences, validating the wisdom of her approach while gently introducing modern techniques that might complement traditional methods. To Linda, she offers reassurance about the compatibility of breastfeeding and career success, sharing statistics about reduced absenteeism among breastfeeding mothers due to healthier babies.

When Tanya expresses concern about potential discrimination at work related to pumping, the nurse provides information about workplace rights for breastfeeding mothers. She also connects Tanya with a local support group for professional mothers who breastfeed, recognizing the importance of peer support in navigating these challenges.

As the delivery approaches, the nurse ensures that Tanya's birth plan, which includes immediate skin-to-skin contact and early breastfeeding initiation, is communicated to the entire health care team. She also arranges for a lactation consultant who specializes in supporting women from diverse backgrounds to visit Tanya after the birth. This more culturally competent and intersectionally aware approach helps alleviate much of the family's anxiety. Tanya feels more confident in her ability to breastfeed while maintaining her career. Linda's concerns are addressed, and she feels more supportive of Tanya's choice. Ruth feels valued for her experiences and is excited to support her granddaughter in this journey.

The contrast between the 2 nurses' approaches highlights the importance of cultural competence and intersectional awareness in health care. While the first nurse's interactions left the family feeling misunderstood and defensive, the second nurse's approach created an environment of support, understanding, and empowerment. This case study demonstrates how health care professionals can develop and apply cultural competence to provide more effective, patient-centered care, regardless of their own background.

Case Study 2: The Williams Family at the Women, Infant, and Children Office

Shanice Williams, a 22-year-old African American mother, visits the WIC office with her 2-month-old son, Jamal. She's accompanied by her mother, Courtney (40), and her aunt Tracy (38). Shanice, who works part-time at a retail store, is struggling to continue breastfeeding while managing work and family responsibilities. She is considering which food package to choose, since she is exclusively breastfeeding her son. She would like to choose the "Fully Breastfeeding" option but is thinking that maybe she should choose the "Mostly Breastfeeding" or "Formula Feeding" package options instead. The thought of not choosing the "Fully Breastfeeding" package option fills her with guilt and anxiety, as she has heard repeatedly about the benefits of breastfeeding but feels torn between her desire to provide the best for Jamal and the realities of her demanding work-family life.

As they wait for their appointment, Shanice notices the posters promoting breastfeeding on the walls, their smiling mothers a stark contrast to her own exhausted reflection. She also sees that many other mothers in the waiting room are using formula, which brings a mix of relief and doubt. The atmosphere is busy and slightly chaotic, with crying babies and toddlers running around, adding to Shanice's stress. When they are called in, the WIC nutritionist, Ms Johnson, greets them professionally but seems rushed, her eyes darting to the clock as she ushers them into her small, cluttered office.

Ms Johnson reviews Shanice's feeding status and explains the different food package options, her words coming out in a practiced, almost mechanical manner. She mentions that the "Fully Breastfeeding package" offers the most food, including canned fish, and lasts for a full year postpartum. As she speaks, she hands Shanice a colorful brochure detailing the packages. However, her tone subtly implies doubt about Shanice's ability to maintain exclusive breastfeeding, her eyebrows rising slightly as she says, "The 'Fully breastfeeding' package is quite demanding, you know?"

Courtney, noticing this subtle perceived judgment, interjects; her voice tight with barely concealed frustration, "Shanice is doing her best, but it's hard with her work schedule. They don't exactly roll out the red carpet for pumping moms at the store." Ms Johnson responds, her tone a mix of resignation and practicality, "Well, the 'Mostly Breastfeeding' package might be more realistic then. It's still a good option." She slides a different brochure across the desk. This comment, while perhaps practical, fails to address the systemic barriers Shanice faces and makes Shanice feel defensive about her efforts. Shanice shrinks a little in her chair, feeling like she has somehow already failed.

Tracy, who successfully breastfed her children while working, sees an opportunity to offer support and change the conversation's direction. She leans forward, her voice warm and encouraging, "You know, I managed to breastfeed while working at the factory. It wasn't easy, but I found some tricks that might help Shanice." Ms Johnson, initially seeming disinterested, her pen poised to move on to the next topic, perks up at this. "Oh? That's interesting. What kind of strategies did you use?" she asks, her tone shifting from clinical to curious, a spark of genuine interest in her eyes.

Encouraged, Tracy shares her experience of using manual expression during short breaks and how she negotiated with her supervisor for pumping time. The nutritionist listens attentively, occasionally nodding, and taking notes. "This is valuable information," she admits. "We don't often hear success stories like this from women in similar work environments." The nutritionist then turns to Shanice, "Would you be comfortable trying some of your aunt's techniques? We could also look into whether your workplace falls under laws requiring pumping accommodations." This collaborative approach, sparked by Tracy's input, creates a more positive and problem-solving oriented discussion.

However, the interaction takes an unexpected turn when the nutritionist adds, "It's refreshing to see such a positive influence in the family. Often, we find that family members can discourage breastfeeding in your community." This comment, though intended as a compliment, carries undertones of stereotyping and makes Shanice and her family uncomfortable.

Tracy, picking up on the tension, diplomatically responds, "Every family is different, just like every mom's breastfeeding journey is unique. We're here to support Shanice in whatever decision works best for her and Jamal." This tactful redirection showcases Tracy's wisdom and her role as an advocate for Shanice.

As they discuss Shanice's work situation further, the nutritionist seems surprised to learn that Shanice's employer does not provide a dedicated space for pumping. "Have you tried talking to your manager?" she asks, not fully grasping the power dynamics at play for a young woman in a low-wage job. When Shanice expresses concern about the cost of a breast pump, the nutritionist informs her about the free pump program but adds, "You'll need to attend a breastfeeding class first." This additional requirement, while intended to be helpful, feels like another barrier to Shanice, who's already struggling to balance work and childcare.

Throughout the appointment, the nutritionist provides factual information but often fails to fully engage with the family's cultural context or the intersectional challenges Shanice faces. Her well-intentioned advice sometimes comes across as judgmental or disconnected from Shanice's reality. As they leave, Shanice feels conflicted. While she appreciates the support WIC provides, she also feels misunderstood and somewhat pressured. Courtney is frustrated by what she perceives as a lack of practical support, although she's glad Tracy's experience was eventually valued. Tracy feels satisfied that she could contribute positively but remains concerned about the underlying assumptions she noticed from the nutritionist.

This case study highlights how even well-meaning programs like WIC can sometimes struggle to provide truly intersectional support. It underscores the need for culturally competent care that considers the complex interplay of race, class, gender, and systemic barriers in shaping a mother's infant feeding decisions and experiences. The interaction also demonstrates the importance of family support and advocacy in navigating these systems. It emphasizes that all health care professionals, regardless of their background, can develop the cultural competence needed to provide more effective, patient-centered care.

IMPLICATIONS FOR HEALTHCARE PROFESSIONALS

To provide effective, culturally sensitive care that addresses the complex intersectional factors influencing breastfeeding among African American women and their families, health care professionals should adopt several key strategies. First and foremost, it is crucial to recognize that each woman's breastfeeding journey is shaped by her unique combination of social identities and life experiences. Health care professionals should avoid making assumptions based on race alone and instead approach each patient as an individual with a distinct background and set of circumstances.

It is crucial to emphasize that cultural competence and sensitivity can and should be developed by all health care professionals, regardless of their own racial or cultural background. The ability to provide culturally congruent care is not inherently tied to one's own identity but is a skill that can be learned, practiced, and continuously improved. Health care organizations should prioritize ongoing cultural competency training for all staff members, focusing on understanding intersectionality, recognizing and addressing implicit biases, and developing skills to provide patient-centered care that respects and responds to diverse cultural perspectives and experiences. By fostering a culture of cultural competence across all levels of health care provision, we can work toward more equitable, effective, and compassionate care for all patients, particularly those from marginalized communities.

This individualized approach should be coupled with an awareness of the historic context of breastfeeding for African American women. The legacy of slavery, forced wet-nursing, and ongoing systemic racism has deeply impacted perceptions of breastfeeding in many African American communities [18]. Discussions about breastfeeding should be approached with sensitivity to this historic trauma, while also emphasizing the empowering aspects of breastfeeding.

Providing culturally congruent care is important for improving breastfeeding outcomes. When possible, patients should be connected with professionals and lactation consultants who share their cultural background or have specific training in culturally diverse care [19]. This can help build trust and improve communication [20]. Additionally, recognizing and respecting the importance of intergenerational family support is crucial. Engaging family members, especially grandmothers and partners, in breastfeeding education and support can be highly effective [10]. Professionals should offer culturally congruent education about breastfeeding to all family members present, acknowledging different generational perspectives, and addressing concerns about work-life balance. Family support is often crucial for breastfeeding success, especially in communities where breastfeeding may not be the norm [11].

Health care professionals should also facilitate connections between patients and local breastfeeding support groups and community organizations that focus on African American maternal health [21]. These resources can offer peer support, culturally relevant information, and a sense of community that may be lacking in traditional health care settings [22]. Health care professionals should offer resources for continued support after discharge, including information about local African American breastfeeding support groups and strategies for successfully combining breastfeeding and work. Moreover, health care professionals have a responsibility to advocate for systemic changes that support breastfeeding [23]. This includes pushing for improved workplace pumping accommodations, advocating for paid family leave policies, or working to increase the diversity of the lactation support workforce in health care settings.

Empowering patients through education is a key role for health care professionals [24]. They should provide evidence-based information about the benefits of breastfeeding while respecting individual choices and circumstances. It is important to discuss the benefits of breastfeeding not just for the baby, but also for the mother's health and potential positive impacts on work performance, such as fewer sick days due to a healthier baby [25]. Professionals should also offer information on workplace rights for breastfeeding mothers and strategies for communicating with employers about pumping needs. When discussing breastfeeding, it is crucial to use inclusive language and culturally relevant examples [26].

Health care professionals should also regularly examine and challenge their own potential biases. Implicit bias can significantly impact patient care, so ongoing self-reflection and cultural competency training are essential for all health care professionals [27]. It is important to be aware of potential biases and avoid making assumptions based on race or appearance. Applying an intersectional framework when assessing and addressing barriers to breastfeeding is crucial. Professionals should consider how race, class, gender, and other social identities intersect to create unique challenges and opportunities for each patient. This approach allows for a more comprehensive understanding of the patient's situation and enables more targeted and effective support.

Lastly, promoting continuity of care throughout the prenatal, perinatal, and postpartum periods is vital [27,28]. This consistent support can help address challenges early and promote long-term breastfeeding success. By implementing these strategies, health care professionals can offer more effective, culturally sensitive care that addresses the complex, intersectional factors influencing breastfeeding among African American women. This approach not only benefits individual mothers and infants but also contributes to broader efforts to achieve health equity in African American communities.

SUMMARY

Intersectionality provides a valuable lens for understanding the complex factors that influence breastfeeding among African American women. By acknowledging how race, gender, class, and generational experiences intersect and influence one another, health care professionals can provide more comprehensive and effective breastfeeding support. This approach benefits individual mothers and infant dyads while contributing to broader efforts to achieve health equity in African American communities. Throughout this article, we have explored how Intersectionality and Black Feminist Thought offer crucial insights into African American women's breastfeeding experiences. Historic contexts, including the legacy of slavery and forced wet-nursing, continue to influence breastfeeding perceptions and practices. Contemporary issues such as workplace discrimination, inadequate support systems, and persistent health care disparities create additional barriers for many African American mothers.

The case studies highlight the real-world implications of these intersecting factors, demonstrating how even well-intentioned health care providers can inadvertently perpetuate harmful stereotypes and fail to address African American mothers' unique needs. These examples underscore the critical need for culturally-competent, intersectionally aware care that recognizes and responds to the multifaceted challenges faced by African American women. Importantly, this care must be provided equitably to all African American women, regardless of their socioeconomic status or insurance type. Health care professionals must consciously reject biases based on perceived class differences and focus on individual needs and experiences, recognizing that disparities persist even among more affluent and educated African American women.

The systemic nature of these challenges calls for advocacy and action at a broader level. Health care professionals should advocate for policy changes that support breastfeeding, such as improved workplace accommodations, paid family leave, and increased diversity in the lactation support workforce. Addressing these structural barriers will create an environment more conducive to successful breastfeeding for all mothers, particularly those from marginalized communities. Health care professionals should develop a nuanced understanding of each patient's unique circumstances, shaped by the intersection of their various social identities. This requires ongoing self-reflection, cultural competency training, and a willingness to challenge one's own biases. Engaging family members and community resources in breastfeeding support is also crucial, recognizing the role of intergenerational knowledge transfer and the potential for both positive and negative family influences.

Moving forward, we must continue research that applies an intersectional framework to understanding breastfeeding disparities, capturing diverse experiences across socioeconomic backgrounds, geographic locations, and family structures. Education and training programs should incorporate intersectionality as a core concept, equipping future providers with the knowledge and skills to offer culturally competent, patient-centered care. As health care professionals, we have the opportunity and responsibility to champion equitable, culturally sensitive care that empowers African American women in their breastfeeding decisions and experiences. By deepening our understanding of intersectionality in the context of breastfeeding and consistently applying these insights, we can improve not just breastfeeding rates, but overall maternal and infant health outcomes in African American communities. This work is essential for advancing health equity and social justice on a broader scale.

CLINICS CARE POINTS

- Apply an intersectional framework when supporting African American mothers by recognizing how race, gender, class, and historical contexts uniquely influence their breastfeeding experiences.
- Recognize that socioeconomic status alone does not shield African American women from health disparities in breastfeeding support (Black's diminished returns).
- Engage family members, especially grandmothers, in breastfeeding education and support, acknowledging their crucial role in infant feeding decisions.
- Provide culturally congruent care by connecting patients with diverse lactation consultants and peer support groups focused on African American maternal health.
- Address workplace barriers by educating mothers about their legal rights for pumping accommodations and providing practical strategies for balancing breastfeeding with work.
- Practice self-reflection to identify and challenge personal biases that may affect the quality of care provided to African American mothers.

Disclosure

The authors declare no commercial or financial conflicts of interest. No funding was received for this work.

References

[1] Gartner LM, Morton J, Lawrence RA, et al. Breastfeeding and the use of human milk. Pediatrics 2005;115(2):496–506.

[2] Chiang KV, Li R, Anstey EH, et al. Racial and ethnic disparities in breastfeeding initiation — United States, 2019. MMWR Morb Mortal Wkly Rep 2021;70(21):769–74.

[3] Centers for Disease Control and Prevention. Rates of any and exclusive breastfeeding by socio-demographics among children born in 2020. National Immunization Survey - child. 2023. Available at: https://www.cdc.gov/breastfeeding/data/nis_data/rates-any-exclusive-bf-socio-dem-2020.htm. Accessed July 28, 2024.

[4] Sriraman NK, Kellams A. Breastfeeding: what are the barriers? why women struggle to achieve their goals. J Womens Health (Larchmt) 2016;25(7):714–22.

[5] Assari S. Health disparities due to diminished return among Black Americans: public policy solutions. Soc Issues Policy Rev 2018;12(1):112–45.

[6] Chinn JJ, Martin IK, Redmond N. Health equity among Black women in the United States. J Womens Health (Larchmt) 2021;30(2):212–9.

[7] Segura-Pérez S, Hromi-Fiedler A, Adnew M, et al. Impact of breastfeeding interventions among United States minority women on breastfeeding outcomes: a systematic review. Int J Equity Health 2021;20(1):72.

[8] Crenshaw K. Traffic at the crossroads: multiple oppressions. In: Morgan R, editor. Sisterhood is forever: the woman's anthology for a new millennium. New York: Washington Square Press; 2003. p. 43–57.

[9] Collins PH. Black feminist thought: knowledge, consciousness, and the politics of empower-ment. 2nd edition. New York: Routledge; 2000. p. 283; https://doi.org/10.4324/9780 203900055.

[10] Muse MM, Morris JE, Dodgson JE. An intergenerational exploration of breastfeeding jour-neys through the lens of African American mothers and grandmothers. J Hum Lactation 2021;37(2):289–300.

[11] Woods Barr AL, Miller E, Smith JL, et al. #Everygenerationmatters: intergenerational percep-tions of infant feeding information and communication among African American women. Breastfeed Med 2021;16(2):131–9.

[12] Hinson TD, Skinner AC, Lich KH, et al. Factors that influence breastfeeding initiation among African American women. J Obstet Gynecol Neonatal Nurs 2018;47(3):290–300.

[13] Bentley ME, Caulfield LE, Gross SM, et al. Sources of influence on intention to breastfeed among AA women at entry to WIC J Hum. J Hum Lactation 1999;15:27–34.

[14] DeVane-Johnson S, Woods-Giscombé CL, Thoyre S, et al. Integrative literature review of fac-tors related to breastfeeding in African American women: evidence for a potential para-digm shift. J Hum Lactation 2017;33(2):435–47.

[15] Woods Barr AL, Austin DA, Smith JL, Schafer EJ. "...[T]his is what we are missing": the value of communicating infant feeding information across three generations of African American women. J Hum Lactation 2021;37(2):279–88.

[16] Handtke O, Schilgen B, Mösko M. Culturally competent healthcare - a scoping review of strategies implemented in healthcare organizations and a model of culturally competent healthcare provision. PLoS One 2019;14(7):e0219971.

[17] Reeves EA, Woods-Giscombé CL. Infant-feeding practices among African American women: social-ecological analysis and implications for practice. J Transcult Nurs 2015;26(3):219–26.

[18] Allers KS. Breastfeeding: some slavery crap? Ebony. 2012. Available at: http://www.ebo-ny.com/wellness-empowerment/breastfeeding-some-slavery-crap#axzz4rGPQhMvh. Ac-cessed August 30, 2017.

[19] Davis C, Villalobos AVK, Turner MM, et al. Racism and resistance: a qualitative study of bias as a barrier to breastfeeding. Breastfeed Med 2021;16(6):471–80.

[20] Ali AM, Young HN. Relationships between key functions of patient-provider communication, trust, and motivation across White, African American, and Hispanic/Latino patients with asthma. Health Commun 2022;37(4):450–6.

[21] Pyles TEH, Umi SA, Madubuonwu S, et al. Breastfeeding sisters that are receiving support: community-based peer support program created for and by women of color. Breastfeed Med 2021;16(2):165–70.

[22] Duncan R, Coleman J, Herring S, et al. Breastfeeding awareness and empowerment (BAE): a black women-led approach to promoting a multigenerational culture of health. Societies 2022;12(1):28.

[23] Lawrence RA, Lawrence RM. Breastfeeding: a guide for the medical professional. Maryland Heights (MO): Elsevier Health Sciences; 2021. p. 508.

[24] Paterick TE, Patel N, Tajik AJ, et al. Improving health outcomes through patient education and partnerships with patients. SAVE Proc 2017;30(1):112–3.

[25] Johnson AM, Kirk R, Muzik M. Overcoming workplace barriers: a focus group study exploring African American mothers' needs for workplace breastfeeding support. J Hum Lactation 2015;31(3):425–33.

[26] Juntereal NA, Spatz DL. Breastfeeding experiences of same-sex mothers. Birth 2020;47(1): 21–8.

[27] Fricke J, Siddique SM, Aysola J, et al. Healthcare worker implicit bias training and education: rapid review. In: Making healthcare safer IV: a continuous updating of patient safety harms and practices. Rockville (MD): Agency for Healthcare Research and Quality (US); 2023.

[28] Fryer K, Reid CN, Cabral N, et al. Exploring patients' needs and desires for quality prenatal care in Florida, United States. Int J MCH AIDS 2023;12(1):e622.

Pediatrics

Advances in Family Practice Nursing 7 (2025) 173–184

ADVANCES IN FAMILY PRACTICE NURSING

Managing the Pressure
Pediatric Blood Pressure Screening and Management in Primary Care

Teresa Whited, DNP, APRN, CPNP-PC*,
Taylor Steele, DNP, RN, CPN

University of Arkansas for Medical Sciences, College of Nursing, 4301 West Markham Street #529, Little Rock, AR 72205, USA

Keywords
- Blood pressure • Hypertension • Cardiovascular • Pediatrics • Children
- Adolescents

Key points

- Screen for blood pressure (BP) beginning at age 3 or sooner if risk factors.
- BP normal values are based on age and gender tables.
- Ambulatory blood pressure monitoring is a key to the diagnosis of hypertension (HTN).
- Evaluation for secondary causes of HTN is essential in children.
- Management includes lifestyle modifications, medication management, and sport participation consideration.

INTRODUCTION

As recommended by the American Academy of Pediatrics (AAP), blood pressure (BP) measurement should begin at the age of 3 years to establish baseline values and detect abnormalities early. BP should be measured in children younger than 3 years of age, if their history indicates risk factors for developing elevated or high BP. Prompt and accurate detection is vital, as hypertension (HTN) in children is often asymptomatic and can lead to serious health issues if left untreated. The incidence of HTN in pediatric populations is rising, largely due to the increasing prevalence of obesity and associated comorbidities

*Corresponding author. E-mail address: tmwhited@uams.edu

https://doi.org/10.1016/j.yfpn.2024.12.005
2589-420X/25/© 2025 Elsevier Inc. All rights are reserved, including those for text and data mining, AI training, and similar technologies.

Abbreviations

AAP	American Academy of Pediatrics
ABPM	ambulatory blood pressure monitoring
ACE	angiotensin converting enzyme
ARB	angiotensin receptor blockers
BP	blood pressure
CKD	chronic kidney disease
DASH	Dietary Approaches to Stop Hypertension
HTN	hypertension
LVH	left ventricular hypertrophy
MI	motivational interviewing
RAAS	renin-angiotensin-aldosterone system

such as type 2 diabetes, dyslipidemia, and obstructive sleep apnea [1,2]. The prevalence of HTN in children ranges from 2% to 5%, with primary HTN being the most common type, particularly in adolescents [3]. Accurate BP measurement and frequent monitoring, especially in high-risk groups, are essential to prevent long-term cardiovascular complications [4].

PREVALANCE

Estimates of pediatric HTN are between 2% and 5% in children and adolescents [1,2]. However, elevated BP without a diagnosis of HTN occurs much more frequently with an estimated occurrence of 13% to 15% in pediatric patients [3]. Risk factors for high BP include obesity, metabolic syndrome, family history of HTN, and health disparities such as lower socioeconomic status [1–3]. Pediatric HTN remains an underdiagnosed condition among many patients and many practices are still not following recommended HTN guidelines. In one study of ~63,000 patients, researchers found that only 13% of practices followed-up on an abnormal BP reading by guidelines within 1 month and only 41% within 6 months [5,6]. Underdiagnoses and lack of guideline follow-up may be due to lack of education, the need for multiple follow-ups to make the diagnosis of HTN, and lack of tools to flag providers on abnormal values based on the BP charts in children [5]. Due to the complications of HTN long-term, it is important for clinicians to diagnose and management HTN in a timely fashion. Long-term pediatric HTN can lead to left ventricular hypertrophy (LVH), carotid artery thickness, microvascular changes, increased risk of kidney disease, proteinuria, decreased executive functioning, and end organ damage [3,4]. It is essential that pediatric HTN be diagnosed and treated in a timely fashion to prevent long-term complications that often result in morbidity or mortality in adulthood.

HISTORY

A comprehensive patient history is crucial for the effective management of pediatric HTN, encompassing the history of present illness, family history, and social history. In evaluating the history of present illness, it is essential to identify risk factors such as obesity, chronic kidney disease (CKD), sleep apnea, and cardiac abnormalities, all of which can contribute to elevated BP in children. Signs and symptoms of HTN can vary; some children may be asymptomatic, while others might experience headaches, dizziness, visual disturbances, or epistaxis. Severe HTN can present with symptoms indicative of end-organ damage, such as LVH, which highlights the importance of early detection and intervention [4].

A detailed family history should be obtained, focusing on first-degree relatives with HTN, cardiovascular diseases, kidney disease, or diabetes, as these conditions can increase the child's risk of developing HTN [2]. The child's social history, including the use of drugs or medications that may influence BP, such as corticosteroids or stimulants, should be reviewed. Additionally, lifestyle factors like diet, physical activity, and participation in sports can impact BP management. For instance, regular physical activity is recommended to help control HTN, whereas the use of tobacco, electronic nicotine delivery systems, or illicit drugs can exacerbate HTN [2–4]. Understanding these aspects can guide interventions aimed at lifestyle modifications and provide a comprehensive approach to managing pediatric HTN.

ASSESSMENT

Pediatric patient assessment for HTN requires adherence to established screening guidelines and proper BP measurement techniques. Accurate measurement involves using an appropriately sized cuff, with the bladder covering 80% to 100% of the arm's circumference and its width covering at least 40% of the arm's circumference. The child should be seated comfortably with their back supported, feet on the floor, and the arm supported at heart level, with measurements taken in the right arm for consistency [4]. It is recommended to take at least 3 readings, averaging the last 2 to confirm elevated BP, and to use automatic *blood pressure measurement devices validated for children*, followed by auscultation for verification if initial readings are high [2]. Additionally, the guidelines recommend ambulatory BP monitoring (ABPM) for certain high-risk patients to identify white coat HTN or masked HTN, providing a more accurate assessment of the child's BP profile over 24 hours [3,4].

Incorrect practices, such as using an improperly sized cuff; measuring BP when the child is anxious or moving; or failing to confirm high readings with repeated measurements, can lead to inaccurate diagnoses and inappropriate management. These guidelines ensure that HTN is identified accurately and managed effectively to prevent long-term cardiovascular complications.

PATHOPHYSIOLOGY

The pathophysiology of pediatric primary HTN, a multifactorial condition, involves complex interactions between genetic, physiologic, and environmental factors. Increased cardiac output, driven by factors such as heightened sympathetic tone and sodium retention, plays a significant role in youth compared to increased vascular resistance seen in adults [3]. Obesity, insulin resistance, renin-angiotensin-aldosterone system (RAAS) dysregulation, and inflammation further contribute to elevated BP and early target organ damage, including

LVH and vascular stiffening [3]. For children and adolescents in the United States, primary HTN is most common. It is generally found in children aged 6 years or older with a positive familial history for HTN [4].

Secondary HTN in children is commonly due to identifiable causes such as renal parenchymal disease, coarctation of the aorta, or endocrine disorders like hyperthyroidism and pheochromocytoma. These conditions often lead to increased RAAS activity and subsequent HTN. Early identification and management of these underlying conditions are crucial for effective treatment and prevention of long-term cardiovascular complications [3]. See Table 1 for pathophysiology of related diagnoses.

DIAGNOSIS

Diagnosis of HTN should be done in the primary care clinic and staged based on age, gender, and height for children less than 13 years of age. The normative values are based on percentiles of BP measurements of a certain age, gender, and height [3]. These tables can be found in the "AAP Clinical Practice

Table 1
Pathophysiology of related diagnoses [3]

Diagnosis	Pathophysiology
Obesity	Excess adiposity increases the risk for hypertension. Higher body mass index in childhood and adolescence is associated with future high blood pressure. Obesity contributes to increased cardiac output, sympathetic tone, and sodium and fluid retention, all of which are mechanisms driving higher blood pressure.
Insulin Resistance	Insulin resistance contributes to adverse cardiovascular phenotypes. It is associated with hypertension-induced target organ injury, which further exacerbates sustained hypertension through mechanisms like cardiac injury, microvascular narrowing, stiffening of larger arteries, and altered baroreceptor activity.
RAAS Dysregulation	RAAS dysregulation contributes to neurohormonal and renal cardiovascular dysregulation, leading to altered baroreflex sensitivity and salt-sensitive blood pressure. These alterations play a role in the development and maintenance of hypertension.
Primary Hypertension	Primary hypertension is multifactorial, involving inherited factors, physiologic traits, and environmental exposures. Increased cardiac output, sympathetic tone, sodium and fluid retention, altered baroreflex sensitivity, and salt-sensitive blood pressure are contributors. It exists on a continuum from childhood to adulthood, leading to cardiovascular disease over time.
Secondary Hypertension	Secondary hypertension often results from identifiable underlying causes, such as rare monogenic forms, or conditions like neurofibromatosis type 1, Turner syndrome, and Williams syndrome. It is more common in younger children and those with more severe hypertension.

Guideline for Screening and Management of High Blood Pressure in Children and Adolescents" or through a variety of tools on the web that will calculate percentile for the clinician [2]. See Box 1 for links to BP tools and tables. Children should be diagnosed with HTN when 3 consecutive BP measures on 3 different days are greater than or equal to the 95 percentile in the office setting [2]. In children 13 years of age or older, the AAP considers HTN at a BP reading of 130/80 or greater [3].

Stages of HTN can be classified based on percentiles above the normal BP for the age, gender, and height of the child. These help to classify the severity of HTN and help the provider know how to intervene. According to the guidelines, when a BP is at the 90th to less than 95th percentile, it is considered elevated BP. When it reaches greater than or equal to the 95th percentile plus 11 mm Hg, it is considered Stage I HTN, and when it is greater than 95th percentile plus 12 mm Hg, this is called Stage II HTN [3].

In children greater or equal to 13 years of age, normal BP should be less than 120 over 80. Elevated BP for this age group is greater than or equal to 121 to 129 over less than 80. At 130 to less than 140 and 80 to less than 90, it is considered Stage I HTN. Stage II HTN is 140 over 90 or greater [3]. See Table 2 for staging and management recommendations.

DIFFERENTIAL DIAGNOSIS

There are several differential diagnoses that must be considered when seeing a child with high BP. Secondary causes of HTN are more common in younger children such as renal or cardiac. HTN children 6 years or younger and those without a positive family history, risk factors for obesity, or physical examination findings indicative of possible secondary HTN should have a workup to evaluate for causes of secondary HTN [2]. The differential diagnoses include primary HTN, cardiac issues, renal issues, and anxiety related HTN [2,3]. See Table 3 for primary and secondary causes of HTN along with examination findings and diagnostics.

DIAGNOSTIC TESTING

When measuring the BP in a child, it is important to select the right cuff size for both diameter and width. The BP cuff should be 80% or greater in length and

---

Box 1: Pediatric blood pressure reference table web-links

AAP Pediatric Hypertension Guidelines Calculator:

   https://www.mdcalc.com/calc/4052/aap-pediatric-hypertension-guidelines

Baylor College of Medicine Age-Based Pediatric Blood Pressure Reference Charts:

   https://www.bcm.edu/bodycomplab/BPappZjs/BPvAgeAPPz.html

Table 2
Staging and management recommendations [2,3]

Stage	BP value	Management
Normotensive	Under 13 years-less than 90% on BP charts. 13 y and older-less than 120/80.	Encourage healthy lifestyle and health promotion strategies.
Elevated BP	Under 13 years-90%–95% on BP charts. 13 y and older-greater than 121–129/<80.	Encourage healthy lifestyle and health promotion strategies.
Stage 1 Hypertension	Under 13 years-greater than 95% plus 11 mm Hg 13 y and older-130–139/80–89.	Initial encourage healthy lifestyle and health promotion strategies. If unsuccessful (6–12 mo) or evidence of end organ damage, initiate pharmacologic therapy.
Stage 2 Hypertension	Under 13 years-greater than 95% plus 11 mm Hg or greater 13 y and older-140 or greater/90 or greater.	Initiate pharmacologic therapy. Encourage healthy lifestyle and health promotion strategies.

37% to 50% of the middle upper arm circumference and position with no more than 2 finger width between cuff and skin (Faulkner, 2023). No matter the cuff size needed, there are 2 methods to measure BP, which are manual and automatic. The child should be seated with feet on the floor in a quiet room for 3 to 5 minutes with the arm supported at heart level with a bare arm (Faulkner, 2017). The automatic BP machine is commonly used to screen BP in primary care offices but must be calibrated for use in pediatric patients. However, if unsure or need to rescreen, it is recommended to use a manual cuff to verify the measurement is accurate. Factors that can increase BP include anxiety, medications, and exercise including walking into the clinic. If concerned about issues such as anxiety or movement interfering with BP readings, you should allow the patient to be seated in a quiet room for few minutes then reattempt the BP.

ABPM is a tool to allow measurement of BP over a 24-h period. This tool allows clear identification of *white coat* or *anxiety* related HTN [3]. ABP should be used for confirmation of HTN in children with elevated BP for 1 year or more, or with stage 1or 2 HTN over 3 visits; in children and adolescents with high-risk conditions for HTN; and to assess treatment effectiveness for those with HTN where BP measures show insufficient response to treatment. The ABPM system allows evaluation of BP over a more prolonged period of time in the child's normal environment and routine [2,3].

If secondary causes of HTN are suspected or there are concerns about end organ damage, more specialized testing should be ordered. First is an echocardiogram, which should be completed on any patient who has a new diagnosis of stage I or stage II HTN or a history or physical examination consistent with end organ damage or risk factors such as coarctation and CKD. It is no longer

Table 3
Causes of hypertension, examination findings, and diagnostics [2–4,7–9]

Cause	Examination findings	Diagnostics
Cardiac (coarctation, congenital heart disease, cardiomyopathy, etc.)	BP differentiation between upper and lower extremities Elevated BP Murmur Extra heart sounds Edema Hepatosplenomegaly Abnormal rhythm Poor growth parameters	ABP monitoring recommended. *Other studies:* Echocardiogram EKG Stress testing Cardiac catheterization Event/Holter monitor
Renal (Chronic Kidney Disease, Renal Artery Stenosis)	Elevated BP Edema Poor growth parameters	ABP monitoring *Other Studies:* Renal ultrasound with doppler VCUG/CT/MRI UA Serum creatinine GFR CMP CBC with reticulocyte count Lipid profile Serum cystatin C Kidney biopsy
Anxiety (White Coat)	Elevated BP in the office setting with normal BP at home or on ABP monitoring.	ABP monitoring recommended to differentiate masked or white coat hypertension. *Other Studies:* Anxiety screening tools
Primary Hypertension	Elevated BP on 3 or more occasions on separate days *May have findings of:* Obesity End organ damage: cardiac or renal findings. Diabetes findings: Acanthus Nigricans, neuropathy, polydipsia, polyuria, polyphagia, vomiting	ABP monitoring *Other Studies:* Echocardiogram for end organ damage No other studies necessary unless concerning findings for end organ damage

recommended to complete an electrocardiogram (EKG) to look for LVH but to immediately go to an echocardiogram for a more definitive evaluation of LVH, left ventricular function, and ejection fraction [3]. Echocardiograms should also be used to monitor cardiac function and LVH every 6 months to 1 year for those with cardiac end organ damage or risk factors [3]. Echocardiograms should be completed annually on any patient who did not have an abnormal echocardiogram but has stage II HTN, uncontrolled stage I HTN, or secondary HTN [3]. Second is a renal ultrasound with Doppler ultrasound for children 6 year or younger or those with a history or physical examination consistent with renal causes of HTN or risk factors for renal disease [2,7–9]. It is no longer recommended that patients over 6 years and risk factors for primary HTN receive an extensive workup for secondary causes of HTN [2,3].

MANAGEMENT
The management of primary HTN in children consists of 3 arms including health lifestyle modifications, pharmacologic management, and limiting or supporting sports participation based on staging. The goal of management in primary HTN is to bring the BP below the 90% or in children 13 years of age or older at or below 130/80 [2]. If complications such as CKD, diabetes, endocrine causes, or evidence of end organ damage, goals for BP management may need to be set significantly lower than the 90% [3,8,9].All children and families should have education on modifiable risk factors, prevention strategies, long-term implications of uncontrolled HTN, and potential risk factors. Certain medications can increase the BP and may need to be modified or discontinued to lower BP such as cold medications, antidepressants, pain, birth control, caffeine, herbal supplements, biologic therapies, stimulants, immunosuppressives, and illegal drugs [10]. Additional education should focus on red flags to seek care for when talking about hypertensive emergencies or significant complications such as stroke. It is recommended to follow-up BP at every visit and to rescreen with ABPM every 6 months to a year [1,2] Referral to specialists should be considered if there are secondary causes of HTN identified, there is evidence of end organ damage, or concerns about uncontrolled HTN despite lifestyle modification and medication management [2,4,7]. Referrals could include cardiology, renal, endocrinology, and optometry depending on underlying concerns.

Lifestyle modifications
Healthy lifestyle behaviors should be recommended in all children to prevent and treat HTN. The current recommendations include the Dietary Approaches to Stop HTN (DASH) diet that is high in fruits, vegetables, low fat dairy, whole grains, fish, poultry, nuts, and lean meats with limited sugar and salt intake; moderate physical activity for 30 to 60 minutes, 3 to 5 days per week; and stress reduction such as mindfulness and meditation [2,3].

Medication management
There is limited research in long-term clinical trials for medication management of primary HTN in children but several short-term clinical trials are there, which lead to a low level of evidence when recommending anti-HTN therapy [2].However, the AAP guidelines recommend initiating pharmacologic management in children who have stage I HTN who have not gotten control with lifestyle modification in 6 to 12 months or those with evidence of end

organ damage [2,3]. Stage II HTN requires pharmacologic therapy initiated at the beginning of treatment plan along with healthy lifestyle recommendations [2,3]. The recommendation for pharmacologic therapy include angiotensin converting enzyme (ACE) inhibitors, angiotensin receptor blockers (ARB), long acting calcium channel blockers, or thiazide diuretics [2,3]. See Table 4 for the most common drugs and medication dosing in pediatrics. If evidence of proteinuria, diabetes, or other kidney complications are seen then ACE inhibitors and ARBs are the recommended treatment modality. [2,3], Typically, the provider should start with 1 agent and maximize that agent prior to adding additional agents to prevent polypharmacy and side effects of multiple medications. In the case of acute severe HTN, it is recommended to initiate immediate treatment with short-acting antihypertensive medications to reduce the BP by no more than 25% over the first 8 hours [2]. This usually takes place in the hospital setting with careful monitoring of BP and other parameters by cardiology or a hospitalist.

Sports/activity participation

While healthy lifestyle modifications include participation in moderate aerobic exercise 3 to 5 times per week, it is important for the provider to understand competitive sports participation and HTN recommendations. Children should be assessed for cardiovascular risks and target organ effects prior to participation in competitive sports [2,3]. If there is no evidence of these risks, participation in competitive sports should be encouraged in those with stage I HTN and below [2,3]. In children with stage II HTN, they should receive treatment to bring their HTN below stage II thresholds prior to participation in competitive sports [2]. Overall, physical activity is important in the management of BP in all children and should be encouraged when safe to allow participation. Even in those with stage II HTN, they should be encouraged to continue to do noncompetitive activities such as walking to promote physical fitness as able. Children with special health care needs may require additional clearance from their specialists prior to competitive sport participation. But many children can participate in Special Olympics, which allows a more inclusive environment even with health conditions [12].

HEALTH PROMOTION

Health promotion for pediatric patients involves a comprehensive approach that includes weight management, regular exercise, and monitoring kidney and heart health. Effective weight management is crucial for reducing the risk of HTN and related cardiovascular issues in children. Intensive weight-loss therapy, which incorporates dietary changes like the DASH diet and vigorous physical activity, is recommended for children with obesity-related risk factors. Motivational interviewing (MI) is also suggested as a useful tool to help pediatric patients adhere to these lifestyle changes. This particular intervention is appropriate for older children and adolescents while younger pediatric patients will require parental involvement and motivation. Although the

Table 4
Common antihypertensive medications and dosing in pediatrics [11]

Class of medication	Medication name	Initial starting dose	Typical dosing	Max dosing
ACE Inhibitors	Captopril	Infants: 0.05–0.1 mg/kg/dose Children: 0.5 mg/kg/dose Adolescents: 12.5mg–25 mg PO q 8 h increase by this amount q 1–2 w.	Infants: 2.5–6 mg/kg/d PO divided q 6–24 h Children: 2.5–6 mg/kg/d PO divided q 8 h Adolescents: 25–50 mg PO q 6–8 h	Infants: 6 mg/kg/d Children: 6 mg/kg/d Adolescents: 450 mg/d
ACE Inhibitors	Enalapril	Infants, children, and adolescents:(1 mth or older): 0.08 mg/kg/d up to 5 mg/d PO divided q 12–24 h.	Infants, children, and adolescents: 0.1–0.5 mg/kg/d PO divided q 12–24 h	Infants, children, and adolescents: 0.58 mg/kg/d up to 40 mg/d
ARB	Valsartan	1–16 y: 1 mg/kg/dose up to 40 mg PO q 24 h 17 y and older: 80–160 mg PO q 24 h	1–16 y: 1.4 mg/kg/dose PO q 24 h 17 y and older: 80–320 mg PO q 24 h	1–16 y: 4 mg/kg/d up to 160 mg/d 17 y and older: 320 mg/d
ARB	Losartan	6 y and older: 0.7 mg/kg/dose PO q 24 h up to 50 mg/day	6 y and older: 0.7–1.4 mg/kg/dose PO q 24 h	6 y and older: 1.4 mg/kg/day up to 100 mg/day
Calcium Channel	Amlodipine	6–17 y and older: 2.5-5 mg PO q 24 h	6 y and older: 2.5-5 mg PO q 24 h	6 y and older: 10 mg/day
Thiazide diuretics	Hydrochlorothiazide	<6 mo: 1-3 mg/kg/d PO divided q 12 h 6 mo to 12 y: 1-2 mg/kg PO divided q 12–24 h	<6 mo: 1-3 mg/kg/d PO divided q 12 h 6 mo to 12 y: 1-2 mg/kg PO divided q 12–24 h	<6 mo to 2 years: 37.5 mg/d 2 y to 12 y: 100 mg/d

efficacy of MI in hypertensive youth is still under study, it has shown promise in addressing childhood obesity by encouraging physical activity and healthy eating habits [1].

Exercise plays a vital role in lowering BP and improving overall cardiovascular health in pediatric patients. Studies suggest that engaging in moderate to vigorous aerobic physical activity for at least 40 minutes, 3 to 5 days a week, can significantly reduce systolic BP and prevent vascular dysfunction. This physical activity regimen is especially beneficial when combined with dietary interventions to manage weight and reduce cardiometabolic risks. These recommendations aim to promote a healthier lifestyle and prevent the onset of serious kidney and heart conditions [1].

SUMMARY

The increasing prevalence of HTN in pediatric patients has significant implications for clinical practice. Screening for HTN should be an integral part of routine pediatric visits, given the association between elevated BP in childhood and the risk of developing adult HTN and cardiovascular diseases [1]. Effective diagnosis relies on accurate BP measurement, which can be challenging due to the variability of normal values related to age, gender, and height percentiles. The use of electronic health records to flag at-risk patients and the implementation of standardized clinic protocols for BP measurement can improve the identification of hypertensive children. Furthermore, training clinic personnel to understand and act on high BP readings is crucial. This includes knowing when to provide counseling, order additional testing, and ensure follow-up visits. Implementing these measures can help overcome common barriers and improve HTN management in the pediatric population [1].

IMPLICATIONS FOR ADVANCED PRACTICE NURSES

Screening for BP should be implemented in all primary care practices beginning at age 3 to promote early detection and management of HTN in children. Diagnosis of HTN can be accomplished through 3 measurements at 3 separate visits or ABPM [2,3]. The cornerstone of management remains modification of risk factors, lifestyle modifications, treatment of underlying conditions contributing to HTN, and medication management [2–4]. Untreated or poorly controlled HTN has long-term health consequences such as LVH, carotid artery thickness, microvascular changes, increased risk of kidney disease, proteinuria, decreased executive functioning, and end organ damage [3,4]. Through screening and guideline management of children and adolescents, the clinician can diagnose and adequately manage HTN in children.

CLINICS CARE POINTS

- Begin measuring blood pressure at 3 years of age for healthy children or sooner if risk factors per the AAP guidelines.

- Blood pressure tables based on sex and size of child help guide the clinician in determining hypertension prior to the age of 13 years of age.
- When children reach 13 years of age, a blood pressure of less than 120/80 is considered normal.
- As in adults, children should have their blood pressures staged to determine the appropriate interventions.
- Children with special healthcare needs that can affect blood pressure should have their blood pressure monitored more frequently and earlier than children without risk factors.
- Health lifestyle and helath promotion strategies remain the cornerstone of hypertension management no matter the staging of hypertension. However, Stage 1-2 hypertension may require pharmacologic management.

Disclosure

T. Whited recieves speaker honoriarum from NAPNAP for the Pediatric Primary Care Review Course and honariarium from NAPNAP for COVID-19 Vaccine Group. Neither of which conflict with this article. T. Steele has no disclosures.

References

[1] Hardy S, Swati S, Jaeger B, et al. Trends in blood pressure and hypertension among US children and adolescents 1999-2018. JAMA 2021;4(4):e213917.
[2] Flynn JT, Kaelber DC, Baker-Smith CM, et al. Clinical practice guideline for screening and management of high blood pressure in children and adolescents. Pediatrics 2017;140(3): 1-15.
[3] Falkner B, Gidding SS, Baker-Smith CM, et al. Pediatric primary hypertension: an underrecognized condition: a scientific statement from the American Heart Association. Hypertension 2023;80:e101-11.
[4] Goknar N, Caliskan S. New guidelines for the diagnosis, evaluation, and treatment of pediatric hypertension. Turkish Archives of Pediatrics 2020;55(1):11-22.
[5] Moin A, Mohanty N, Tedla Y, et al. Under-recognition of pediatric hypertension diagnosis: examination of 1 year of visits to community health centers. J Clin Hypertens 2021;23(2): 257-64.
[6] Rose J, Krishnan-Sarin S, Exil V, et al. Cardiopulmonary impact of electronic cigarettes and vaping products: a scientific statement from the American Heart Association. Circulation 2023;148(8):708-28.
[7] Cheung A, Chang T, Cushman W, et al. Executive summary of the KDIGO 2021 clinical practice guideline for the management of blood pressure in chronic kidney disease. Kidney Int 2021;99:559-69.
[8] Stabouli S, Beropouli S, Goulas I, et al. Diagnostic evaluation of the hypertensive child. Pediatr Nephrol 2024;39:339-43.
[9] Benenson I, Waldron F, Porter S. Pediatric hypertension: a guideline update. Nurse Pract Am J Prim Health Care 2020;45(5):16-23.
[10] Vitarello J, Fitzgerald C, Cluett J, et al. Prevalence of medications that may raise blood pressure among adults with hypertension in the United States. JAMA Intern Med 2022;182(1): 90-3.
[11] Epocrates. Drugs. Available at: https://www.epocrates.com/online/.
[12] Centers for Disease Control (CDC). CDC and special Olympics: inclusive health. Available at: https://www.cdc.gov/ncbddd/disabilityandhealth/features/special-olympics-heroes.html.

Advances in Family Practice Nursing 7 (2025) 185–197

ADVANCES IN FAMILY PRACTICE NURSING

Updated (New) Hyperbilirubinemia Guidelines for the Primary Care Provider

Check for updates

Mary E. Flynn, DNP, PPCNP-BC, CPNP-AC[a,b,*]

[a]Conway School of Nursing, The Catholic University of America, 620 Michigan Avenue, Northeast, Washington, DC 20064, USA; [b]Children's National Hospital, Washington, DC, USA

Keywords

• Hyperbilirubinemia • Jaundice • Newborn • Infant • Phototherapy

Key points

• Most newborns will develop jaundice in the first week of life that self-resolves within 1 to 2 weeks.

• Newborns discharged from the hospital need a follow-up appointment within 1 to 3 days to monitor for jaundice.

• Assess infant's weight, elimination patterns, and adequacy of feedings at each visit.

• Monitor bilirubin levels, as appropriate, based on the infant's history, risk factors, and assessment.

• Initiate the appropriate treatment when infants meet or exceed the phototherapy threshold.

INTRODUCTION

It is estimated that approximately 80% of all infants will have some level of jaundice within the first week of life [1]. Most cases are caused by physiologic jaundice and typically self-resolves in the first few weeks of life. The American Academy of Pediatrics recently updated and replaced their 2004 clinical practice guideline for the management and treatment of hyperbilirubinemia in infants aged greater than or equal to 35 weeks gestation [2].

The new guideline includes 25 Key Action Statements that focus on:

• Prevention
• Risk assessment

*Conway School of Nursing, The Catholic University of America, 620 Michigan Avenue, Northeast, Washington, DC 20064. E-mail address: flynna@cua.edu

https://doi.org/10.1016/j.yfpn.2024.12.006
2589-420X/25/© 2025 Elsevier Inc. All rights are reserved, including those for text and data mining, AI training, and similar technologies.

- Monitoring
- Treatment [2]

Both guidelines focused heavily on hospital management of significant hyperbilirubinemia especially during the newborn's birth hospitalization. Most are routinely discharged home for follow-up with an advanced practice provider (APP), this updated guideline adds key recommendations for timely bilirubin follow-up, plus management and treatment after hospital discharge. Although, most newborns will have physiologic jaundice, it is the APP who will encounter the rare case of significant hyperbilirubinemia after discharge, making it important to understand which newborns are at greater risk for significantly elevated bilirubin levels and how to manage them in an outpatient setting.

PATHOPHYSIOLOGY

Bilirubin is a byproduct of hemoglobin catabolism. Newborns naturally have a higher hematocrit at birth, elevated red blood cells, an immature process of bilirubin metabolism through the liver, and a shorter red blood cell life span that can contribute to jaundice in a newborn [3]. Elevation of the serum bilirubin level causes jaundice in the newborn, noted by a yellow appearance to the newborn's mucous membranes and skin tone. Unconjugated bilirubin (indirect bilirubin) is lipid soluble and can cross the blood–brain barrier. Unconjugated bilirubin binds to albumin and is transported to the liver where it is conjugated (direct bilirubin) with glucuronic acid. Once conjugated, it is water-soluble and transported through the bile duct system where it can be excreted through bile, urine, or stool. Bilirubin that is not excreted may be unconjugated in the intestines and reabsorbed through the enterohepatic circulation [3].

If unconjugated bilirubin is elevated enough, it will cross the blood–brain barrier and settle in the basal ganglia and brainstem nuclei. This excessive accumulation of bilirubin in the brain can lead to kernicterus [4]. Although rare, kernicterus is a severely debilitating neurotoxic disorder, which is characterized by the yellow staining of the infant's brain tissue causing acute or chronic bilirubin encephalopathy and is often fatal [5,6]. Infants with kernicterus have a 5% [7] to 10% mortality rate [8] and an estimated 70% [9] to 88% morbidity rate [7]. Newborns diagnosed with kernicterus that survive have the potential of developing athetoid cerebral palsy, dental dysplasia, sensorineural hearing loss, paralysis of upward gaze, and/or cognitive or intellectual deficits [2,6]. Despite substantial evidence to support the management and treatment of hyperbilirubinemia, there still lacks a consensus on a specific bilirubin level that may result in kernicterus [2].

Full-term newborns with a gestational age greater than or equal to 38 weeks will have a peak bilirubin level of 6 to 8 mg/dL by their third day of life [10]. A preterm newborn with a gestational age between 35 weeks and 36 6/7 weeks will typically reach a peak bilirubin level of 10 to 12 mg/dL around day 5 of life [10]. These bilirubin levels are consistent with physiologic jaundice of the newborn.

DIAGNOSIS

Hyperbilirubinemia is an excess of bilirubin in the blood and presents as jaundice. Physiologic jaundice is the most common cause of hyperbilirubinemia, but it is a diagnosis of exclusion [3]. Pathologic causes of hyperbilirubinemia may be due to an increase in bilirubin production or decrease in its clearance.

Hemolysis, the destruction of red blood cells, is the most common and considered pathologic in infants when it leads to a rapid rise in transcutaneous bilirubin (TcB) or total serum bilirubin (TSB) levels, or when the infant requires phototherapy during their birth hospitalization [11]. In the United States, the most prevalent hemolytic disorders include ABO/Rh blood group incompatibility, whether or not it is accompanied by a positive direct antiglobulin test (DAT) screen, and glucose-6-phosphate dehydrogenase (G6PD) deficiency [11].

See Table 1 for additional conditions to consider with an increase in bilirubin production.

See Table 2 for a list of conditions to consider with a decrease in bilirubin elimination.

PREVENTION OF HYPERBILIRUBINEMIA

Prevention starts during pregnancy with the recommendation of routine maternal screening that includes blood group typing, Rh(D) typing, and antibody screening for every mother during the pregnancy. If a mother gives birth without prenatal care or maternal screenings prior to delivery, she should be screened immediately. If the mother is not screened, the newborn should have blood drawn for a DAT and a blood type to evaluate for early hemolysis [2].

If maternal laboratories are available, the newborn should be screened with a DAT and blood type if the maternal antibody is positive or the maternal Rh(D) is negative. It is optional to screen newborns whose mother's blood type is O+ if the hospital has established guidelines to monitor the newborn for jaundice during the stay. These newborns will require either a TcB or a TSB evaluation prior to discharge.

Newborns who are DAT positive are considered to have a neurotoxic risk factor that places them at greater risk for developing hyperbilirubinemia [2].

Table 1
Causes of increased bilirubin production [12]

Iso-immune disorders	Red blood cell membrane defects	Erythrocyte defects	Infection	Other causes
ABO incompatibility	Hereditary spherocytosis	G6PD deficiency	Sepsis/urinary tract infection	polycythemia
Rh incompatibility	Hereditary elliptocytosis	Pyruvate kinase deficiency	Cytomegalovirus (CMV)	Enclosed hemorrhage (ie, hematomas)
Positive maternal antibody screen	—	Congenital erythropoietic porphyria	Other perinatal congenital infections	—

Table 2
Causes of decreased bilirubin elimination [12]

Suboptimal intake	Crigler–Najjar syndrome	Panhypopituitarism
Breast milk jaundice	Congenital hypothyroidism	α1-antitrypsin deficiency
Gilbert syndrome	Galactosemia	Transient familial hyperbilirubinemia

The APP must take the positive DAT into consideration as a neurotoxic risk factor when evaluating an outpatient bilirubin level to determine the need for phototherapy treatment or escalation of care. In addition, it is not known if a newborn has G6PD deficiency, thus a positive family history in a first-degree relative may be considered a positive neurotoxic risk factor. All levels of treatment are lowered when newborns are known to have neurotoxic risk factors [2].

See Box 1 for a list of relevant neurotoxic risk factors in the outpatient setting.

After delivery, prevention begins with encouraging breastfeeding. Breast milk is the optimal nutrition for infants, yet there is an association with exclusive breastfeeding and hyperbilirubinemia. Mothers should be encouraged to breastfeed their infants 8 to 12 times a day and encourage lactation consultations to support their breastfeeding effort [2]. With frequent feedings, the infant should receive an increase in fluid and caloric intake, but this intake is likely less than a formula-fed infant [12].

RISK ASSESSMENT

Many infants have risk factors for the development of hyperbilirubinemia that will require closer observation. Most newborns are discharged from their birth hospitalization between 24 and 48 hours of life; thus, a routine follow-up should occur within 1 to 3 days after hospital discharge. It is important to review the risk factors for the development of significant hyperbilirubinemia at these early visits.

See Box 2 for a list of risk factors that may contribute to the development of significant hyperbilirubinemia.

Box 1: Neurotoxic risk factors relevant in the outpatient setting [2]

- Gestational age <38 weeks (already considered in the treatment graphs)
- Positive DAT
- G6PD deficiency (may consider a positive family history)
- Sepsis
- Any other known hemolytic conditions

Box 2: Significant hyperbilirubinemia risk factors [2]

- Lower gestational age (ie, risk increases with each additional week <40 weeks)
- Jaundice in the first 24 hours of life
- Predischarge TcB or TSB level near PTT
- Any cause of hemolysis: a rapid ROR of 0.3 mg/dL per hour within the first 24 hours after birth or 0.2 mg/dL per hour after the initial 24 hours of life
- Phototherapy during birth hospitalization
- Parent or sibling requiring phototherapy or exchange transfusion
- Family history or genetic ancestry suggestive of inherited red blood cell disorders, including G6PD deficiency
- Exclusive breastfeeding with suboptimal intake
- Cephalohematoma or significant bruising
- Down syndrome
- Macrosomia infant of a diabetic mother [2]

Reproduced with permission from Journal Pediatrics. 150(3). doi: 10.1542/peds.2022-058859. Copyright © 2022 by the AAP.

DIAGNOSTIC TESTING AND MONITORING

Screening or testing for jaundice is completed with either a TcB or a TSB measurement. A TcB is a painless, noninvasive method of obtaining a bilirubin measurement by a superficial reading of the bilirubin-stained skin of an infant. It provides an instantaneous reading and is a valid substitute for evaluating the risk of significant hyperbilirubinemia in newborns [13]. Even though a TcB measurement may be used to effectively estimate a TSB level, if the TcB measurement either exceeds or is within 3 mg/dL of the phototherapy threshold (PTT) or 15 mg/dL or greater, a TSB should be drawn to confirm the bilirubin level [2]. A TSB is a precise measurement of the total bilirubin level from the blood obtained from a heel stick of the infant.

All newborns should be monitored for jaundice and have either a TcB or a TSB obtained prior to discharge or within the first 24 to 48 hours of life, whichever occurs first. Each bilirubin level is plotted on a gestational age-specific graph. To graph the bilirubin, you must know the gestational age of the infant, age in hours of life, the date and time the bilirubin level was measured, and if there are any neurotoxic risk factors. The most likely neurotoxic risk factors seen in the outpatient setting is an infant who is DAT positive or has a family history of G6PD deficiency. These data can be entered in either bilitool.org or peditools.org to determine next steps for treatment or follow-up.

If more than one bilirubin measurement was obtained on an infant, the rate of rise (ROR) between the 2 levels may be calculated and useful to identify high-risk infants and determine the need for additional follow-up evaluations

(Calculate ROR: Current bilirubin level – previous bilirubin level (or discharge bilirubin)/the number of hours between the 2 measurements = ROR). A rapid ROR is 0.3 mg/dL per hour within the first 24 hours after birth or 0.2 mg/dL per hour after the initial 24 hours of life [2]. It is important to remember that the initiation of treatment, either escalation of care or phototherapy, must be based on a TSB measurement only [2].

COMMON CAUSES OF HYPERBILIRUBINEMIA

The most common cause of physiologic jaundice in infants is due to suboptimal intake, formally referred to as "breastfeeding jaundice" [2]. This typically appears within 2 to 5 days after birth and seen in both breast-fed and formula-fed infants. In breast-fed infants, this may be due to delayed maternal breastmilk production or feeding fewer than 8 times a day, or poor intake in formula-fed infants. Generally, jaundice due to suboptimal intake will resolve by 2 weeks of life, but APPs must assess the infant's weight, adequacy of feeding, urine output, and stooling at each follow-up visit. Infants with suboptimal intake will frequently continue to lose weight after discharge, have fewer wet diapers (minimum of 6 wet diapers per day) and may have uric acid crystals (brick dust urine) noted in the diaper, and small loose dark green or black stools [12]. Parents may also report a fussy infant who does not calm easily after feeding or is difficult to wake for feedings. Infants born at a gestational age of less than 38 weeks have a greater risk of presenting with the clinical findings of suboptimal feeding [12].

Jaundice may be persistent in some breast-fed infants for up to 3 months of life. This is recognized as breastmilk jaundice and the cause of this prolonged duration of jaundice is unknown. These babies will have an appropriate weight gain at each follow-up visit, 6 to 8 saturated wet diapers, and many yellow seedy stools per day. The infant will spontaneously wake for feeding every 2 to 3 hours. Persistent jaundice may be considered normal in breast-fed infants, but if breast fed infants are still jaundiced at 3 to 4 weeks of age, or formula-fed infants at 2 weeks of age, a total and direct reacting bilirubin concentrations should be obtained to identify jaundice due to possible pathologic cholestasis [12].

The leading cause of hazardous hyperbilirubinemia globally is the x-linked recessive disorder known as G6PD deficiency [2]. Identifying infants with this disorder is challenging since many families are unaware of the disorder or that they may be carriers. Black infants were found to have a disproportionately higher risk for G6PD deficiency compared to the general population, which led to delays in recognizing acute hemolysis caused by G6PD deficiency. This delay was associated with many cases of kernicterus [14]. Asking families about their genetic ancestry may be more helpful in identifying infants at greatest risk. G6PD deficiency is prevalent in Sub Saharan Africa, Middle East, Mediterranean, Arabian Peninsula, and Southeast Asia. Making a conscious effort to identify these infants early can improve health outcomes in this population [2].

HOSPITAL MANAGEMENT

The goal of phototherapy treatment is to prevent the bilirubin level from reaching the level that could lead to escalation of care or kernicterus [15]. The evidence presented in the new guidelines highlight that bilirubin neurotoxicity occurs at bilirubin levels above the 2004 exchange transfusion thresholds, which allowed for a slight increase in the phototherapy treatment thresholds [15]. Newborns who reach the PTT threshold during their birth hospitalization are treated with intense phototherapy until their bilirubin level meets criteria to discontinue treatment. Once phototherapy treatment is discontinued, depending on a risk factor assessment, a newborn may be discharged home to follow-up with their provider for a repeat bilirubin level on the following day or a "rebound" bilirubin level may be obtained prior to discharge. Newborns who receive phototherapy during their birth hospitalization are at greater risk for readmission thus require close observation by their APP once discharged home. If adequate follow-up is not established, the recommendation is to delay discharge until an appropriate follow-up appointment is secured.

The guidelines recommend intensive phototherapy for newborns who reach the phototherapy treatment threshold, especially during their birth hospitalization and/or if there are any neurotoxic risk factors. The goal of intensive phototherapy is to decrease the bilirubin level quickly with a shorter duration of treatment. Intensive phototherapy is provided with a narrow spectrum light-emitting diode (LED) blue light irradiance to as much of the infant's surface area as possible [2]. Thus, to maximize the infant's skin exposure requires the infant to only wear a diaper while under phototherapy.

There is not a standardized phototherapy device used for the treatment of hyperbilirubinemia, but the guideline recommends "an irradiance of at least 30 mW/cm^2 per nm at a wavelength around 475 nm. The light outside the 460 to 490 nm range provides unnecessary heat and potentially harmful wavelengths" [2][(p7)]. APPs treating infants with phototherapy should be aware that each phototherapy device for inpatient and outpatient use may provide a different irradiance and wavelength and may affect how quickly the bilirubin level decreases after initiating treatment.

One addition to the new guidelines is the recommendations regarding the timing for postdischarge follow-up. The follow-up recommendations established within this guideline are specific for evaluation of jaundice only. Infants may require earlier follow-up due to other clinical factors noted at discharge that may not be directly related to jaundice or hyperbilirubinemia [2].

See Table 3 for discharge follow-up recommendations adapted from the hyperbilirubinemia guideline.

OUTPATIENT MANAGEMENT

When an infant's outpatient bilirubin level is at or above the PTT, initiation of treatment should begin as soon as possible. It is important to obtain a thorough history and perform a risk factor assessment on the infant before making treatment decisions. When an infant needs phototherapy, it may be delivered as an

Table 3
Predischarge or postdischarge bilirubin [2]

Predischarge or postdischarge bilirubin		Recommendations
<2 mg/dL below PTT	—	TcB: Obtain a TSB TSB: Consider phototherapy or re-measure a TSB in 4–8 h
2–3.4 mg/dL below PTT	—	TcB: Obtain a TSB TSB: Measure TSB or TcB in 4–24 h
3.5–5.4 mg/dL below PTT	—	TcB/TSB: Measure TcB or TSB in 1–2 d
5.5–6.9 mg/dL below PTT	<72 h of life	TcB/TSB: Follow-up within 2 d and measure TcB or TSB based on clinical judgment
	>72 h of life	TcB/TSB: Clinical judgment if additional measurements are needed
≥7 mg/dL	<72 h of life	TcB/TSB: Follow-up within 2 d and measure TcB or TSB based on clinical judgment
	>72 h of life	TcB/TSB: Clinical judgment if additional measurements are needed

inpatient, which will likely require an overnight hospital admission. There is a possibility to provide outpatient or at home phototherapy, but the APP must assess the infant's risk factors before making this decision. If the infant meets all the criteria listed in Box 3, then home phototherapy is a management option.

Home phototherapy is more affordable and promotes maternal–infant bonding in a comfortable setting. However, its effectiveness depends on the

Box 3: Criteria below must be met for home LED-based phototherapy [2]

- Gestational age ≥38 weeks
- ≥48 hours old
- Clinically well with adequate feeding
- No known hyperbilirubinemia neurotoxicity risk factors (see Table 1)
- No previous phototherapy
- TSB concentration no more than 1 mg/dL above the phototherapy treatment threshold
- An LED-based phototherapy device will be available in the home without delay
- TSB can be measured daily

quality of the device and the family's ability to use it properly. The APP should prioritize safety and recommend hospital admission for treatment if there are concerns about any of the following: the infant's clinical condition, delays in acquiring a home LED device, the quality of the equipment, the parents' ability to use it correctly, or issues with obtaining daily TSB during treatment. Home phototherapy may be beneficial for some families, and shared decision-making should involve the family in the infant's care whenever possible.

IMPLICATIONS FOR ADVANCE PRACTICE NURSES

- At each visit during the first few months of life, evaluate:
  - Weight: Compare the current weight to the birth and previous weights.
  - Feedings: For breast-fed infants assess the number of feedings per day (8–12 per day), duration of each feeding, and maternal milk production.
  - Elimination: Number of voids and stools. Volume of urine, any evidence of brick dust (uric acid crystals) in diaper, stool numbers and if it has started to transition from meconium to yellow seedy stools.
  - Activity level: Does the infant wake for feeding and calms or appears satisfied after each feeding.
  - For jaundice: Review the discharge TcB or TSB level. Account for any neurotoxic risk factors and plot the bilirubin level on the appropriate gestational age graph, or enter the appropriate data into bilitool.org or peditools.org. See Box 4 for a list of resources.
- Bilirubin testing in the outpatient setting:
  - All infants who received inpatient phototherapy during their birth hospitalization and discharged home after discontinuation of phototherapy will need a follow-up with their provider within 1 day of discharge and obtain a bilirubin level [2].
  - Infants who were readmitted for phototherapy and who also received phototherapy during their birth hospitalization will need a follow-up appointment with a bilirubin level 1 day after discontinuation of phototherapy [2].

Box 4: Resources and guideline for bilirubin management

- Bilitool: (bilitool.org)
- Peditools: (2022) Hyperbilirubinemia management guidelines (peditools.org)
- Graphs are included in the AAP guidelines:
  - Clinical Practice Guideline Revision: Management of Hyperbilirubinemia in the Newborn Infant 35 or More Weeks of Gestation | Pediatrics | American Academy of Pediatrics (aap.org) [2].
    - Phototherapy threshold graph for newborns without neurotoxic risk factors. (Lines for gestational ages 35, 36, 37, 38, 39, and ≥40 weeks)
    - Phototherapy threshold graph for newborns with one or more neurotoxic risk factors. (Lines for gestational ages 35, 36, 37, and ≥38 weeks.) [2]

- o A TSB should be obtained after infants receive phototherapy. A TcB may be obtained, only if the infant was off phototherapy for 24 hours prior to testing, but there is evidence that a TcB obtained after phototherapy may not be as accurate as a TSB [2].
  - o Infants who were readmitted for phototherapy, but did not receive phototherapy during their birth hospitalization, as well as infants treated with home phototherapy who surpassed the threshold, should have their bilirubin levels checked 1 to 2 days after stopping phototherapy.
  - o When making this decision, it is important to consider risk factors for rebound hyperbilirubinemia, including the TSB level at the time phototherapy was discontinued and the infant's gestational age [2].
- Support breastfeeding: If possible, observe feeding during the outpatient visit and refer to a lactation consultant for additional support as needed.
- If breast-fed infants are still jaundiced at 3 to 4 weeks of age, or formula-fed infants at 2 weeks of age, a total and direct reacting bilirubin concentrations should be obtained to identify jaundice due to possible pathologic cholestasis [2]. Consultation with a gastroenterologist or other clinical expert may be warranted.
- Involve the family in shared decision-making whenever possible.
- Anticipatory guidance for parents:
  - o Jaundice is a common finding in most newborns.
  - o Jaundice appears in the face then moves down the body to chest, abdomen, arms, and legs as the level rises and may be difficult to accurately visualize in darker toned skin.
  - o Notify your APP if you see any of the following in your infant:
    - Skin turns darker yellow.
    - Abdomen, arms, and legs turn yellow.
    - Gums or whites of the eyes turn yellow.
    - Difficult to wake for feedings, is fussy, or not feeding well.
    - A decrease in wet diapers or there is an orange or brick dust color (urate crystals) in diaper after 3 days of life.

SUMMARY

- Close follow-up after discharge from the birth hospitalization is important. Most infants should be seen within 1 to 3 days after discharge.
- A thorough history and physical examination are important to evaluate the health of the infant as well as to assess for jaundice.
- Monitor urine and stool outputs for adequacy of intake. A well-hydrated infant will void at least 6 times per day and will saturate a diaper with light or colorless urine. By day 5 to 7, the stools should be loose and yellow approximately 3 to 4 times a day [16].
- Provide breastfeeding support. Encouraging frequent feedings (minimally 8–12 feedings per day) and encourage lactation consultations as necessary.

CLINICS CARE POINTS

- Infants should have a follow-up appointment with their APPs within 1 to 3 days after hospital discharge.

- Follow-up appointments are not based solely on the recommendations of the bilirubin guidelines, there may be other clinical indications requiring an earlier appointment.
- Perform a thorough prenatal and postnatal history on the infant to include neurotoxic risk factors. See Table 3.
- Asking families about their genetic ancestry may be more helpful in identifying infants at greatest risk. G6PD deficiency is prevalent in Sub Saharan Africa, Middle East, Mediterranean, Arabian Peninsula, and Southeast Asia [2].
- Monitor the infant's screening results because some conditions detected through newborn screenings can lead to persistent jaundice.
- Newborn metabolic screening tests will vary by state. Review your state's approved screenings here: Newborn Screening in Your State | Newborn Screening (hrsa.gov)
- A TSB should be obtained if the TcB is within 3 mg/dL of the PTT or if the TcB measurement is greater than 15 mg/dL [2].
- Each bilirubin level is plotted on a gestational age-specific graph. You must know the gestational age of the infant, age in hours of life, the date and time the bilirubin level was measured, and if there are any neurotoxic risk factors [2].
- These data can be entered in either bilitool.org or peditools.org to determine next steps for treatment or follow-up.
- A TSB should be used as the standard test to guide all treatment decisions.
- A TSB should be obtained after infants receive phototherapy and the timing will be based on infant's risk factors.
- A TcB may be obtained after an infant receives phototherapy *only* if the infant was off phototherapy for 24 hours prior to testing, but there is evidence that a TcB obtained after phototherapy may not be as accurate as a TSB [2].
- Persistent jaundice may be considered normal in breast-fed infants, but if breast-fed infants are still jaundiced at 3 to 4 weeks of age, or formula-fed infants at 2 weeks of age, total and direct reacting bilirubin concentrations should be obtained to identify jaundice due to possible pathologic cholestasis [12].
- Consider consultation with a gastroenterologist or other specialist if any infant has prolonged jaundice.
- Considered shared decision-making with the family as appropriate.
- Before recommending home phototherapy, make sure the infants meet all listed requirements in Box 3.
- Repeat bilirubin measurement after phototherapy is based on the risk of rebound hyperbilirubinemia.
- Close outpatient follow-up is important to trend adequacy for feeding and jaundice. A telephone consultation may be valuable between scheduled follow-up visits.

Disclosure
No disclosures.

References

[1] Bhutani VK, Stark AR, Lazzeroni LC, et al. Predischarge screening for severe neonatal hyper-bilirubinemia identifies infants who need phototherapy. J Pediatr 2013;162(3):477.

[2] Kemper AR, Newman TB, Slaughter JL, et al. Clinical practice guideline revision: management of hyperbilirubinemia in the newborn infant 35 or more weeks of gestation. Pediatrics 2022;150(3); https://doi.org/10.1542/peds.2022-058859.

[3] Marcdante KJ, Kliegman RM, Schuh AM, et al. Nelson essentials of pediatrics. 9th edition. Philadelphia: Elsevier; 2023.

[4] Bottu A, Manzar S. Phototherapy threshold: changes between 2004 and 2022 AAP guidelines. Neonatology Today 2024;19(4):25–8.

[5] IP S, Lau J, Chung M, et al. Hyperbilirubinemia and kernicterus: 50 years later. Pediatrics 2004;114(1):263–4.

[6] Screening of infants for hyperbilirubinemia to prevent chronic bilirubin encephalopathy: US preventive services task force recommendation statement. Pediatrics 2009;124(4): 1172–7.

[7] Bhutani VK, Johnson LH, Schwoebel A, et al. A systems approach for neonatal hyperbilirubinemia in term and near-term newborns. J Obstet Gynecol Neonatal Nurs 2006;35(4): 444–55.

[8] Burke BL, Robbins JM, Bird TM, et al. Trends in hospitalizations for neonatal jaundice and kernicterus in the United States, 1988-2005. Pediatrics 2009;123(2):524–32.

[9] Management of hyperbilirubinemia in the newborn infant 35 or more weeks of gestation. Pediatrics 2004;114(1):297–316.

[10] Mishra S, Agarwal R, Deorari AK, et al. Jaundice in the newborns. Indian J Pediatr 2008;75(2):157–63.

[11] Kaplan M, Bromiker R, Hammerman C. Hyperbilirubinemia, hemolysis, and increased bilirubin neurotoxicity. Semin Perinatol 2014;38(7):429–37.

[12] Flaherman VJ, Maisels MJ. ABM clinical protocol #22: guidelines for management of jaundice in the breastfeeding infant 35 weeks or more of gestation-revised 2017. Breastfeed Med 2017;12(5):250–7.

[13] Okwundu CI, Olowoyeye A, Uthman OA, et al. Transcutaneous bilirubinometry versus total serum bilirubin measurement for newborns. Cochrane Database Syst Rev 2023;5: CD012660.

[14] Wright JL, Trent ME. Applying an equity lens to clinical practice guidelines: getting out of the gate. Pediatrics 2022;150(3); https://doi.org/10.1542/peds.2022-058918.

[15] Slaughter JL, Kemper AR, Newman TB. Technical report: diagnosis and management of hyperbilirubinemia in the newborn infant 35 or more weeks of gestation. Pediatrics 2022;150(3); https://doi.org/10.1542/peds.2022-058865.

[16] Maaks DLG, Starr NB, Brady MA, et al. Burns' pediatric primary care. St Louis (MO): Elsevier; 2020.

Advances in Family Practice Nursing 7 (2025) 199–214

ADVANCES IN FAMILY PRACTICE NURSING

Caring for Children with Trisomy 18 in the Primary Care Setting

Ann Marie Ramsey, MSN, CPNP-PC*,
Lauren Nichols, DNP, CPNP-AC

Pediatric Home Ventilator Program C.S. Mott Children's Hospital, University of Michigan Health

Keywords

- Trisomy 18 • Multiple congenital anomalies • Cardiac defect
- Central sleep apnea

Key points

- Due to increasing lifespan, there is a growing need for comprehensive primary care services to coordinate the complex care children with Trisomy 18 require.
- Children with trisomy 18 have multiple congenital anomalies effecting almost every organ system with the most severe including cardiac malformations, central and obstructive sleep apnea, and seizures.
- Small stature and poor growth are common findings associated with feeding intolerance, gastroesophageal reflux, and constipation.
- Routine surveillance monitoring is required to prevent known complications including formation of solid tumors, hematologic abnormalities, airway anomalies, hearing, and vision impairments.

INTRODUCTION

Trisomy 18, also known as Edwards syndrome, is a rare chromosomal abnormality with 3, rather than 2, copies of the 18th chromosome, occurring in one of every 5000 live-born infants [1]. Trisomy 18 prevalence has risen, related to increase in maternal age [2] and number of surviving children has increased due to families choosing full treatment including surgical and other life-prolonging care. This supports a paradigm shift from palliative care to full treatment resulting in greater numbers of children who will require long-term primary care [3].

*Corresponding author. L2221 Women's Hospital, 1500 East Medical Center Drive, Ann Arbor, MI 48109-5212. E-mail address: amramsey@med.umich.edu

https://doi.org/10.1016/j.yfpn.2025.01.008
2589-420X/25/© 2025 Elsevier Inc. All rights are reserved, including those for text and data mining, AI training, and similar technologies.

Abbreviations

CHD   congenital heart disease
ECHO   echocardiogram
GERD   gastroesophageal reflux disease
H2RA   histamine-2 receptor antagonist
OSA   obstructive sleep apnea
PPI   proton pump inhibitor

DIAGNOSTICS

Trisomy 18 can be either complete or mosaic. Complete trisomy 18 occurs when all cells contain 3 copies of the 18th chromosome [4]. Mosaicism occurs when more than 1 cell line is present in the same child. These individuals carry both a trisomy 18 and a euploid cell line that may result in wide phenotypic variation [4].

Prenatal diagnostic testing is recommended if maternal screening identifies risk factors including advanced maternal age [2] and ultrasound abnormalities [4]. If abnormalities are present, then an amniocentesis or chorionic villus sampling is recommended to confirm the diagnosis. Noninvasive prenatal screening is another emerging diagnostic method that is recommended by the American College of Medical Genetics and Genomics [5]. Early confirmation of diagnosis allows for termination which is the intervention families choose in 86% of cases [2]. For children born with trisomy 18 features who were not prenatally diagnosed, karyotyping, a blood test evaluating for chromosomal abnormalities, is the preferred method to confirm diagnosis [4].

PATHOPHYSIOLOGY AND DEVELOPMENT

Cardiac defects are the most prevalent occurring anomaly [6]. Central and obstructive sleep apnea (OSA) occur frequently due to risk for neurologic impairment in central control of breathing, craniofacial anomalies, and overall low muscle tone [7–9]. Central sleep apnea is cited as the most common cause of death in children aged less than 1 year [10–13]. Scoliosis, congenital hip dislocation, and joint contractures can occur due to abnormal muscle tone [4]. Common abdominal wall defects include umbilical and inguinal hernia [14]. Renal defects include horseshoe kidney and hydronephrosis [4,14]. Neurologic abnormalities are manifested in brain malformations that are associated with cognitive impairment, and hearing and visual deficits [4,14] (refer to Figs. 1 and 2 for summary of congenital malformations and Table 1 for frequency of occurrence).

While most children with trisomy 18 function in the severe to profound developmental disability range, many can achieve meaningful skills and demonstrate the ability to continue to learn throughout life [15]. Studies report that most children achieve a maximum developmental level of 18 month [15]. Social development is the area of greatest strength with many children demonstrating social development aged between 7 and 24 months. Communication

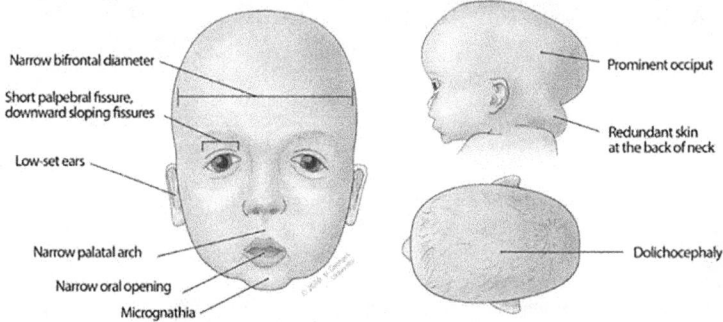

Fig. 1. The classical craniofacial presentation of trisomy 18. The combination of low-set ears; short, downward slanting palpebral fissures; prominent occiput combined with a decrease in the following features: oral opening, jaw, and bifrontal diameter are typical of trisomy 18. © 2016. St. George's University. (Roberts W, Zurada A, Zurada-ZieliŃSka A, Gielecki J, Loukas M. Anatomy of Trisomy 18. Clinical anatomy. 2016;29(5):628–32. doi.org/10.1002/ca.2272. Used with permission.)

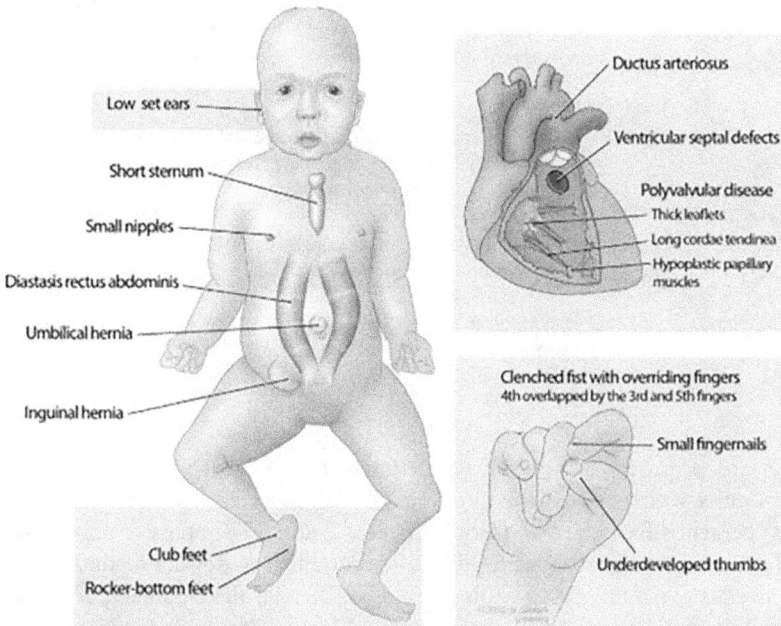

Fig. 2. The classical trisomy 18 phenotype. That is, the illustrated anatomic defects are seen in greater than 50% of patients diagnosed with trisomy 18. The diagram highlights the most common defects that are seen in trisomy 18: low-set ears, rocker bottom feet, clenched fists, and ventricular septal defect. These anatomic findings may occur with other defects such as small nipples, short sternum, hernias, and diastasis rectus abdominis. © 2026. St. George's University. (Roberts W, Zurada A, Zurada-ZieliŃSka A, Gielecki J, Loukas M. Anatomy of Trisomy 18. Clinical anatomy. 2016;29(5):628–32. doi.org/10.1002/ca.2272. Used with permission.)

Table 1
Anomalies and conditions associated with trisomy 18 [13]

System	Anomaly	Frequency of occurrence
Cardiac	Ventricular septal defect	Over 90%
	Atrial septal defect	50%–75%
	Coronary artery anomalies transposition of the great vessels, tetralogy of Fallot coarctation of the aorta dextrocardia an aberrant subclavian artery	<10%
Otolaryngology	Retrognathia and micrognathia	25%–50%
	Tracheobronchial defects	<25%
	Obstructive sleep apnea	25%–50%
	Cleft lip and/or palate	<25%
Musculoskeletal	Overriding fingers and clenched hands	Over 90%
	Club feet	25%–50%
	Scoliosis	25%–50%
Neurologic	Cerebellar hypoplasia, agenesis of the corpus callosum, spina bifida	<25%
	Seizure disorder	25%–50%
	Central apnea	50%–75%
	Cognitive impairments and developmental delay	>90%
Gastrointestinal	Feeding difficulties and gastroesophageal reflux	Over 90%
	Omphalocele, esophageal atresia tracheoesophageal fistula pyloric stenosis Meckel diverticulum	<25%
	Hernia	<50%
Ophthalmologic	Anopthalmos, microphthalmos, bilateral retinal dysplasia optic nerve hypoplasia congenital glaucoma, and congenital cataracts	<25%
Audiological	Hearing loss	>50%
	Small pinna, unfolded helix, and cryptotia	<25%
Renal	Horseshoe kidney, ectopic kidney, double ureter, and hydronephrosis	<25%
Genitourinary	Cryptorchidism	>50%
	Hypospadias, bifid scrotum bifid uterus ovarian hypoplasia	<25%

skills are acquired at a very rudimentary level between the age of 6 and 12 months with maximum communication skills at an 18 month level [15]. Fifty percent of children function between 7 and 12 months in motor skills and approximately 20% were able to accomplish a developmental level of 12 months for daily living skills (Healey PJ. Social development of children with Trisomy 18 and 13 in the context of family and community. Doctoral Dissertation, Boston College [unpublished]. 2003).

MANAGEMENT
Cardiac
The treatment of congenital heart disease (CHD) is controversial and may include observation or surgery (Table 2 for surgical trends). Trends in offering

Table 2	
Surgical trends [40,41]	
Most reported cardiac surgeries Numbers of procedures reported	Other frequently reported surgeries Numbers of procedures reported
Atrial Septal Defect Repair 56 Patent Ductus Arteriosus Repair 85 Ventricular Septal Defect Repair 85	Gastrostomy Tube Placement 295 Tracheostomy 73 Spinal Fusion 34 Myringotomy and Ear Tubes 30 Hernia Repair 28 Chemotherapy 21 Cleft lip/palate repair 20

cardiac repair surgery have changed dramatically, with increasing numbers of families seeking cardiac repair surgery [16]. The success of cardiac surgery can be related to extra-cardiac factors including other congenital anomalies [17], presence of pulmonary vascular disease and pulmonary hypertension [18], history of chronic mechanical ventilation [18–20], and lower weight at time of surgery with the majority of studies describing weight as the most important factor in contributing to long-term survival [18,21]. To minimize risk and maximize benefit, a subgroup of children with CHD will not undergo full repair in early life and may undergo palliative procedures in an effort to allow for growth and medical stabilization prior to full repair [18,21].

When prenatally diagnosed, a fetal echocardiogram (ECHO) is done to identify congenital heart defects. All children with trisomy 18 should undergo an ECHO in the first few days of life even in the absence of prenatal findings [4,12]. Routine outpatient care should include screening for heart failure with referral to a pediatric cardiologist for any abnormal cardiac findings [22].

Respiratory

Craniofacial deformities, such as micrognathia, and narrow palatal arch in combination with low muscle tone contribute to the development of upper airway obstruction and OSA [14]. In a single-center report of anesthesia experiences among 165 children, the investigators identified children with trisomy 18 having a 30 fold higher risk of difficult intubation compared with other children with orofacial abnormalities [23]. Any concern for upper airway obstruction should prompt referral to a pediatric otolaryngologist.

Based on these findings, children with trisomy 18 should be routinely evaluated for OSA symptoms including snoring, bradycardia during sleep, hypoxia during sleep, and pauses in breathing. Most children will have had a polysomnogram by the age of 4 years; however, if a polysomnogram has not been done by this age, a routine surveillance polysomnogram should be scheduled [22].

Treatment is based on the type of sleep apnea. Children with OSA with large tonsils and adenoids benefit from adenotonsillectomy [7,13]. Children with complex OSA or central sleep apnea benefit from positive-pressure ventilation which has been associated with improved long-term survival [9]. The prevalence of tracheostomy with positive-pressure ventilation has been increasing (see Table 2 for surgical trends) [13]. Mild central sleep apnea may be treated with long-term home oxygen therapy. Children with tracheostomy and ventilator requirements, noninvasive ventilation, and/or home long-term oxygen needs will require long-term follow-up with a pulmonologist [22].

Children with trisomy 18 are at risk for pneumonia secondary to the high prevalence of dysphagia, aspiration, and gastroesophageal reflux [13]. In addition, hypotonia reduces the child's ability to clear secretions from the airway in the setting of an acute infection and may result in development of atelectasis and subsequent pneumonia. Parents should be counseled on the signs and symptoms of pneumonia including persistent cough, fever, and chest congestion and should seek evaluation as soon as possible. Due to the considerable risk for severe outcomes associated with RSV infection, children with trisomy 18 are recommended to receive RSV prophylaxis as part of routine primary care [4,13].

Musculoskeletal

Due to the high prevalence of both congenital and developmental orthopedic conditions, primary care surveillance should include yearly evaluation of hips and spine, and spinal radiographs. Orthopedic examinations should begin at the age of 2 years and continue annually [4,13]. Referral should be made to orthopedic surgery for any abnormal findings [22]. Children with trisomy 18 are at risk for the development of contractures and have poor motor function and benefit from physical and occupational therapy. Referral to speech therapy should be made to promote all oral and speech skill development [13].

Gastrointestinal

Gastroesophageal reflux disease (GERD) is a common finding and presents with symptoms of inconsolable irritability, respiratory compromise including hypoxic spells, and in cases of aspiration, it can contribute to choking, gagging, and the development of pneumonia [12,13]. It is important to recognize gastroesophageal reflux can also be silent. In situations in which the earlier symptoms are suspected to be secondary to GERD, it is reasonable for the primary care provider to initiate first-line interventions for reflux. The American Academy of Pediatrics guideline on management of GERD in pediatric patients published in 2013 [24] endorses lifestyle changes as a first-line intervention including upright positioning for infants when receiving feedings. Medical management includes the use of antacids that fall into two classes: acid suppressants histamine-2 receptor antagonists (H2RAs), and proton pump inhibitors (PPIs) and prokinetic agents [25]. H2RAs are noted to be highly effective acid suppressants; however, use is limited by a short time to development of tolerance and has shown to be less effective for severe GERD and erosive esophagitis then PPIs. PPIs have a unique characteristic of reducing acid in relation to a meal, and therefore, timing of 30 minutes before a meal is extremely important to efficacy. They do not have the tachyphylaxis as noted with H2RA agents; however, they are associated with an increased risk for lower respiratory infections [25]. A referral to a pediatric gastroenterologist should be considered for children with complex GERD that is not responsive to first-line therapies. Referral to pediatric surgery is indicated for children with any type of congenital malformation including omphalocele, Meckel's diverticulum, and malrotation [22].

Constipation is a frequently occurring problem that is associated with abdominal distention, pain, vomiting, and failure to thrive. This problem is difficult to manage due to the lack of evidence on effective methods of management in this specific population; however, clinically, children with trisomy 18 have been managed with pediatric-based protocols with success [13]. Polyethylene glycol 3350 is a highly effective agent for both disimpaction and maintenance [24,26]. Other osmotic agents, such as lactulose, and stimulant agents, such as senna and bisacodyl, have successfully been used in long-term constipation management [26]. Referral to a pediatric gastroenterologist should be considered for children with complex constipation who are not responsive to first-line therapies.

Growth and nutrition

Small stature and growth retardation are a hallmark finding that continues throughout life [4]. Many newborns have a diagnosis of intrauterine growth retardation and plot below the third percentile for height and weight relative to gestational age [27]. Growth should be tracked on the trisomy 18 height and weight chart [28] (Growth charts can be found: https://Trisomy.org/resources/surgeries-ggrowth-charts/#/). In addition to genetic predisposition to small stature, difficulty feeding secondary to poor suck swallow, muscle weakness, feeding intolerance, slow gastric motility, and GERD present significant challenges to weight gain and overall growth and development [13]. Only a small subset of children are able to take in enough nutrition orally to sustain appropriate growth. Frequent office checks are indicated to confirm ongoing appropriate oral intake as measured by appropriate growth [4]. An even smaller subset of children with trisomy 18 can breastfeed. Breastfeeding can be extremely challenging, and these families benefit from consultation with the lactation consultant [13].

Many children are unable to take in enough calories orally and require supplemental tube feedings. Initial tube feedings can be delivered by nasogastric method; however, most children will undergo placement of a gastrostomy tube (see Table 2 for surgical trends) [29]. Common complications of tube feedings include recurrent vomiting, worsening symptoms of gastroesophageal reflux, and abdominal distension, and pain often manifested by worsening respiratory status and cyanotic spells. An important clinical pearl is to evaluate for feeding intolerance as an underlying cause of abdominal pain/discomfort, respiratory decompensation, hypoxic spells, and long-term inconsolability.

Enteral nutrition should be managed by a dietitian experienced in managing tube feedings in this population. Typically, infants initiate tube feedings with breast milk, or an intact infant formula (eg, Similac, Enfamil). In cases in which infants require higher calories than a standard 20 kcal/oz formula, breast milk can be enriched with commercial powder formulas, or an intact formula preparation recipe can be adjusted to produce higher calorie concentration. Tube feeding schedules are also critical in managing feeding intolerance. Many infants are not able to tolerate bolus feedings early in life and benefit from a continuous feeding schedule. Gastric and intestinal gases are a frequent problem, resulting in abdominal distension and pain. A method of feeding utilizing a "chimney" allows feedings to be delivered into an open 60 mL syringe then infused via gravity that allows for expulsion of gastric gas (Fig. 3 of chimney set up). Persistent feeding intolerance may require the use of alternative formulas such as peptide-based formulas (eg, Pediasure Peptide) or elemental formulas (eg, Elecare Infant).

As children grow, their nutritional needs will change, requiring advancement from infant formula to pediatric formulas. As with infant formulas, pediatric formulas are available as food-based, intact, peptide, and elemental preparations. The pediatric formulas are more concentrated than infant formulas, requiring consideration of not only calories, but also total fluid requirements. Recently, families have developed an interest in providing food-based blended diet utilizing food and a high-efficiency blender. Laboratory analysis including complete blood count, renal function panel, iron studies including iron-binding capacity, and percent transferrin as well as vitamin-D levels will be important for total nutritional management. Some children will develop skills necessary for oral feeding. Before beginning oral feeding, it is important to ensure an intact swallow and absence of aspiration. Video fluoroscopic swallow study is the gold standard for evaluating swallow efficacy and safety [22].

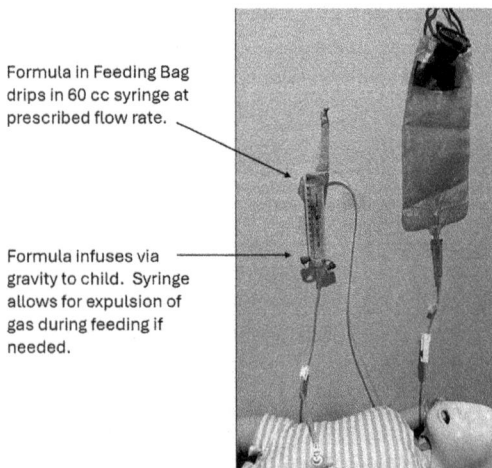

Formula in Feeding Bag drips in 60 cc syringe at prescribed flow rate.

Formula infuses via gravity to child. Syringe allows for expulsion of gas during feeding if needed.

Fig. 3. Chimney gravity feeding system.

Renal and genitourinary

Abdominal ultrasound to evaluate for renal abnormalities is recommended 48 to 72 hours after birth and referral to pediatric urology and/or pediatric nephrology should be initiated if abnormalities are noted [22]. Recurrent urinary tract infections should trigger additional investigation including voiding cystourethrogram and referral to urology if not already in place [30]. Prophylactic antibiotics are often used for congenital urologic defects that result in or place children at risk for recurrent urinary tract infections [13].

Neurologic vision and hearing

Seizures are common and typically present in the first year of life [12,31] and continue to be a common finding in older children [32]. Seizure morphology varies from tonic-clonic seizures to partial complex seizures. Postnatal cranial ultrasound is recommended, even in the absence of prenatal findings, to identify intracranial anomalies and determine whether additional imaging is required. Keep in mind that a negative cranial ultrasound does not exclude structural anomalies. If significant defects are identified, referral to pediatric neurology and/or neurosurgery is indicated [22].

Significant ocular manifestations include cataracts and corneal opacities, and older children may develop photophobia [32]. An ophthalmologic examination should be completed in the first year of life and then annually. In addition, children should wear sunglasses to reduce discomfort associated with photophobia [32].

Cerumen impaction or middle-ear effusions, particularly if a cleft palate is present, are risk factors for conductive hearing loss [32,33]. Older children are at risk for moderate-to-severe sensorineural hearing loss [32]. Audiologic evaluation should begin at birth and repeated at 6 months of life and then annually. If hearing deficits are noted, the child should be referred to an audiologist and otolaryngologist [22].

Neoplastic and hematologic

Hepatoblastoma is the most common solid tumor and typically presents between the ages of 3 months and 4 years [34]. Other less frequently occurring tumors include Wilms, renal, and tricuspid aortic tumors [4]. Screening abdominal ultrasounds and serum alpha-fetoprotein are recommended every 3 months from birth until the age of 4 years [22]. Screening for Wilms tumor should begin after the age of 1 year, with renal ultrasound every 3 to 6 months until the age of 5 years [4,13]. Hematologic abnormalities have been reported including thrombocytopenia, neutrophilia, and anemia; [35] therefore, a complete blood count with differential should be obtained in all newborns and any child prior to surgical intervention and when managing acute illness [22,36].

Puberty and gynecology

Historically short life spans limit the experience to report puberty trends. Those who do reach the age of puberty are at risk for delayed puberty, amenorrhea, and premature ovarian failure. Children with decreased growth velocity should be

Box 1: Staying on track with trisomy 18

Trisomy 18 is a chromosomal abnormality that causes multiple medical morbidities. While some abnormalities will be present at birth, or apparent with a thorough history and physical examination, others might require careful monitoring and surveillance. The following is a checklist of surveillance tests to ensure that medical issues are identified and treated promptly.

Birth

☐ Cranial ultrasound or MRI

☐ Echocardiogram

☐ Ophthalmologic examination

☐ Abdominal ultrasound

☐ Serum alpha-fetoprotein (AFP)

☐ Complete blood count with differential

☐ Audiologic examination

☐ Occupation and physical therapy consultation

☐ Early on referral

☐ Polysomnogram

　　○ If any clinical concerns for obstructive or central apnea

　　○ If patient is in neonatal intensive care unit (NICU) and blood gas shows P_{CO_2} greater than 50 mm Hg

1 month

☐ Abdominal ultrasound to assess for renal abnormalities.

　　○ Only done at 1 month if abnormalities are seen on prenatal, but not postnatal ultrasound.

3 months

☐ Abdominal and renal ultrasound

☐ Serum AFP

☐ Physical medicine and rehabilitation evaluation

6 months

☐ Abdominal and renal ultrasound

☐ Serum AFP

☐ Audiologic evaluation

9 months

☐ Abdominal and renal ultrasound

☐ Serum AFP

12 months

☐ Abdominal and renal ultrasound

☐ Serum AFP

☐ Ophthalmologic exam

☐ Dental exam

Starting at age 1 year

☐ Abdominal and renal ultrasounds every 3 months

- Until age 4

☐ Serum AFPs every 3 months

- Until age 4

☐ Annual orthopedic exam and spinal x-rays

- Starting at age 2

☐ Annual ophthalmologic evaluations

☐ Renal ultrasounds every 3 months

- Between ages 4 and 7

☐ Renal ultrasounds every 6 months

- Between ages 7 and 12

☐ Abdominal ultrasounds every 6 months

- From age 7-12

☐ Baseline polysomnogram by age 4 or sooner if concerns for obstructive or central sleep apnea

Puberty

☐ Monitor growth and pubertal development.

In addition, all well child visits for children with Trisomy 18 should include the following:

☐ Assessment of growth, nutrition, and swallowing

☐ Growth should be measured using a Trisomy 18 growth chart.

☐ Assessment of psychomotor motor, social, verbal, and cognitive development

- Referral to Early On/physical therapy/occupational therapy/speech therapy

☐ Development of seizures or other neurological or ophthalmological concerns

☐ Assessment for scoliosis, hand, or foot deformities

☐ Assessment of respiratory illnesses, airway clearance, and noisy breathing

☐ Assessment of sleep concerns including snoring and excessive daytime sleepiness

☐ Dental assessment every 6 months

☐ Routine vaccinations as well as Palivizumab and 23-valent pneumococcal vaccine

☐ Assessment of psychological, social, educational, and emotional needs of the child and family

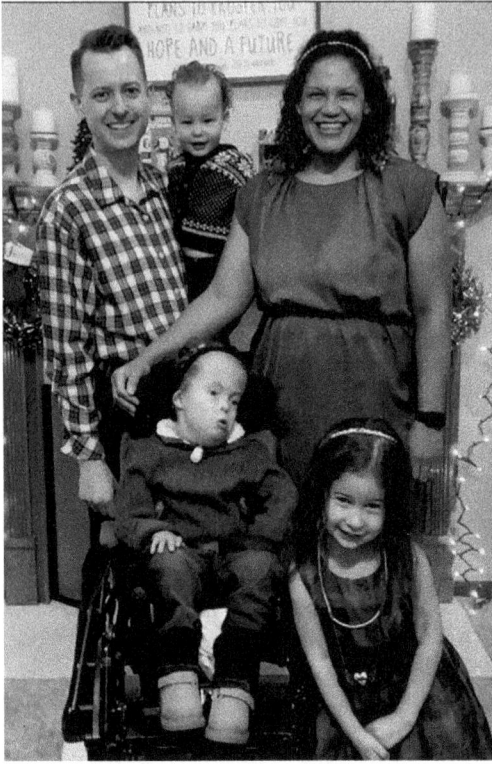

Fig. 4. Children with trisomy 18 are members of loving families.

referred to a pediatric endocrinologist, and those with amenorrhea should be referred to a gynecologist [22].

IMPLICATIONS FOR ADVANCED PRACTICE NURSES

As the lifespan increases, children with trisomy 18 will require comprehensive primary care to order and follow up on results of surveillance testing, and to help families coordinate subspeciality and community-based care consistent with the American Academy of Pediatrics definition of a medical home. Discuss with parents the importance of vaccinations and provide reassurance vaccines that are not associated with increased risk to their child due to the diagnosis of trisomy 18. Children should receive both routine childhood vaccines and annual vaccinations including influenza and RSV vaccines. Routine audiologic and ophthalmologic screenings are important. Due to the specific musculoskeletal, neurologic, and developmental pathophysiology, all children with trisomy 18 should receive physical therapy, occupational therapy, and speech therapy.

Alongside routine primary care considerations, children with trisomy 18 require other routine screenings that include surveillance laboratories and

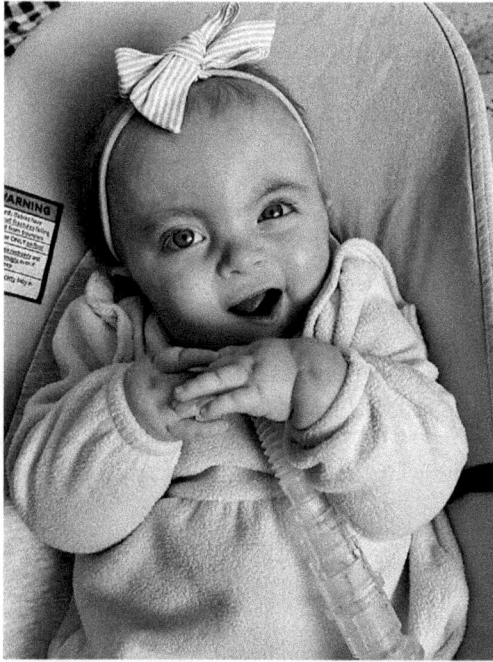

Fig. 5. A child with trisomy 18 with an endearing personality and charm.

imaging studies. Refer to Box 1 "Staying on track with trisomy 18" checklist that is designed as a "quick reference" of the recommended screenings. Additional screening may be indicated based on the child's specific medical needs.

Finally, it is important to offer support to the families. Many families report feeling judged regarding their decision to continue the pregnancy and to advocate for full medical intervention [37,38]. In a 2020 survey of 332 parents, 88% identified trust as a vital component of a positive provider relationship. Simple interventions, such as addressing the child by name, commenting on the positive such as gaining weight or making developmental gains, and commenting to parents on the excellent job they are doing caring for their child, are critical to building trust [39]. Parents reported taking care of a disabled child who was harder than expected, however, despite the severe disabilities, describing their child as happy, and an important and integrated member of their family [38] (Fig. 4).

SUMMARY

Children with trisomy 18 are a rapidly expanding population who will require extensive and comprehensive care coordination. Due to the multiple congenital anomalies and significant medical interventions, they are at risk for complications and death. Risk reduction occurs through appropriate screening, referral, and prompt attention to change in their status. Despite their fragility, children with trisomy 18 have the potential to grow, thrive, and develop endearing personalities and charm and be a source of joy for both families and the medical professionals on their care teams (Fig. 5).

CLINICS CARE POINTS

- Plan for frequent primary care evaluations in early life to closely monitor feeding, growth and to order and monitor recommended screening and surveillance testing.
- Suspect feeding intolerance if child demonstrates persistent irritability and or worsening respiratory event such as apena or cyanotic events.
- Recommend full routine childhood immunizations, respiratory syncytial virus prophylaxis and annual flu and COVID vaccinations.
- Recognize respiratory infections can quickly progress to pneumonia and need for hospitalization. Children should be evaluated in the primary care office at the onset of respiratory symptoms.
- Obtain video fluoroscopic swallow study before progressing to any type of oral feedings.
- Refer to occupational, physical and speech therapy to promote optimal development.
- Approach families in a supportive and non judgemental fashion to promote trust and establish a mutually respectful long-term care relationship.

Disclosure

No disclosures.

References

[1] National Library of Medicine. Trisomy 18. Medline plus. 2021. Available at: https://medlineplus.gov/genetics/condition/Trisomy-18/#synonyms. Accessed May 20, 2024.

[2] Irving C, Richmond S, Wren C, et al. Changes in fetal prevalence and outcome for trisomies 13 and 18: a population-based study over 23 years. J Matern Fetal Neonatal Med 2011;24(1): 137–41.

[3] Carey JC. Management of children with the trisomy 18 and trisomy 13 syndromes: is there a shift in the paradigm of care? Am J Perinatol 2021;38(11):1122–5.

[4] Cereda A, Carey JC. The Trisomy 18 syndrome. Orphanet J Rare Dis 2012;7(1):81.

[5] Dungan JS, Klugman S, Darilek S, et al. Noninvasive prenatal screening (NIPS) for fetal chromosome abnormalities in a general-risk population: an evidence-based clinical guideline of the American College of Medical Genetics and Genomics (ACMG). Genet Med 2023;25(2):100336.

[6] Bruns DA, Martinez A. An analysis of cardiac defects and surgical interventions in 84 cases with full Trisomy 18. Am J Med Genet 2016;170(2):337–43.

[7] Benson J, Stewart C, Kenna MA, et al. Otolaryngologic manifestations of Trisomy 13 and Trisomy 18 in pediatric patients. Laryngoscope 2023;133(6):1501–6.

[8] Kettler EB, Bhattacharjee R, Lesser D, et al. Sleep disordered breathing in children with Trisomy 13 and Trisomy 18. Am J Otolaryngol 2020;41(6):102555.

[9] Taira R, Inoue H, Sawano T, et al. Management of apnea in infants with Trisomy 18. Dev Med Child Neurol 2019;62:874–8.

[10] Root S, Carey JC. Survival in trisomy 18. Am J Med Genet 1994;49:170–4.

[11] Embleton ND, Wyllie JP, Wright MJ, et al. Natural history of trisomy 18. Arch Dis Child Fetal Neonatal Ed 1996;75(1):F38–41.

[12] Carey J. Trisomy 18 and trisomy 13 syndromes, . Management of genetic syndromes. Third edition. Hoboken (NJ): Wiley Blackwell; 2010. p. 807–23.

[13] Barnes A, Carey J. Care of the infant and child with trisomy 18 or trisomy 13. Support Organization for Trisomy. 2018. Available at: https://Trisomy.org/wp-content/uploads/2023/03/Carebook-3-22-2018-English.pdf.

[14] Roberts W, Zurada A, Zurada-ZieliŃSka A, et al. Anatomy of trisomy 18. Clin Anat 2016;29(5):628–32.

[15] Baty BJ, Jorde LB, Blackburn BL, et al. The natural history of Trisomy 18 and Trisomy 13: II psychomotor development. Am J Med Genet 1994;49:189–94.

[16] Fick TA, Sexson Tejtel SK. Trisomy 18 trends over the last 20 years. Pediatrics 2021;147(3_MeetingAbstract):405–6.

[17] Jacobs JP, O'Brien SM, Pasquali SK, et al. The society of thoracic surgeons congenital heart surgery database mortality risk model: Part 2-clinical application. Ann Thorac Surg 2015;100(3):1063–70.

[18] Peterson R, Calamur N, Fiore A, et al. Factors influencing outcomes after cardiac intervention in infants with Trisomy 13 and 18. Pediatr Cardiol 2018;39(1):140–7.

[19] Graham EM, Bradley SM, Shirali GS, et al. Pediatric cardiac care consortium. Effectiveness of cardiac surgery in trisomies 13 and 18 (from the pediatric cardiac care consortium). Am J Cardiol 2004;93(6):801–3.

[20] Cooper DS, Riggs KW, Zafar F, et al. Cardiac surgery in patients with Trisomy 13 and 18: an analysis of the society of thoracic surgeons congenital heart surgery database. J Am Heart Assoc 2019;8(13):e012349.

[21] Kosiv KA, Gossett JM, Bai S, et al. Congenital heart surgery on in-hospital mortality in Trisomy 13 and 18. Pediatrics 2017;140(5):e20170772.

[22] Kepple JW, Fishler KP, Peeples ES. Surveillance guidelines for children with Trisomy 18. Am J Med Genet 2021;185(4):1294–303.

[23] Bai W, Klumpner T, Zhao X, et al. Difficult airway management in children with Trisomy 18: a retrospective single-centre study of incidence, outcomes, and complications. Br J Anaesth 2023;130(6):e471–3.

[24] Tabbers MM, DiLorenzo C, Berger MY, et al. Evaluation and treatment of functional constipation in infants and children: evidence-based recommendations from ESPGHAN and NASPGHAN. J Pediatr Gastroenterol Nutr 2014;58(2):258–74.

[25] Lightdale JR, Gremse DA. Section on Gastroenterology, Hepatology, and Nutrition. Gastroesophageal reflux: management guidance for the pediatrician. Pediatrics 2013;131(5):e1684–95.

[26] Mutyala R, Sanders K, Bates MD. Assessment and management of pediatric constipation for the primary care clinician. Curr Probl Pediatr Adolesc Health Care 2020;50(5):100802.

[27] Kosho T, Kuniba H, Tanikawa Y, et al. Natural history and parental experience with children with Trisomy 18 based on questionnaire given to Japanese Trisomy 18 parental support group. Am J Med Genet 2013;161(7):1531–42.

[28] Baty BJ, Blackburn BL, Carey JC. Natural history of Trisomy 18 and Trisomy 13: I. Growth, physical assessment, medical histories, survival, and recurrence risk. Am J Med Genet 1994;49(2):175–88.

[29] Bruns D, Campbell E. Twenty-two survivors over the age of 1 year with full Trisomy 18: presenting and current medical conditions. Am J Med Genet 2014;164A(3):610–9.

[30] Becker AM. Postnatal evaluation of infants with an abnormal antenatal renal sonogram. Curr Opin Pediatr 2009;21(2):207–13.

[31] Verrotti A, Carelli A, di Genova L, et al. Epilepsy and chromosome 18 abnormalities: a review. Seizure 2015;32:78–83.

[32] Carey JC. Trisomy 18 and trisomy 13 syndromes. Cassidy and Allanson's Management of Genetic Syndromes 2021. p. 937–56.

[33] National Organization for Rare Disorders. Trisomy 18. National organization for rare disorders. 2024. Available at: https://rarediseases.org/rare-diseases/Trisomy-18-syndrome/. Accessed June 2, 2024.

[34] Farmakis SG, Barnes AM, Carey JC, et al. Solid tumor screening recommendations in Trisomy 18. Am J Med Genet 2019;179(3):455–66.

[35] Wiedmeier SE, Henry E, Christensen RD. Hematological abnormalities during the first week of life among neonates with Trisomy 18 and Trisomy 13: data from a multi-hospital healthcare system. Am J Med Genet 2008;146A(3):312–20.

[36] Kalish JM, Doros L, Helman LJ, et al. Surveillance recommendations for children with overgrowth syndromes and predisposition to wilms tumors and hepatoblastoma. Clin Cancer Res 2017;23(13):e115–22.

[37] Guon J, Wilfond BS, Farlow B, et al. Our children are not a diagnosis: the experience of parents who continue their pregnancy after a prenatal diagnosis of Trisomy 13 or 18. Am J Med Genet 2014;164(2):308–18.

[38] Janvier A, Farlow B, Wilfond BS. The experience of families with children with Trisomy 13 and 18 in social networks. Pediatrics 2012;130(2):293–8.

[39] Janvier A, Farlow B, Barrington KJ, et al. Building trust and improving communication with parents of children with Trisomy 13 and 18: a mixed-methods study. Palliat Med 2020;34(3):262–71.

[40] Support for families with trisomy website cardiac surgeries. Available at: https://trisomy.org/resources/cardiac-surgeries-or-procedures-by-diagnosis/#/.

[41] Support for families with trisomy website non-cardiac surgeries. Available at: https://trisomy.org/non-cardiac-surgeries-or-procedures-performed/#/.

Advances in Family Practice Nursing 7 (2025) 215–225

ADVANCES IN FAMILY PRACTICE NURSING

Diagnosing and Treating Disorders of the Gut–Brain Interaction in Pediatric Patients

Charlotte C. Rensberger, MSN, APRN, PNP-PC

Bronson Children's Hospital, 601 John St. MOP Suite M-351, Kalamazoo, MI 49007, USA

Keywords

- Abdominal pain • Constipation • Diarrhea • Nausea • Dyspepsia
- Irritable bowel syndrome

Key points

- There are true disorders that can have an impact on the function of the gastro-intestinal tract but display no correlating abnormal test results, such as disorders of gut-brain interaction or DGBIs.
- Previously referred to as functional GI disorders, now called DGBIs because the underlying abnormality is impaired nervous system communication from gut to brain and brain to gut.
- DGBI diagnosis and management is routinely not given a lot of attention in clinical training, which can lead to costly unnecessary testing and treatment modalities that has associated risks to the patient.
- The symptoms of DGBIs can overlap with other GI diseases, making it challenging to know what diagnostic testing is indicated, and when it should be done, and ultimately when a consultation with a GI specialist is indicated.

INTRODUCTION

It is estimated that up to 50% of visits to pediatric gastroenterologists across the country may be due to disorders of the gut–brain interaction (DGBIs) [1]. Referred to, in the past as functional gastrointestinal (GI) disorders, some examples of these conditions include functional dyspepsia, chronic diarrhea, Rumination syndrome, cyclic vomiting syndrome, and irritable bowel syndrome (IBS) [2]. Over the years, research has proven that the gut and the brain (nervous system) are so well connected with one another that any distress experienced by one can result in minor to life altering symptoms in the other. For example, as much as anxiety and depression can contribute to the symptoms of IBS, the

E-mail address: Rensberc@bronsonhg.org

https://doi.org/10.1016/j.yfpn.2025.01.006

Abbreviations

DGBI   disorders of gut–brain interaction
GI   gastrointestinal
HRQOL   health-related quality of life
IBS   irritable bowel syndrome

symptoms of IBS can also contribute to a patient's mental health status. The symptoms of these conditions can range from mild to severe, which can cause delays in diagnosis, and result in costly and sometimes traumatic examinations and testing. Many times, the symptoms they are experiencing negatively impact their quality of life, often limiting their ability to attend school, participate in sports and other extracurricular activities, and have healthy enjoyable relationships with food.

Typically, by the time patients arrive at a GI specialist, they have already been on a long and frustrating journey looking for answers and a diagnosis, or they have been told that their symptoms are a DGBI, but it is not explained therapeutically, and they feel like their symptoms are "all in their head." However, by using Rome IV criteria, developed in 2016 (the most recent edition), practitioners can accurately diagnose these patients and begin a treatment plan to help restore their quality of life and daily function, as well as coping strategies to deal with the symptoms we are not able to improve [3,4]. The Rome IV criteria can be found online by following this link: https://theromefoundation.org/rome-iv/rome-iv-criteria/.

PATHOPHYSIOLOGY

It is not always known why DGBIs affect certain patients and not others, and that alone can be a source of frustration. Over the years, there has been a perception that DGBIs are less valid than those disorders that have a clear organic cause, and there has been a misconception that they are psychiatric in nature. Physical symptoms can occur without an organic disease process and can be caused by many factors [2].

Genetics, culture, and environment impact a patient's psychosocial development and physiology. These factors also influence a patient's susceptibility to dysfunction within their gut. Some patients may experience a heightened pain response to stimulus that did not incite pain in the past which we refer to as visceral hypersensitivity, an example of this would be pain experienced due to a full stomach after eating, or even the act of motility and digestion. Another component could be a brain that is in a hyper-responsive state when signals from the gastrointestinal tract are being received by the brain [2].

The mechanism of these disorders is not well defined, as there can also be physiologic processes that also cause GI symptoms, causing an overlap with other diseases or disorders, which can delay diagnosis and make the condition difficult to manage, further contributing to frustration for patients, their families, and their medical team [3]. An example is a patient being seen for nausea, who is also diagnosed with anxiety and is medicated with an SSRI. In taking the history, the nurse practitioner learns that this is the third medication that they have tried for the mental health in the last 2 months, and they miss doses frequently, leading the nurse practitioner to question if her nausea could be related to medication changes and poor adherence to dosing regimens.

PREVALENCE

A study published in the *Journal of Pediatrics* in 2018 evaluated the prevalence of disorders of the gut–brain interaction in the pediatric patient population [5]. This study revealed that using Rome IV criteria, DGBI are common in the pediatric population and contribute to decreased quality of life. To complete the study, the researchers recruited mothers of children ages 0 to 18 years old to participate in online surveying. The resulting response was 1515 completed questionnaires, 368 included information regarding children from birth to 3 years, and 1147 for the age of 4 to 18 years. There were questionnaires excluded due to preexisting medical conditions or from parents who only had custody of their children for less than half of the time. This left a remaining 1255 surveys. The survey contained questions related to quality of life and health conditions. When comparing the responses of the Rome IV criteria, 24.7% of those with children aged 0 to 3 years and 25% of those with children aged 4 to 18 years met the symptom-based criteria for diagnosis of a disorder of the gut–brain interaction [6]. Not surprisingly, there was a correlation between diminished quality of life in those who met criteria for DGBI, as well as a DGBI in the child of a parent of with a DGBI [5].

Another study published just a few years earlier in 2014, sought to compare health-related quality of life (HRQOL) in pediatric patients diagnosed with DGBI to patients with organic gastrointestinal diagnosis [7]. The study was completed using The Pediatric Quality of Life Inventory 4.0 Generic Score Scales and consisted of 689 responses from 9 clinical sites. Patients included in the surgery were diagnosed with chronic constipation, functional abdominal pain, functional dyspepsia, IBS, gastroesophageal reflux, or inflammatory bowel disease. In addition to the HRQOL, they also sought information related to school attendance, occurrence of inability to get out of bed or need additional care, missed guardian workdays, and health care resource utilization. As expected, results showed that both groups of patients reported less HRQOL than the healthy patients in the control group in all dimensions. However, the patients diagnosed with a DGBI revealed lower HRQOL than those with an organic diagnosis [7].

CLINICAL PRESENTATION

Contributing to the challenge of diagnosing these conditions is that every patient can report a multitude of GI symptoms in varying intensity occurring intermittently, or constantly. Each patient can have their own unique constellation of symptoms.

A thorough and complete history is the best way to get the details needed to determine if additional tests are indicated, or to make a diagnosis. To get accurate information, it is important to ask the right questions so that you can get a good picture of each patient's unique symptoms. Rather than yes or no questions, it can be helpful to ask open-ended questions. Refer to Box 1 for examples of open-ended questions that can be used in taking a patient's history.

It is also important to ask clarifying questions to get a full picture of your patients' symptoms. It is helpful to repeat what you have heard the patients say and then ask additional questions, such as the clarifying questions listed in Box 2.

By asking effective questions, the nurse practitioner will have all the needed information to determine if the patient has any concerning symptoms that could indicate an organic cause for the patients' symptoms, prompting additional testing and referral to GI specialist. Box 3 contains a list of symptoms for which a referral to a GI specialist would be indicated.

HEALTH EQUITY

Social determinants of health as outlined by Healthy People 2020 encompasse 5 key domains: economic, education, social and community context, health and health care, and neighborhood and built environment [8]. Specifically digestive health can be negatively impacted by factors like decreased access to healthy food, lack of social/emotional support contributing to poor mental health, lack of transportation causing missed health care visits. It is important to examine current health care inequities that exist in our country today and focus on mitigating these disparities in the future [9].

DIAGNOSIS

There are no diagnostic tests for the various DBGIs. Rather, diagnosis is based on symptom-based criteria, The Rome Criteria. The most recent update to *criteria* was completed in 2016, Rome IV [3]. Making these diagnoses can be

---

Box 1: Examples of open-ended questions

Can you tell me what your pain feels like?

Is your pain there all the time, or does it come and go?

When you have pain, how long does it last?

What time of day do you feel like your pain is the worst?

Where is your pain located?

What symptoms are the most bothersome to you?

What things make your symptoms worse? What things make your symptoms better?

Box 2: Examples of clarifying questions

You have said you have abdominal pain and nausea, do they always come at the same time, or can they occur separately?

You said you throw up every morning, do you throw up repeatedly until your stomach is empty, or just once?

You have been having these symptoms for 6 months, did the symptoms all come at the same time, or one after the other? Can you walk me through the timeline of symptoms occurring?

You said you have tried everything, what specific things have you tried and what response did you notice to them?

challenging because often patients and families want testing done to confirm the presence of an underlying issue that can be cured, and they are discouraged by negative/normal testing. The diagnosis of a DGBI is satisfied by meeting a criterion of symptom characteristics and is not a diagnosis of exclusion. What ends up happening frequently is that testing confirms that there is no underlying issue that needs to be "fixed" or treated. It can be challenging because patients and their families must wrap their heads around the diagnosis and can often feel like the diagnosis of a DBGI means that the symptoms are psychological and not factual. The nurse practitioner should prepare patients and families that DBGI could be a diagnosis, trying to validate their symptoms and emotions related to their diagnostic journey at each check point.

To accurately diagnose a DBGI, the provider must be familiar with the Rome Criteria for the various DBGIs and the red flags that would necessitate additional testing [3,4]. Additional information for warning signs indicating the need for referral can be found here:

Box 3: Symptoms that warrant referral to gastrointestinal specialist

Unexplained, recurrent fevers that have no clear source and accompany abdominal pain, diarrhea, and/or nausea and vomiting.

Intractable vomiting, especially if the vomitus contains blood and/or occurs in the night repeatedly waking them from sleep.

Chronic diarrhea, more than 3x a day for 3 weeks, especially if the stool contains blood and/or mucus or wakes them in the night.

Jaundice, or the presence of elevated liver enzymes.

Unintentional weight loss or continued poor growth.

Family history of celiac disease, peptic ulcer disease, or inflammatory bowel disease.

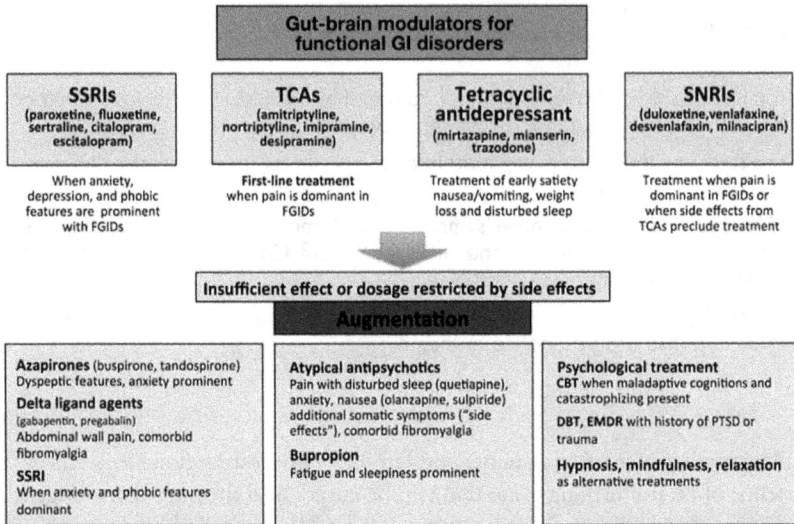

Fig. 1. Demonstrates selection of pharmacotherapy focused on neuromodulation of the gut–brain interaction, by considering clinical characteristics. Summary of the clinical characteristics that can be considered when selecting gut–brain neuromodulating pharmacotherapy to treat FGIDs. The medications listed those drugs in the top of the figure can be considered as first-line options. At the bottom, there are pharmacologic options most often used to augment treatment effects are depicted, as well as some nonpharmacologic treatment alternatives [12].

https://www.contemporarypediatrics.com/view/gastrointestinal-disorders-red-flags-and-best-treatments.

MANAGEMENT

The goal for treating DBGI effectively is to reduce symptoms, restore function, and improve quality of life. This looks different for each patient, because their symptoms, their anatomy, function, and microbiome are unique [8]. While the approach is similar, the treatment plan is unique for every patient. Treatment plans are developed to include pharmaceutical, dietary, supplemental, psychological, and/or alternative interventions.

Pharmacologic treatment

There are medications that can help ease pain, or calm nausea and vomiting. It is not recommended to use narcotics for pain relief. Sometimes low dose antidepressants are prescribed to calm the nerve cells in the gut and help quiet symptoms. Antiemetics can be used for short-term nausea and vomiting. Antimuscarinics, formerly known as anticholinergics, can be used for cramping abdominal pain because they reduce intestinal motility (Fig. 1).

Dietary modifications/eliminations

In some pediatric patients, dietary habits play a key role in GI symptoms and the health of their GI tract. Patients who eat more whole foods and avoid processed foods have better gut health overall than those patients who eat foods that are high in sugar and fat [10]. Referral to a registered dietician who specializes in pediatric nutrition can be helpful in ensuring that patients are still meeting nutritional needs while restricting their diet as necessary to avoid those that cause GI upset.

Supplements

Herbal supplements, specifically peppermint and ginger, have been helpful in decreasing GI symptoms. Also, probiotics either in the supplemental form or in dietary sources can also improve gut health overall [11]. A study published in 2020 explored herbal supplements and their role as complementary and/or alternative medicine for the symptoms associated with functional gastrointestinal disorders (FGIDs) [11]. The article specifically assessed herbal therapies considered to have an evidence base, Iberogast (STW-5) and peppermint oil, and Rikkunshito and Motilitone (DA-9701), which are extracted from natural substances in traditional medicine. These herbal medications have multitarget pharmacology like the etiology of FGIDs, such as altered intestinal sensory and motor function, inflammation, neurohormonal abnormality, and have displayed comparable efficacy and safety in controlled trials [11]. The role of herbal therapies in FGIDs is still unclear but appears promising. The active ingredients and mechanisms of action have not been fully identified and well-designed clinical trials are insufficient. There is a place for herbal therapies to supplement the treatment plan in refractory patients [11].

Trigger identification and avoidance

Sometimes patients can identify patterns of symptoms after eating certain foods, lack of sleep, or change in schedule or structure. A brief period of journaling symptoms can be helpful in identifying these patterns as they emerge. Once triggers are identified, the provider can assist the patient in developing a plan to avoid triggers when possible. Patients should journal for a brief period and not constantly to prevent hypervigilance. Some examples of information to be gathered in symptom journals are listed in Box 4.

Box 4: Symptom journal information

What symptoms occur-when do they start, stop, and how severe are they?

What foods were eaten in the prior 12 to 24 hours?

What other symptoms are present?

Is this a school day or not?

How was the quality of sleep the night before the episode?

When was the last bowel movement-what was the amount and texture?

Cognitive behavioral therapy

Focused psychological therapy can help soften the interactions between the brain and the gut [8]. This approach can also improve a patient's depression and anxiety, which has been shown to also decrease GI symptoms. Patients should be referred to a therapist who specializes in Cognitive Behavioral Therapy in their area.

Promotion of physical activity

Exercise can improve function and mobility; and help restore activity that may have been deconditioned over times of prolonged symptomatic illness and decreased physical activity [8]. If the family lacks the means for the patient to join a gym, or play organized sports, low impact exercise, such as walking, or bike riding should be explored.

Acupuncture and neuromodulation

In acupuncture, small needles are placed on the specific pressure points on and around the ear (or other parts of the body). There are also newer, noninvasive devices that deliver timed impulses to the auricular pressure points, calming the nerve impulses between the brain and the gut [13].

A DGBI treatment plan that is multifaceted has a better chance of long-term success; rarely will a patient show improvement with only one intervention [8]. When possible, triggers for symptoms should be identified and strategies to mitigate response put in place. Remaining symptoms can then be managed accordingly. Table 1 provides examples of triggers, and interventions that could be considered.

Cognitive behavioral approaches can be used to help patients cope with symptoms and psychosocial stressors that cannot be controlled. There should be a plan in place for patients to resume daily activity and a sense of normalcy which often includes school attendance and participation in extracurriculars.

TREATMENT CHALLENGES

Getting back to life and regaining normal function looks different for every patient. Patient goals may vary, from the need to alleviate debilitating belly pain when studying for finals or to be able to play their favorite sport, while another might need help to eat, gain weight and have enough energy to get back to school and extracurriculars. A therapeutic rapport between patients and their providers is a key to establishing a successful treatment plan, realistic expectations, and mutual goal setting. It can take time to effectively manage the symptoms of DGBIs, and the progress is not always longitudinal [14,15]. It is critical to continue to follow the patient with routine appointments to assess current symptoms, and the success or failure of treatment plans. There should be a strong emphasis on improving the quality of life and the ability to function, not to cure the condition or resolve all pain and discomfort. Families should be actively involved in appointments and agreeable to the plan developed because if they are not unified, they could unintentionally halt or reverse any potential for progress.

Table 1
Examples of symptoms and interventions

Trigger and resulting symptoms	Proposed interventions
Spicy foods cause heartburn	Decrease intake of spicy foods.
	Do not eat spicy foods within 2 h of bedtime.
	If spicy foods cannot be avoided, a dose of short acting antacid could decrease symptoms.
Lack of sleep causes nausea and abdominal pain	Move bedtime up an hour to allow for a full night's sleep.
	Decrease electronic use before bedtime, turn all sources of 2 h before bed.
	Discuss a delayed start with school to allow patient to wake up more slowly.
Early morning nausea causes patient to not want to eat breakfast and often miss school	Consider peppermint oil capsules at bedtime or first thing in the morning.
	Consider small snacks upon waking before getting out of bed.
	Consider smoothies for breakfast that they can sip on frequently before leaving for school.
	Discuss a delayed start schedule with school.

IMPLICATION FOR ADVANCED PRACTICE NURSES

It is important for every member of a patient's care team to validate their experience and symptoms. Often patients report being told that symptoms "are all in their head" which can lead to an undercurrent of mistrust in the medical community. At each encounter with a patient who has been diagnosed with or is suspected to have DGBI it can be beneficial to reassure them that:

- Their symptoms are real and occurring the cause is related to dysfunction between how the gut is working and how the brain is communicating.
- Pain is hurtful, but not an indication of harm being done to their body.
- Learning to cope with symptoms is an important part of management.
- Treatment plans that are multimodal are more likely to bring about symptom relief.
- Their team of providers wants to help them and restore their function, and the best way to do that is with routine follow-up and open 2-way communication.

CASE STUDY

Carly is an 11-year-old female patient who is seen by the primary care provider today for abdominal pain and intermittent diarrhea. Carly reports that her abdominal pain occurs daily, happens at various times of the day, and varies in severity, but is worse after eating. She sometimes feels nauseated but does not throw up. They have not noticed that it is worse after eating any specific food groups. She has diarrhea a few times a week, but also has days when her stools are normal. Her abdominal pain improves after passing stool. She has not been seeing blood or mucus in her stool, and she is not waking up in the night to have a bowel movement. Her appetite is normal, though mom notes that she is a very picky eater, and her weight has been stable since symptoms began. She is otherwise a happy, healthy child. Her birth was unremarkable, and she passed meconium on the day she was born. She has good bowel sounds, and a soft abdomen. An abdominal XR was normal.

Based on the information earlier, the nurse practitioner can make a diagnosis of Irritable Bowel Syndrome using the Rome IV criteria discussed earlier. The initial treatment plan should focus on digestive health and should include education regarding appropriate hydration and water intake, as well as the importance of dietary fiber and physical activity. The patient should keep a log of bowel movements tracking frequency and consistency, and diet to allow for the identification of any dietary triggers. Next steps to consider would be removing any identified dietary triggers, a course of probiotics, cognitive behavioral therapy, or peppermint oil. Only one intervention should be implemented at a time to determine which are effective. If there is no improvement in symptoms after various interventions, then the patient should be re-evaluated, and other etiologies could be entertained.

SUMMARY

DGBIs are commonly encountered by nurse practitioners who care for pediatric patients in the primary care setting and acute care. A positive diagnosis can be made based on signs and symptoms using Rome IV Criteria, and any diagnostic work up done is usually normal or negative. Treatment is tailored to each patient's constellation of symptoms, with a multifaceted approach focused on improving quality of life and daily function. Effective management depends on providers achieving a therapeutic alliance with the patient and their caregivers and working together to develop a treatment plan agreeable to all parties.

CLINICS CARE POINTS

- DGBIs are real disorders that negatively impact patients and their quality of life.
- Appropriate diagnosis and management of a DGBI is key to the success in treatment.

Disclosure

The author has nothing to disclose.

References

[1] Graham KMD. What are disorders of the Gut-Brain interaction? Cincinnati Children's Blog. 2024. Available at: https://blog.cincinnatichildrens.org/rare-and-complex-conditions/what-are-disorders-of-the-gut-brain-interaction/.

[2] Tome J, Kamboj A, Loftus C. Mayo Clinic proceedings: disorders of the gut-brain interaction. 2022. Available at: https://www.mayoclinicproceedings.org/article/S0025-6196(22)00618-8/fulltext;. Accessed April 21, 2024 https://www.mayoclinicproceedings.org/article/S0025-6196(22)00618-8/fulltext.

[3] Drossman DA, Hasler WL. Rome IV—functional GI disorders: disorders of gut-brain interaction. Gastroenterology 2016;150(6):1257–61.

[4] Vernon-Roberts A, Alexander I, Day AS. Systematic review of pediatric functional gastroin-testinal disorders (Rome IV criteria). J Clin Med 2021;10(21):5087.

[5] Van Tilburg MAL. Pediatric functional gastrointestinal disorders. New York (NY): Elsevier eBooks; 2020. p. 557–63.

[6] Lewis ML, Palsson OS, Whitehead WE, et al. Prevalence of functional gastrointestinal dis-orders in children and adolescents. J Pediatr 2016;177:39–43.e3.

[7] Varni JW, Bendo CB, Nurko S, et al. Health-related quality of life in pediatric patients with functional and organic gastrointestinal diseases. J Pediatr 2014;166(1); https://doi.org/10.1016/j.jpeds.2014.08.022.

[8] Velez CMD. Recognizing and treating disorders of the gut-brain interaction. 2022. Available at: https://www.health.harvard.edu/blog/recognizing-and-treating-disorders-of-gut-brain-interaction-202204202730;. Accessed April 25, 2024 https://www.health.harvard.edu/blog/recognizing-and-treating-disorders-of-gut-brain-interaction-202204202730.

[9] Daniel R, Jimenez J, Pall H. Health equity and social determinants of health in pediatric gastroenterology. Pediatr Clin 2021;68(6):1147–55.

[10] Rosa D, Zablah RA, Vazquez-Frias R. Unraveling the complexity of Disorders of the Gut-Brain Interaction: the gut microbiota connection in children. Front Pediatrics 2024;11:1283389.

[11] Kim YS, Kim J-W, Ha N-Y, et al. Herbal therapies in functional gastrointestinal disorders: a narrative review and clinical implication. Front Psychiatr 2020;11; https://doi.org/10.3389/fpsyt.2020.00601.

[12] Drossman DA, Tack J, Ford AC, et al. Neuromodulators for functional gastrointestinal disor-ders (disorders of gut–brain interaction): A Rome Foundation Working Team Report. Gastro-enterology 2018;154(4); https://doi.org/10.1053/j.gastro.2017.11.279.

[13] Kundu A, Tassone RF. Acupuncture for the treatment of functional disorders in children. New York (NY): Springer eBooks; 2014. p. 331–42.

[14] Williams SE, Bursch B. Diagnostic and treatment approaches associated with functional gastrointestinal disorders in children and adolescents. Milton Park, Abingdon, Oxfordshire: Routledge eBooks; 2017. p. 207–18.

[15] Black CJ, Drossman DA, Talley NJ, et al. Functional gastrointestinal disorders: advances in understanding and management. Lancet 2020;396(10263):1664–74.

Advances in Family Practice Nursing 7 (2025) 227–238

ADVANCES IN FAMILY PRACTICE NURSING

A Dose of Prevention is Worth a Pound of Cure

Respiratory Syncytial Virus Immunity for a Safer Community

Ann Mattison, MSN, CPNP- PC, CPNP-AC, APRN*,[1],
Cristy Toburen, MSN, CPNP- PC, APRN[1]

Well Baby Nursery, Children's Mercy Kansas City, Children's Mercy Hospital, 2401 Gillham Road, Kansas City, MO 64108, USA

Keywords
- Respiratory syncytial virus (RSV) • Bronchiolitis • Beyfortus (Nirsevimab)
- Abrysvo (RSV preF) • Synagis (Palivizumab)

Key points

- Respiratory syncytial virus (RSV) is the leading cause of hospitalization of infants in the United States. Symptoms range from cold-like illness to lower respiratory tract disease such as pneumonia and bronchiolitis.
- Clinical studies have shown that Abrysvo can reduce the risk of severe RSV disease by 81.8% at 90 days after birth and 69.4% at 180 days after birth.
- Beyfortus reduced the risk of hospitalization from RSV-associated lower respiratory tract infection by 80% and intensive care unit admission by 90%.

INTRODUCTION

Respiratory syncytial virus (RSV) is the leading cause of lower viral respiratory tract infection in infants and young children worldwide [1]. Most of the population will become infected by the age of 2 years and reinfection is common throughout life [2]. Of infants who are infected, the majority will experience upper respiratory symptoms, while 20% to 30% will develop lower respiratory symptoms such as pneumonia or bronchiolitis. Recurrent infection is common and typically manifests as upper respiratory symptoms and rarely involves the lower respiratory tract [3]. Hospitalization due to RSV-associated illness is a

[1]Each author contributed equally to this manuscript.

*Corresponding author. E-mail address: amattison@cmh.edu

https://doi.org/10.1016/j.yfpn.2025.01.009

Abbreviations

AAP	American Academy of Pediatrics
CPAP	continuous positive airway pressure
DFA	direct fluorescence assay
FDA	Food and Drug Administration
HFNC	high-flow nasal cannula
IV	intravenous
NAAT	nucleic acid amplification test
RADT	rapid antigen detection test
RSV	respiratory syncytial virus
rRT-PCR	real-time reverse transcription-polymerase chain reaction
SIADH	syndrome of inappropriate secretion of anti-diuretic hormone

substantial burden on the health care system [4]. Most infants and children recover in a week or two, but RSV can be serious. Prevention strategies have been limited despite high infant and childhood morbidity and mortality. Treatment of this disease is supportive. In 2023, the US Food and Drug Administration (FDA) approved 2 immunization products to decrease the disease burden.

HISTORY
As reported in multiple studies, the RSV virus was first discovered in 1956 by Dr Morris Hilleman in chimpanzees that were showing cold symptoms. Scientists initially called the newly discovered virus "chimpanzee coryza agent". In 1957, it was isolated from children and the virus was renamed RSV. Its name is derived from the fact that F proteins on the surface of the virus cause neighboring cell membranes to merge, creating large multinucleated "syncytia." Syncytial formation is the virus causing cell-to-cell fusion or sticking together of the cells lining the respiratory tract [5].

VIROLOGY
The universal viral taxonomy system classifies viruses into taxa placed into hierarchical ranks. The primary ranks for viral identification include realm (viria), kingdom (virae), phylum (varicota), class (viricetes), order (virales), family (viridae), subfamily (virinae), genus (virus), and species. RSV is the type species of genus Orthopneumovirus hominis, subfamily Pneumovirinae, family Paramyxoviridae, order Mononegavirales, Class Monjiviricetes, phylum Negarnaviricota, kingdom Orthonavirae, and realm Riboviria [6,7].

Viruses within the Mononegavirales order consist of negative-strand RNA viruses that have nonsegmental genomes. Some of the most well-known pathogenic viruses in this group include the Ebola virus, mumps virus, and rabies virus. The virus replicates intracellularly [7]. Unlike influenza, RSV has a negative-sense, non-segmented genome that makes it impossible for it to have antigenic shifts that could lead to a viral pandemic [7]. Additionally, the virus contains 3 surface glycoproteins: glycoprotein G, fusion protein F, and a small hydrophobic protein (SH). The F (fusion) protein and the G (attachment glycoprotein) protein are the major viral antigens that play a critical role in the virulence of RSV. The G protein facilitates attachment to the host cell followed by the F protein enabling fusion to the host that allows viral plasma membranes to permit viral passage into the host cell. The F protein also promotes the aggregation of multinucleated cells through fusion of their plasma membranes, producing the syncytia from which the virus derives its name and allows transmission of virus from cell to cell [5]. The F and G proteins are important because they stimulate the production of protective immune responses. Responses to the F protein include humoral and cytotoxic T-lymphocyte responses. The G protein is recognized by neutralizing antibodies but does not stimulate significant cytotoxic T-lymphocyte responses. The function of the hydrophobic protein SH is not well understood [7].

Pathophysiology and antigenic subtypes
RSV has 2 distinct antigenic subtypes, A and B, with multiple genotypes within them. Both are usually circulated simultaneously within local epidemics. Controversy continues to exist whether subtype A is more virulent, which is thought to be possibly related to higher viral loads and faster transmission time. The 2 antigenic subgroups differ in glycoproteins G and F. The prefusion form of RSV glycoprotein F (pre-F) is the key to vaccine success [1].

Transmission of RSV infection occurs through inoculation of the nasopharyngeal or conjunctival mucosa with respiratory secretions from infected people via respiratory droplets from coughing, sneezing, kissing, etc. [1] The virus remains viable on hard surfaces for up to 6 hours, on rubber gloves for 90 minutes, and on skin for 20 minutes. This prolonged survival highlights the need for handwashing and contact precautions to decrease the spread of infection. The incubation period ranges from 2 to 8 days, while immunocompetent hosts can shed the virus anywhere from 8 days up to 3 weeks [2].

RSV infection starts in the nasopharyngeal epithelium and spreads rapidly to the lower airways reaching the bronchioles. Viral replication is the most efficient in this area. The influx of polymorphonuclear neutrophils into the airways is rapidly replaced by predominantly lymphomononuclear infiltration of peribronchiolar tissues and increased microvascular permeability, leading to submucosal edema, and swelling. The mucus secretions increase in quantity and viscosity and tend to pool because of the loss of ciliated epithelium resulting in widespread mucous plugging. Acute inflammatory changes in the bronchioles leads to airway obstruction and air trapping, producing the classic clinical triad of wheezing, patchy atelectasis, and bilateral hyperinflation [8].

Epidemiology
In the United States, RSV is the primary cause of lower respiratory tract infection (LRTI) among infants and young children globally and a primary reason for hospitalization [9]. In infants and young children, a primary RSV infection may cause severe bronchiolitis that could be life-threatening. In older children and adults without comorbidities, recurrence is common with varying degrees

of symptoms [10]. Reinfection occurs at a rate of 10% to 20% per epidemic often as early as a few weeks after initial infection since the immune response is usually poor [7]. Each year in the United States, RSV leads to approximately 2.1 million outpatient visits, up to 80,000 hospitalizations, and 100 to 300 deaths to children younger than 5 years [1]. Increased morbidity and mortality are noted in infants less than 6 months, preterm infants, and infants with congenital heart disease or chronic lung disease [1]. In addition to the pediatric burden, RSV is increasingly being recognized as an important pathogen in older adults, with infection leading to an increase in hospitalization rates among those aged 65 years and over [1].

RSV is a seasonal disease and typically coincides with influenza [7]. RSV severity and peaks vary from country to country and year to year. In the United States and other areas with similar climates, RSV typically peaks during the winter months; however, circulation patterns were disrupted during the coronavirus disease 2019 (COVID-19) pandemic of 2020 [6]. Prior to 2020, RSV patterns were very consistent [11]. Studies outside the United States in the post-COVID-19 pandemic period have also demonstrated shifts of RSV season. Other countries such as France, Germany, Finland, Israel, and England have also seen delays in RSV seasons [11]. Additionally, increased RSV severity has been noted in New York in the youngest populations, whereas severity and age distribution remained typical to pre-pandemic RSV seasons in France [11]. Literature suggests that pandemic disruption created increased susceptibility among older children who have had no prior exposures. In addition to seasonality changes in RSV, demographic shifts have been noted as well with severity and frequency being higher in boys as compared to girls in pediatric populations globally [12].

DIAGNOSIS

RSV symptoms can vary from mild to severe. The majority of cases are mild. The symptoms vary from rhinorrhea, pharyngitis, cough, wheezing, headache, fever, and anorexia. Very young infants may only have irritability, lethargy, or difficulty breathing. Severe cases can lead to bronchiolitis or pneumonia [7]. It occurs most commonly in children under the age of 2 years, peaking between the age of 3 and 6 months. RSV symptoms typically peak on days 3 to 5 from onset of illness. This is likely due to the time it takes for the virus to infect the lower airway after the initial nasal infection.

Bronchiolitis can be diagnosed clinically in a child with 1 to 3 days of rhinorrhea followed by persistent cough, tachypnea, and wheezes or crackles in the lungs. Around 30% of patients have fevers up to 39 C [7]. If fever is higher than 39 C or localized crackles, pneumonia should be considered. Infants aged under 6 weeks may present with apnea without other clinical signs. This may be due to RSV affecting the sensitivity of the laryngeal chemoreceptors and exacerbating reflex apnea. This is thought to be associated with sudden infant death syndrome [7]. Reinfections occur frequently in children. Disease severity typically declines with each reinfection. RSV is more likely to cause ear infections compared to other viruses [7]. RSV symptoms are similar to other common respiratory viral illnesses, such as COVID-19, influenza, and the common cold. Table 1 depicts the symptoms associated with each virus (see Table 1).

DIAGNOSTIC TESTING

Since clinical symptoms of RSV overlap with many other viral and bacterial infections, laboratory tests are available to confirm RSV infection. Commonly used tests include real-time reverse transcription-polymerase chain reaction (rRT-PCR), viral culture, and rapid antigen testing [13]. The American Academy of Pediatrics (AAP) does not routinely recommend the use of laboratory testing to diagnose RSV bronchiolitis as treatment is largely supportive. Laboratory confirmation testing should be pursued if identification of RSV will affect clinical treatment such as affecting decisions about antimicrobial therapy, additional work-up, and infection control. Testing is often used to increase confidence in a viral cause of the respiratory symptoms. Specimen samples include nasal wash, nasopharyngeal swab, mid-turbinate nasal swab, tracheal aspirate, and bronchoalveolar lavage. Due to the thermolability of RSV, specimens should be processed immediately [7].

Though viral culture was once considered the gold standard, due to the lengthy turnaround time of viral culture identification taking anywhere from 3 days to 2 weeks, it is not very useful for diagnosis within the therapeutic window to affect treatment [7]. Viral culture is more common in research settings and less commonly used for clinical patient care.

Antigen testing involves detection of fragments (pieces of molecular viral structures) of the RSV virus. This can be accomplished by direct fluorescence assay (DFA) in a laboratory with a microscope or using commercially available rapid antigen detection tests (RADT). Enzyme immunoassay is the most widely used rapid detection test and is cost-effective [7]. Sensitivity of RSV antigen detection tests generally ranges from 80% to 90% in infants and children

Table 1
Comparing respiratory syncytial virus, flu, coronavirus disease 2019, and the common cold

Symptoms	RSV	Flu	COVID-19	Common cold
Fever	X	X	X	
Cough	X	X	X	X
Sore throat		X	X	X
Loss smell/taste			X	
Fatigue		X	X	X
Body aches		X	X	
Wheezing	X			
Nausea/Vomiting		X	X	
Headache		X	X	
Diarrhea		X	X	
Loss of appetite	X	X	X	
Nasal congestion	X	X	X	

aged less than 5 years. Antigen tests are not sensitive for older children and adults due to having lower viral loads in their respiratory specimens; therefore, rRT-PCR assays should be used in this population [3]. Antigen tests are also more sensitive to false-positive rates outside of the peak RSV season. RADT is commonly used as point-of-care testing and provides a very quick turn-around time, often less than 30 minutes. One should be aware that some RADTs may be affected by palivizumab prophylaxis, resulting in false-negative readings [7].

Molecular assays such as nucleic acid amplification tests (NAATs) allow detection of very small amounts of virus from specimens. NAAT assays such as PCR detect virus-specific genetic material rather than viral antigens. A very small sample of genetic material can be rapidly amplified into millions of copies for study. PCR is more sensitive than antigen and viral culture testing. They have a sensitivity and specificity greater than 95%. These tests are more expensive and require more complex equipment than antigen tests. The testing may be more useful in individuals with lower viral loads and shedding such as older children and adults. Due to the sensitivity of PCR testing, results may remain positive for prolonged periods after infection has clinically resolved [7]. Additionally, some commercially available molecular diagnostic tests can identify multiple respiratory viruses from a single nasopharyngeal sample. As many as 30% of symptomatic children will test positive for 2 or more respiratory viruses at the same time. The implication of the severity of disease with coinfections is still unknown [3] (Table 2).

Routine imaging is not recommended by the AAP for infants or children with presumed RSV bronchiolitis. Chest radiograph images may mimic pneumonia and should not be used to determine the need for antibiotics. Alternatively, radiographs may be normal or show nonspecific viral infection abnormalities such as perihilar opacities, hyperinflation, or patchy atelectasis. Imaging can be considered in a very sick child to determine the extent of illness or to rule out other etiology [7].

RESPIRATORY SYNCYTIAL VIRUS MANAGEMENT
RSV prevention is of the utmost importance. Good hand hygiene is imperative. Cough etiquette is also crucial. High-risk children should be kept away from exposure, including other children during RSV season.

RSV vaccine for pregnant women was approved in the United States on August 21, 2023 [13]. Abrysvo (RSVpreF) was developed by Pfizer. It is a bivalent vaccine. The prefusion structure of the RSV F protein is considered the primary target of the neutralizing antibodies against RSV [13]. The vaccine is approved in the United States to be given to pregnant women at 32 through 36 weeks gestation for the prevention of lower respiratory tract disease caused by RSV in infants from birth through 6 months of age. In clinical trials of women 24 to 36 weeks pregnant, more preterm births were observed in the group that received RSVpreF versus placebo, but this was not statistically significant. It is a single-dose vaccine and is to be given seasonally from September

Table 2
Respiratory syncytial virus testing methodology comparison

Test method	Advantages	Disadvantages	Age
Antigen Test-RADTs	• Quick turnaround time (<30 min) • On-site test completion • 80%–90% sensitivity and specificity	• Not recommended for adults and older children due to lower sensitivity/specificity • False-negative results are possible	• Infants and children aged <5 y
Antigen Test-DFA	• Shorter turnaround than PCR or viral cultural	• Requires laboratory to perform test • Lower sensitivity than PCR • Specimen sample collection must be adequate test accuracy	• Infants and children aged <5 y
PCR	• Sensitivity and specificity >95% • Detects coinfection • Low likelihood of false-positive or false-negative result	• More expensive • Require complex lan equipment • Longer turnaround that DFA • May detect virus after the infection has been cleared	• Any age
Viral culture	• Viruses can be stored for diagnostic studies • High specificity • Detects coinfection	• Long turnaround time of 3 days 2 weeks • Lower sensitivity	• Any age

through January in the continental United States. There was a 57.3% decrease in medically attended RSV visits through 180 days of life when the vaccine was given between 32 and 36 weeks [14]. The most common adverse reactions were pain at injection site, headache, nausea, and muscle pain. RSVpreF can be given with other recommended vaccines such at tetanus, diphtheria, and pertussis, influenza, and COVID-19. There are currently no data on need or safety of additional doses in subsequent pregnancies [14].

Beyfortus (Nirsevimab) is a recombinant monoclonal antibody that is manufactured by AstraZeneca/Sanofi. It was approved for use in the United States by the US FDA in July 2023 for use in infants and young children to prevent RSV-associated LRTIs. It is given intramuscularly as a single dose. It is recommended for all infants aged less than 8 months born during or entering their first RSV season whose mother did not receive RSVpreF (Abrysvo) vaccine or if they were born less than 14 days after maternal vaccine [11]. It is also recommended that children aged 8 to 19 months who are at increased risk for severe disease and are entering their second RSV season receive another dose (Box 1).

A 50 mg dose is given if infant weighs less than 5 kg and 100 mg if greater than or equal to 5 kg. In clinical trials, there was a 79% decrease in medically attended RSV associated with LRTIs, 80% decrease in hospitalization, and 90% decrease in intensive care unit admission [15]. Nirsevimab was well tolerated with no increase in adverse events compared to placebo. Another randomized, double-blind trial was done that enrolled 925 preterm infants with chronic lung disease of prematurity or congenital heart disease, and results supported the use of Nirsevimab in children up to 24 months as a significant cost-saving intervention [16].

Synagis (Palivizumab) in 1998 was the first successful monoclonal antibody developed and licensed for RSV prophylaxis [16]. It provides passive, short-term immunity with a half-life of 18 to 21 days. It requires monthly intramuscular injections, up to a maximum of 5 doses per season (October–March in the continental United States). The recommended dose is 15 mg/kg [16]. There are no statistically significant adverse reactions compared to placebo. A recent

---

Box 1: Children who qualify for second dose of Beyfortus (Nirsevimab) [14]

- Children who have chronic lung disease of prematurity required medical support (chronic corticosteroid therapy, diuretic therapy, or supplemental oxygen) any time during the 6 month period before the start of second RSV season.
- Children with severe immunocompromise
- Children with cystic fibrosis with severe disease
- American Indian and Alaska Native Children

Cochrane review suggests that Palivizumab has a 56% reduction in RSV hospitalization in premature infants, 22% reduction in hospitalization from any respiratory illness, and reduced number of wheezing days at 1 year follow-up [16]. There is no difference in RSV mortality, adverse events, rate or duration of mechanical ventilation, or length of hospital stay [17]. It is very expensive, so its use is limited to very high-risk infants (Box 2).

If any infant or young child receiving palivizumab experiences an RSV hospitalization, monthly prophylaxis should be discontinued because of the extremely low likelihood of a second RSV hospitalization in the same season (<0.5%) [18].

TREATMENT

RSV treatment consists of supportive care as no effective antiviral treatment is currently available. The goal is preventing severe disease with RSV vaccination of pregnant women or monoclonal antibodies of infants under the age of 8 months.

Treatment of RSV with or without bronchiolitis is supportive care with close monitoring. Hydration is imperative. If the child is unable to drink enough fluids orally, they should receive fluids via nasogastric or orogastric tube. Isotonic intravenous (IV) fluids should only be given if impending respiratory

---

Box 2: High-risk infants who may qualify for Palivizumab (Synagis) [12]

- Infants born before 29 weeks, 0 day gestation who are younger than 12 months at the start of the RSV season. It is not recommended in the second year of life based on prematurity alone.

- Preterm infants who develop chronic lung disease of prematurity defined as gestational age less than 32 weeks, 0 days, and a requirement for greater than 21% oxygen for at least the first 28 days after birth. During the second year of life, consideration of recommended only for infants with chronic lung disease of prematurity continues to require medical support (chronic corticosteroid therapy, diuretic therapy, or supplemental oxygen) during the 6 month period before the start of the second RSV season. Prophylaxis is not recommened for infants with chronic lung disease who do not continue to require medical support in the second year of life.

- Infants with hemodynamically significant congenital heart disease (infants with acyanotic heart disease who are receiving medication to control congestive heart failure and will require cardiac surgical procedures and infants with moderate-to-severe pulmonary hypertension).

- Infants with neuromuscular disease or congenital anomaly that impairs the ability to clear secretions from the upper airway because of ineffective cough.

- Children aged under 24 months who are profoundly immunocompromised during RSV season.

failure. There is a risk of syndrome of inappropriate anti-diuretic hormone se-crection (SIADH) and fluid shift to the lungs so avoidance of excessive IV fluids is recommended. It is not the intention of this article to define SIADH. The reader is referred to a pathophysiology book for detail on this syndrome.

Oxygen supplementation is recommended for saturation that is persistently below 90% for infants aged over 6 weeks and 92% if infant is aged less than 6 weeks [7]. High-flow nasal cannula (HFNC) can be used as respiratory support for those with persistent oxygen desaturation as a way to provide constant oxy-gen and washout of the nasopharyngeal dead space. It humidifies and hydrates the inspired air leading to decreased work of breathing. It also creates positive end-expiratory pressure. HFNC has been shown to have respiratory failure rates that are significantly lower than those on oxygen alone [7]. HFNC serves as an intermediate form of respiratory support between supplemental oxygen and continuous positive airway pressure (CPAP). Studies have shown that 70% of patients failing HFNC have been successful on CPAP. HFNC does not decrease length of hospital stay in children with bronchiolitis [7].

Upper airway clearance with suctioning is not routinely recommended. However, it can be done in children with respiratory distress or feeding diffi-culties due to secretions in the nasal passages.

Ribavirin is the only antiviral approved for the treatment of documented RSV infection in immunocompromised patients. The AAP recommends against the routine use of this medication. It should only be given to immuno-compromised patients with severe RSV infection due to its questionable bene-fits if not given early in the disease and its high cost [7].

It is not recommended to use antibiotics or systemic steroids in children with bronchiolitis. There is no evidence to show efficacy of inhaled adrenaline, albu-terol, ipratropium, corticosteroids, or hypertonic saline. RSV immunoglobulin and palivizumab should not be used to treat bronchiolitis [7].

SUMMARY

LRTIs are the leading cause of death in children aged less than 5 years outside of the neonatal period worldwide [19]. The majority of these are caused by vi-ruses (60%) with 31% of them being caused by RSV [19]. Previous attempts to create a vaccine proved to be either ineffective or expensive. RSV immuniza-tion prophylaxis is recommended to be used seasonally (September–January). Abrysvo (RSV preF) is to be given to pregnant women between 32 and 36 weeks gestation. Beyfortus (Nirsevimab) is given if mother did not receive Abrysvo 14 days prior to delivery until the infant is 8 months of age. RSV pre-vention can change the course of RSV disease for all infants. This is an oppor-tunity to decrease the RSV burden in vulnerable populations.

IMPLICATIONS FOR ADVANCED PRACTICE NURSES

These new preventive measures are very important in decreasing the burden of severe RSV disease. Advanced Practice Nurses are on the front lines providing parental education regarding health prevention and will have great influence on educating the community about RSV immunization opportunities. Anticipatory guidance should be provided to all new parents and caregivers on the importance of hand hygiene and avoiding kissing infants to prevent the spread of disease both in the nursery and at well-child checks. Infants should be kept home and out of crowded areas as much as possible, especially in peak viral season. Infants can attend daycare as long as they are afebrile.

If infants become infected with RSV caregivers need to be educated on the expected duration of illness and signs and symptoms of worsening disease. Parents should expect peak symptoms on days 3 to 5 and should gradually improve over the next 2 to 3 weeks. It is important for families to understand that infants have potential to get worse before symptoms improve. It is imperative that parents are aware of how to suction the nose and the importance of maintaining hydration. It can be difficult for infants to feed when the nose is congested; therefore, use of saline drops in the nose and a suction device is often helpful to maintain oral intake and comfort. If sunken fontanelle, decreased wet diapers, dry mucus members, or increased heart rate is noted, they should seek additional follow-up. Since the care for infants and children with RSV is supportive, they only need to be seen by a health care provider if there are concerns for respiratory distress or dehydration.

Families should avoid over-the-counter medications such as cough suppressants as these have not proven to be beneficial and have the potential to cause harm. Over the counter, anti-pyrectics can be administered as fever has potential to cause increased respiratory rates. Ibuprofen should be avoided in infants aged less than 6 months and acetaminophen can be used for this age group. Aspirin should never be given to infants or children. Lastly, caregivers need to be acutely aware of respiratory distress symptoms (nasal flaring, grunting, retractions, and increased respiratory rates) and know how to seek additional follow-up care emergently if needed. Providers should always consider differential diagnoses or the possibility of a secondary superimposed illness such as bacterial pneumonia when infants present with acute respiratory symptoms [20].

CLINICS CARE POINTS

- Symptomatic treatment only.
- Avoid Ibuprofen in infants less than 6 months.
- Avoid cough suppressants in all children.
- Monitor for signs of respiratory distress.

Disclosures
The authors have nothing to disclose.

References
[1] Joseph N, Kuller J, Louis J, et al. Society for Maternal Fetal Medicine Statement: clinical considerations for the prevention of respiratory syncytial virus disease in infants. Am J Obstet Gynecol 2024;230(2):B41–9.

[2] Respiratory Syncytial Virus (RSV). CDC website. 2024. Available at: https://www.cdc.gov/rsv/about/index.html. Accessed June 10, 2024.

[3] Kimberlin D, Banerjee R, Barnett ED, et al. Red book: 2024–2027 report of the committee on infectious diseases: respiratory syncytial virus. Boston (MA): American Academy of Pediatrics; 2024.

[4] Srikantiah P, Vora P, Klugman KP. Assessing the full burden of respiratory syncytial virus in young infants in low- and middle-income countries: the importance of community mortality studies. Clin Infect Dis 2021;73:S177–9, PMID.

[5] J. Kaler, A. Hussains, K. Patel, et al., Respiratory syncytial virus: a comprehensive review of transmission, pathophysiology, and manifestation-PMC. nih.gov Available at: 2023. ncbi.nlm.nih.gov/PMC/articles/PMC10111061. (Accessed 23 May 2024).

[6] Kuhn J. Virus Taxonomy. nih.gov. 2021. Available at: ncbi.nlm.nih.gov/pmc/articles/PMC7157452. Accessed May 15, 2024.

[7] Soni A, Kabra SK, Lodha R. Respiratory syncytial virus infection: an update. Indian J Pediatr 2023;90:1245–53.

[8] Piedimonte G, Perez MK. Respiratory syncytial virus infection and bronchiolitis. Pediatr Rev 2014;35(12):519–30.

[9] McLaughlin JM, Khan F, Schmitt HJ, et al. Respiratory syncytial virus-associated hospitalization rates among US infants: a systematic review and meta-analysis. J Infect Dis 2022;225(6):1100–11.

[10] Respiratory syncytial virus (RSV) disease. World Health Organization; 2024. Available at: https://who.int/teams/health-product-policy-and-standards/standards-and-specifications/vaccine-standardization/respiratory-syncytial-virus-diease#:~:text=Respiratory%20syncytial%20virus%20(RSV)%belongs,RSV%20and%20murine%20pneumonia%20virus. Accessed May 27, 2024.

[11] Surveillance of RSV. CDC.gov. 2024. Available at: https://www.cdc.gov/rsv/research/index.html. Accessed June 10, 2024.

[12] Suss RJ, Simoes EAF. Respiratory syncytial virus hospital-based burden of disease in children younger than 5 years, 2015-2022. JAMA Netw Open 2024;7(4):e247125.

[13] Syed Y. Respiratory syncyctial virus prevusion F subunit vaccine: first approval of a maternal vaccine to protect infants. Pediatr Drugs 2023;25:727–34.

[14] Fleming-Dutra K, Jones J, Roper EM, et al. Use of the pfizer respiratory syncytial virus vaccine during pregnancy for the prevention of respiratory syncytial virus- associated lower respiratory tract disease in infants: recommendations of the advisory committee on immunization practices- United States. Morbidity and Mortality Weekly Report 2023. Available at: Cdc.gov/mmwr/volumes/72/wr7241e1.htm?s_cid=mm7241e1_w.

[15] Rzymsk P, Gwenzi W. Respiratory syncytial virus immunoprophylaxis: novel opportunities and a call for equity. J Med Virol 2023;96:e29453.

[16] O'Hagan S, Galway N, Shields MD, et al. Review of the safety, efficacy and tolerability of palivizumab in prevention of severe respiratory syncytial virus (RSV) disease. Drug Healthc Patient Saf 2023;15:103–12.

[17] Drysdale S, Cathie K, Flamein F, et al. Nirsevimab for prevention of hospitalizations due to RSV in infants. N Engl J Med 2023;389(26):2425–35.

[18] Brady M, Byington C, Davies HD, et al. Updated Guidance for Palivizumab Prophylaxis Among Infants and Young Children at Increased Risk of Hospitalization for Respiratory Syncytial Virus Infection. Pediatics 2014;134(2):415–20.

[19] Verwey C, Dangor Z, Madhi S. Approaches to the prevention and treatment of respiratory syncytial virus infections in children: rationale and progress to date. Pediatr Drugs 2024;26:101–12.

[20] RSV in infants and young children. Cdc.gov. 2024. Available at: https://www.cdc.gov/rsv/infants-young-children/index.html. Accessed June 18, 2024.

Advances in Family Practice Nursing 7 (2025) 239–247

ADVANCES IN FAMILY PRACTICE NURSING

Common Pediatric Ears, Nose, and Throat Referrals

Trisha Williams, MSN, CPNP- PC*, Sara Ray, MSN, FNP-C

Department of Otolaryngology, Children's Mercy Kansas City, Kansas City, MO, USA

Keywords
- Acute otitis media • Tympanostomy tubes • Strep throat • Tonsil hypertrophy
- Sleep-disordered breathing • Obstructive sleep apnea • Epistaxis

Key points
- Ears, nose, and throat (ENT) is a common surgical specialty in which primary care providers (PCPs) refer.
- Health care costs for chronic and acute ENT conditions, such as otitis media, tonsillitis, tonsil hypertrophy, and epistaxis, substantially impact the US population and overall health care cost.
- Medical management for these conditions prior to referral, understanding indications for ENT referrals, and surgical indications by PCP may decrease the health care burden.

INTRODUCTION

In the United States, specialty clinic visits account for over 50% of outpatient clinic visits [1]. One of the leading specialty clinics within that 50% is pediatric otolaryngology/ears, nose, and throat (ENT). Pediatric ENT is a surgical subspecialty that provides services for children with health concerns of the ENT, neck, and airway and is considered a highly sought after surgical specialty for outpatient pediatric referrals. Health care costs for chronic and acute ENT conditions, such as otitis media, pharyngitis, tonsil hypertrophy, and epistaxis, substantially impact the US population due to clinic visits, medical management, and possible need for surgical intervention [2]. Referring patients to a surgical specialty for surgery that may not meet indication for surgical intervention could lead to added cost for the family and health care institution. This may

---

Each author contributed equally to this manuscript.

*Corresponding author. Children's Mercy Hospital, 2401 Gillham Road, Kansas City, MO 64108. *E-mail address:* twilliams@cmh.edu

https://doi.org/10.1016/j.yfpn.2025.01.010
2589-420X/25/© 2025 Elsevier Inc. All rights are reserved, including those for text and data mining, AI training, and similar technologies.

Abbreviations

AOM	acute otitis media
ENT	ears, nose, and throat
GAS	group A streptococcus
OME	otitis media with effusion
PCP	primary care provider
TM	tympanic membrane
TT	tympanostomy tube

also lead to an overloaded clinic and add to the delay in patient access to specialty care [3].

Primary care providers (PCPs) are responsible for providing comprehensive care including the management and care of common ENT conditions. There are recommended management strategies that PCPs may utilize prior to recommending a specialty referral that may eliminate patient symptoms and need for actual referral. This article guides the reader through the overall health care burden, reasons ENT referral, PCP treatment strategies prior to referral that may migrate symptoms, and surgical indications and risks for the most common pediatric ENT conditions [4].

COMMON EARS, NOSE, AND THROAT REFERRALS
Suppurative and Non-suppurative Otitis Media

Acute otitis media (AOM) is defined as "the rapid onset of signs and symptoms of inflammation in the middle ear" [5]. Recurrent otitis media is defined as episodes of AOM on 3 separate occasions in a period of 6 months or 4 or more occasions in the last 12 months [6]. Otitis media with effusion (OME) is defined as liquid in the middle ear space without the signs and symptoms of AOM [5]. Tympanostomy tube (TT) insertion and myringotomy are the most frequently implemented surgical interventions [7]. AOM and OME are the leading cause of acute care visits and oral antibiotic prescriptions in the pediatric population. Approximately 50% of all children will have an ear infection by the age of 2 years [8]. *Streptococcus pneumoniae* accounts for 25% of the bacterial associated with otitis media [8]. Complications of AOM and/or OME include tympanic membrane (TM) rupture, temporary conductive hearing loss due to infected or noninfected fluid in the middle ear space, speech delay due to temporary hearing loss, and infections involving the intracranial region such as mastoiditis [7].

Prior to a pediatric ENT referral for AOM or OME, PCPs will often treat AOM with oral antibiotics and should review guidelines and indications for TT placement. It is important to discuss with patients and families the guidelines and indications for TT placement and provide reassurance and explanation if ENT referral is not indicated. Children with developmental delay or disorders (Box 1) may not fall within the recommended clinic practice recommendations and the PCP may consider an earlier referral to ENT for surgical

> **Box 1: Developmental risk factors**
>
> Hearing loss without evidence of middle ear dysfunction
>
> Patient with sensorineural hearing loss
>
> Children with genetic conditions such as (Coloboma, Heart defects, atresia choanae, retardation of growth and development, genital abnormalities, ear abnormalities, including deafness [CHARGE]) association
>
> Children with craniofacial disorders
>
> Visual impairment
>
> Developmental delay related to speech and/or learning
>
> Intellectual disabilities
>
> (*Adapted from* Rosenfeld [10])

consideration [8]. PCPs are in a position to reduce the burden of AOM or OME with discussion and management of vaccine compliance, smoking cessation, and treatment of allergies (seasonal or chronic).

Consideration of TT placement is the most common reason for pediatric ENT referral [8,9]. Guidelines for consideration of TT insertion include recurrent acute suppurative otitis media that is defined as 3 or more well-documented episodes of AOM in a 6 month time frame, or at least 4 well-documented AOM in a 12 month time frame or child with persistent OME for at least 3 months, and experiences conductive hearing loss [8,9]. ENT providers may also consider antibiotic intolerance/allergic reaction to antibiotic treatment choice, TM rupture, speech delay, febrile seizures associated with AOM, and/or the need for Rocephin as indications for TT [8].

TT placement is a relatively short surgical procedure; however, there are risk factors associated. Anesthesia-related death is lower in pediatric patients who undergo TT placement due to short duration of anesthetic agents and a low risk for intubation [8]. The most common sequel from TT placement includes TT otorrhea, myringosclerosis (scaring of the TM), persistent perforation of the TM, TT retention, early TT extrusion, and possible cholesteatoma (inner ear skin cyst) [8].

The recommended treatment plan for patients with TT who have otorrhea should include otic antibiotic drops and aural hygiene (ear wicking the otorrhea from the ear canal prior to eardrop placement) [10,11]. Understanding the different presentations for children with concerns for otitis media with TT versus no TT is important to drive clinic decision-making when treating otitis media [11] (Table 1).

Strep Throat/Tonsillitis

Recurrent pharyngitis infections often lead to an ENT evaluation for tonsillectomy. Group A streptococcus (GAS) is the most common bacteria responsible

Table 1
Acute otitis media symptoms without or with tympanostomy tubes

	AOM without TT	AOM with TT
Otalgia	Yes	No
Otorrhea	No (unless perforation of TM)	Yes
Oral antibiotic use	Often	Rarely if otic drops do not resolve
Otic drop use	No (unless perforation of TM)	Yes
Risk of tympanic membrane (TM) perforation	Yes	No (unless TT plugged)

(*Adapted from* Rosenfeld[10].)

for acute pharyngitis. It accounts for 20% to 30% of all pediatric pharyngitis cases. It is also one of the most common complaints seen in ambulatory care with roughly 12 million visits yearly [12]. GAS pharyngitis is most common in school-age children [13]. The known complications of untreated GAS pharyngitis include acute rheumatic fever, poststreptococcal reactive arthritis, scarlet fever, streptococcal toxic shock syndrome, acute glomerulonephritis, pediatric autoimmune neuropsychiatric disorder associated with group A streptococci, cellulitis, and abscess [14].

A throat infection or pharyngitis is a sore throat with at least one other symptom including fever greater than 100.9 F, cervical lymphadenopathy, tonsil exudate, and positive strep test [15]. Before an ENT referral, the primary care physician (PCP) should evaluate a patient with a sore throat to determine whether antibiotic therapy is indicated, or if the cause is viral. GAS infections are unlikely in the presence of cough, congestion, or diarrhea. If a viral infection is suspected, it should be treated symptomatically without antibiotics. There are several screening tools available to aid the PCP in determining whether rapid strep testing should be considered. The most used is the Centor tool [16]. This tool looks at the age of the patient, if tonsil swelling or exudate is present, if lymphadenopathy is appreciated, and if they are febrile and have a cough. Based on the results, the provider has a better idea of strep testing that could be beneficial. PCP should treat bacterial pharyngitis with oral antibiotics.

Box 2: Paradise criteria

Seven well-documented throat infections in a 12 month timeframe

Five well-documented throat infections each year for 2 consecutive years

Three well-documented throat infections each year for 3 consecutive years

(*Adapted from* Mitchell [15])

A patient would benefit from an ENT evaluation when they have met Paradise criteria (Box 2). Paradise criteria are defined as 7 throat infections in 1 year, 5 infections each year for 2 consecutive years, and 3 infections each year for 3 consecutive years. A throat infection as defined earlier is a sore throat with at least one other symptom including fever greater than 100.9, cervical lymphadenopathy, tonsil exudate, and positive strep test[15]. For a patient who has not met the earlier criteria, watchful waiting would be most appropriate, and the PCP should reassure the family that the surgical criteria have not yet been met. Additional indications that would warrant consideration of tonsillectomy are multiple antibiotic allergies that would limit treatment options, a history of periodic fever, aphthous stomatitis, pharyngitis, and adenitis and more than one peritonsillar abscess[15]. When placing a referral to ENT for evaluation and possible tonsillectomy for recurrent pharyngitis, the PCP should provide documentation of these episodes with dates, clinical examination findings, and antibiotic treatment that was provided to help support surgical intervention. For a patient who has not met the earlier criteria, watchful waiting would be most appropriate, and the PCP should reassure the family that the surgical criterion has not yet been met.

It is important to remember that episodes of pharyngitis can still occur post-tonsillectomy but typically not as often. If a patient continues to get frequent strep throat infections after a tonsillectomy has been performed, an evaluation of infectious diseases could be considered by the PCP.

Tonsil Hypertrophy

Snoring with observed tonsil hypertrophy is another common reason for a pediatric patient to be referred for evaluation by an ENT specialist. The palatine tonsils are lymphatic tissue in the lateral oropharynx. The primary role of the tonsils is to aid in immune response to inhaled or ingested pathogens. The tonsils are most active in the age between 3 and 10 years. There is currently no study showing less of an immune response after tonsillectomy [17].

A complication of tonsil hypertrophy includes symptoms of sleep-disordered breathing. Symptoms of sleep-disordered breathing include snoring with witnessed pausing or gasping, restless sleep, frequent nighttime waking, daytime

---

Box 3: Symptoms of sleep-disordered breathing

Snoring with pausing/gasping

Restless sleep

Frequent nighttime waking

Difficult to wake/tired in the morning

Daytime fatigue/somnolence

Nocturnal enuresis

fatigue, poor focus at school, nocturnal enuresis, and frequently falling asleep after school or in the car (Box 3). Before placing an ENT referral, a trial of nasal steroid spray and montelukast has been shown to reduce the symptoms of mild sleep apnea and can be initiated by the PCP [18]. There is a black box warning regarding the use of this medication. Montelukast can cause mental health problems including depression or suicidal thoughts. The patient should be monitored closely, and if any changes in mood or behavior are noticed, the medication should be stopped immediately, and the provider notified. This risk should be discussed with the patient and their guardian at the time of initiating therapy [19]. If a trial of medication is completed and there is no resolution or improvement in symptoms, a referral to the ENT specialist for evaluation should be completed.

In patients who are younger than 2 years or have a history of obesity, Down syndrome, craniofacial abnormalities, neuromuscular disorders, sickle cell disease, or mucopolysaccharidoses, an overnight polysomnogram (sleep study) is recommended before surgical intervention [15]. A sleep study can be ordered by the PCP before referring to the ENT specialist or at the time of the referral. Having the sleep study completed before seeing the ENT specialist can help expedite getting the patient scheduled for surgery sooner as there can often be a wait for the sleep study to be completed. If a patient continues to have symptoms of sleep-disordered breathing after tonsillec-tomy, an overnight sleep study should be ordered or repeated if one has already been done preoperatively.

Complications of tonsillectomy either for pharyngitis or sleep-disordered breathing include uncontrolled pain, dehydration, and postsurgical hemor-rhage. Due to significant throat pain after tonsillectomy, a patient may have decreased oral fluid intake leading to dehydration. This can also be compli-cated by nausea and vomiting from anesthesia. Post-tonsillectomy hemorrhage can occur an average of 3% of the time [20]. It is important for patients and families to know to seek emergency care if bleeding is noted after tonsillectomy. Admitting for observation is recommended for post-tonsillectomy hemorrhage with some patients requiring intervention in the operating room to control the bleeding [20].

Epistaxis

Epistaxis is a common issue affecting up to 60% of pediatric patients [21]. Bleeding is often due to superficial blood vessels in the anterior nasal septum. In most cases, epistaxis can be treated with direct pressure to the anterior septum and hydration to the mucosa lining of the nose. Interventions including chemical and mechanical cautery are often utilized in the outpatient ENT setting when medical management fails [21].

Before ENT referral for surgical consideration, PCPs should reassure fam-ilies and educate them on appropriate anterior nasal septum pressure. This is performed by squeezing both nares together and holding pressure for 5 to 10 minutes, without releasing pressure. Saline spray/gel or petroleum jelly

Table 2
Common ENT referrals with PCP treatment options and reasons to refer to ENT

	Acute suppurative/ nonsuppurative otitis media	Recurrent strep tonsillitis	Tonsil hypertrophy/snoring	Epistaxis
Interventions prior to referral	Ensure vaccination status Smoking cessation Monitor nonsuppurative otitis media Family reassurance Strict diagnostic criteria for suppurative otitis media Obtain audiogram or tympanograms	Treat positive strep infection with antibiotics Monitor number of infections to meet Paradise criteria. Encourage supportive care while acutely ill	If medically complex, severe obesity consider obtaining a sleep study Initiate nasal steroid spray and montelukast	Education on pinch at the nares during bleeding Humidification in sleeping area at least 3 foot or closer to sleep space Saline or petroleum jelly twice daily (BID) to inside both sides of nose Mupirocin ointment twice a day for 7–10 ds inside both sides of nose
Criteria to refer to ENT	3 or more well-documented episodes of AOM in a 6 mo time 4 well-documented AOM in a 12 mo time frame Presence of serous otitis media for >3 mos Hearing loss associated with otitis media Speech delay Febrile seizures with acute suppurative otitis media History of tympanic membrane ruptures	Paradise criteria have been met for number of infections Antibiotic limitations due to allergies History of peritonsillar abscess Periodic fever, aphthous stomatitis, pharyngitis and adenitis (PFAPA)	Tonsil hypertrophy with signs and symptoms of sleep-disordered breathing Start medication (nasal steroid spray and montelukast) prior to referral	Failed medical management Known bleeding disorder such as hemophilia or von Willebrand

should be used frequently for hydration of the anterior septal wall. It may be warranted to have humidification with an over-the-counter warm/cool air humidifier within the child's home and/or sleep space, keeping it closer than 3 feet from the sleeping child. In some cases when there is extensive crusting on the septal wall, it is important to treat this with topical mupirocin twice a day for 7 to 10 days (about 1 and a half weeks) as this is typically an infection caused by the *Staphylococcus aureus* bacteria [22].

If epistaxis is frequent, prolonged, or in large volume, a patient could experience anemia or gastric upset due to swallowing blood. ENT will often perform nasal cautery in cases where medical therapy fails. This may be performed in the clinical setting with chemical cautery or in the operating room. Risk factors of surgical interventions for epistaxis include pain, bleeding, failure to obtain hemostasis, and nasal septal perforation. An extensive laboratory workup to evaluate coagulation studies or referral to a hematologist to rule out underlying bleeding disorders may be considered if epistaxis continues to occur after surgical intervention with medical management [23].

SUMMARY
Specialty clinic visits account for over 50% of outpatient clinic visits with pediatric ENT being a top referral surgical specialty. It is impactful to patient care for PCPs to understand referral guidelines; medical management strategies of ENT diagnoses (AOM, OME, recurrent strep pharyngitis, snoring and tonsil hypertrophy, and epistaxis) recommend appropriate medical management strategies before referral, indications for surgical intervention, and risks associated with pediatric ENT surgeries. Table 2 provides a quick reference guide for PCP management before ENT referral. Providing comprehensive patient care eliminates unnecessary referrals in reflection and decreases the health care burden.

IMPLICATIONS FOR ADVANCED PRACTICE NURSING
When considering an ENT referral, as with all patients, it is important to obtain a thorough history of present illness and examine the ENT. This includes documenting findings such as middle ear effusions, enlarged tonsils, vascularity of the nasal septal wall, and symptoms associated with examination findings. If abnormal examination findings are present, determine whether there are clinical indications for surgical consideration and refer to ENT if the patient meets those indications. Preventative measures and medical management before referral allow advanced practice providers to be good stewards of the health care system.

Acknowledgments
A special thanks to Gretchen Curtis FNP for her leadership and amazing editorial skills.

Disclosure
The authors have nothing to disclose.

References

[1] Mehrotra A, Forrest CB, Lin CY. Dropping the baton: specialty referrals in the United States. Milbank Q 2011;89(1):39–68.

[2] Ruthberg JS, Khan HA, Knusel KD, et al. Health disparities in the access and cost of health care for otolaryngologic conditions. Otolaryngology-Head Neck Surg 2020;162(4):479–88.

[3] Lesperance MM. Cummings pediatric otolaryngology. Elsevier Health Sciences; 2021.

[4] Harahsheh AS, Hamburger EK, de Winter JP. Empowering pediatric providers more: mastering management of common complaints. Eur J Pediatr 2023;182:4767–70.

[5] Lieberthal AS, Carroll AE, Chonmaitree T, et al. The diagnosis and management of acute otitis media. Pediatrics 2013;131:0–99.

[6] Dowell SF, Marcy SM, Phillips WR, et al. Otitis media—principles of judicious use of antimicrobial agents. Pediatrics 1998;101:165–71.

[7] Nguyen LH, Manoukian JJ, Yoskovitch A, et al. Adenoidectomy: selection criteria for surgical cases of otitis media. Laryngoscope 2004;114:863–6.

[8] Tan TQ. Textbook of pediatric care: otitis media and otitis externa. American Academy of Pediatrics; 2017.

[9] Jamal A, Alsabea A, Tarakmeh M, et al. Etiology, diagnosis, complications, and management of acute otitis media in children. Cureus 2022;14(8):e28019.

[10] Rosenfeld RM, Tunkel DE, Schwartz SR, et al. Clinical practice guideline: tympanostomy tubes in children (update). Otolaryngology-Head Neck Surg 2022;166:S1–55.

[11] Rosa-Olivares J, Porro A, Rodriguez-Varela M, et al. Otitis media: to treat, to refer, to do nothing: a review for the practitioner. Pediatr Rev 2015;36(11):480–8.

[12] Ashurst JV, Edgerley-Gibb L. Streptococcal pharyngitis. National Library of Medicine; 2023. Available at: https://www.ncbi.nlm.nih.gov/books/NBK525997/. Accessed August 10, 2024.

[13] Wald E. Group A streptococcal tonsillopharyngitis in children and adolescents: clinical features and diagnosis. In: Connor RF, editor. UpToDate. Wolters Kluewer; 2024. Accessed May 31.

[14] Pichichero M. Complications of streptococcal tonsillopharyngitis. In: Sexton D, Kaplan S, editors. UpToDate. 2024. Accessed August 9.

[15] Mitchell RB, Archer SM, Ishman SL, et al. Clinical practice guideline: tonsillectomy in children (Update). Otolaryngology-Head Neck Surg 2019;160:S1–42.

[16] Mustafa Z, Ghaffari M. Diagnostic methods, clinical guidelines, and antibiotic treatment for group a streptococcal pharyngitis: a narrative review. Front Cell Infect Microbiol 2020;10:563627.

[17] Meegalla N, Downs BW. Anatomy, head and neck, palatine tonsil (faucial tonsils). National Library of Medicine; 2023. Available at: https://www.ncbi.nlm.nih.gov/books/NBK538296/. Accessed August 10, 2024.

[18] Liming BJ, Ryan M, Mack D, et al. Montelukast and nasal corticosteroids to treat pediatric obstructive sleep apnea: a systematic review and meta-analysis. Otolaryngol Head Neck Surg 2019;160(4):594–602.

[19] Messner A. Tonsillectomy (with or without adenoidectomy) in children: postoperative care and complications. UpToDate 2022. Available at: https://www.uptodate.com/contents/tonsillectomy-with-or-without-adenoidectomy-in-children-postoperative-care-and-complications. Accessed August 29, 2024.

[20] Montelukast. UpToDate lexidrugs. 2021. Available at: http://online.lexi.com. Accessed August 29, 2024.

[21] Lucas JP, Shaffer A, Rushchak M, et al. Environmental impact on pediatric epistaxis and the utility of diagnostic studies: a single-institutional review. Int J Pediatr Otorhinolaryngol 2024;176:111827.

[22] Tunkel DE, Anne S, Payne SC, et al. Clinical practice guideline: nosebleed (epistaxis) executive summary. Otolaryngology-Head Neck Surg 2020;162(1):8–25.

[23] Clinical practice guideline: nosebleed (epistaxis). Pediatrics 2022;145(4).

Moving?

Make sure your subscription moves with you!

To notify us of your new address, find your **Clinics Account Number** (located on your mailing label above your name), and contact customer service at:

Email: journalscustomerservice-usa@elsevier.com

800-654-2452 (subscribers in the U.S. & Canada)
314-447-8871 (subscribers outside of the U.S. & Canada)

Fax number: 314-447-8029

Elsevier Health Sciences Division
Subscription Customer Service
3251 Riverport Lane
Maryland Heights, MO 63043

*To ensure uninterrupted delivery of your subscription,
please notify us at least 4 weeks in advance of move.

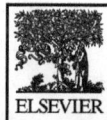

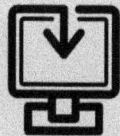

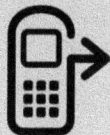

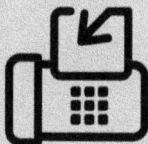

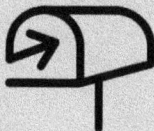

ELSEVIER